CAMBRIDGE PUBLIC HEALTH SERIES

UNDER THE EDITORSHIP OF

G. S. Graham-Smith, M.D. and   J. E. Purvis, M.A.

University Lecturer in Hygiene and Secretary to the Sub-Syndicate for Tropical Medicine	University Lecturer in Chemistry and Physics in their application to Hygiene and Preventive Medicine, and Secretary to the State Medicine Syndicate

SEWAGE PURIFICATION

AND

DISPOSAL

SEWAGE PURIFICATION

AND

DISPOSAL

by

G BERTRAM KERSHAW, M.Inst.C.E.

Consulting Engineer

Late Engineer to the Royal Commission on Sewage Disposal: Member of the
American Society of Civil Engineers: Fellow of the Royal Sanitary Institute:
Fellow and Past-President of the Institution of Sanitary Engineers.

SECOND EDITION

Cambridge:

at the University Press

1925

CAMBRIDGE
UNIVERSITY PRESS

University Printing House, Cambridge CB2 8BS, United Kingdom

Cambridge University Press is part of the University of Cambridge.

It furthers the University's mission by disseminating knowledge in the pursuit of
education, learning and research at the highest international levels of excellence.

www.cambridge.org
Information on this title: www.cambridge.org/9781107494725

© Cambridge University Press 1925

First edition 1915
Second edition 1925
First published 1925
First paperback edition 2015

A catalogue record for this publication is available from the British Library

ISBN 978-1-107-49472-5 Paperback

EDITORS' PREFACE

IN view of the increasing importance of the study of public
hygiene and the recognition by doctors, teachers, administrators and members of Public Health and Hygiene Committees
alike that the *salus populi* must rest, in part at least, upon a
scientific basis, the Syndics of the Cambridge University Press
have decided to publish a series of volumes dealing with the
various subjects connected with Public Health.

The books included in the Series present in a useful and
handy form the knowledge now available in many branches
of the subject. They are written by experts, and the authors
are occupied, or have been occupied, either in investigations
connected with the various themes or in their application and
administration. They include the latest scientific and practical
information offered in a manner which is not too technical.
The bibliographies contain references to the literature of each
subject which will ensure their utility to the specialist.

It has been the desire of the editors to arrange that the
books should appeal to various classes of readers : and it is
hoped that they will be useful to the medical profession at home
and abroad, to bacteriologists and laboratory students, to municipal engineers and architects, to medical officers of health and
sanitary inspectors and to teachers and administrators.

Many of the volumes will contain material which will be
suggestive and instructive to members of Public Health and
Hygiene Committees ; and it is intended that they shall seek
to influence the large body of educated and intelligent public
opinion interested in the problems of public health.

AUTHOR'S PREFACE

IN writing this book it has been the endeavour of the author to present the most recent knowledge relating to sewage disposal and purification as concisely as possible, giving a bibliography at the end of each chapter which may be referred to by those who are desirous of detailed information on any particular point in which they are specially interested.

Methods of treatment which are in the first stages of experiment have not been dealt with in detail, as this would often tend to mislead. It is unfortunately the case with many of these processes, when they come to be impartially investigated, that the initial and working costs are not infrequently found to be lacking ; conversely, when these figures are forthcoming, reliable data as to the real efficiency of the process are often absent. Again, a method of treatment which yields satisfactory results on a small scale may fail when called upon to cope with the conditions met with in actual practice on sewage works.

In the treatment of sewage so as to yield a satisfactory degree of purification, the cost must always be the predominant factor ; any degree of purification can be obtained if the expense is no object.

The disposal of sewage or sewage liquors by dilution is not discussed in this book, as this aspect of the question is being dealt with by Dr W. E. Adeney in a separate volume of the Cambridge Public Health Series.

The author has been engineer to the Sewage Disposal Commission since its inception some 16 years ago, and he has therefore had somewhat exceptional opportunities for investigating the various sewage treatment processes in use at the present day, and frequent references are made to the reports of the Commission.

The valuable reports of the Massachusetts State Board of Health have been freely drawn upon, and it may not be out of place to express the hope that, some day in the near future, the matter in these volumes exclusively devoted to sewage may be extracted and issued separately by the Board.

In the chapter upon sludge disposal, many quotations have been made from Mr Kenneth Allen's book *Sewage Sludge*, by the courtesy of Mr Allen, and it is believed that due acknowledgment has been made in the case of all other quotations. To facilitate reference, American and Continental practice in sewage treatment has been printed in smaller type.

The writer's thanks are due to Messrs S. H. Johnson for the loan of the blocks used in Figs. 26 and 27 ; to Mr W. Clifford, A.M.I.C.E., for permission to reproduce the table and diagram given on pages 169 and 170 relating to the Wolverhampton sewage farm ; to Messrs Crossley Bros., Ltd., for the photograph showing their spent tan plant ; and to Mr J. Radcliffe for lending the block reproduced on Fig. 56 ; also to Mr Owen Travis for the plan and photograph of the Luton hydrolytic tank shown on Figs. 18 and 19; to Dr Ing. Karl Imhoff for photographs of the Wanne-Nord Imhoff tank installation, and to Messrs Ames Crosta and Co. for permission to reproduce the plan and section of the Fieldhouse tank. I am also indebted to the Controller of His Majesty's Stationery Office for permission to reproduce diagrams from the reports of the Sewage Disposal Commission (Figs. 4, 37, 38 and 46).

I owe a debt of gratitude to Mr J. E. Purvis—one of the editors of the Cambridge Public Health Series—for many kind suggestions and help, and I also wish to express my indebtedness to Mr F. O. Moore for valuable assistance in the preparation of the drawings and diagrams.

G. B. K.

9, VICTORIA STREET,
    WESTMINSTER, S.W.
    October, 1914.

PREFACE TO SECOND EDITION

WHEN this book was first written in 1915, the activated sludge process of sewage treatment was in its infancy, and only the work of Dr Fowler was available. Since then much work has been done in connection with this process by various experimenters, both at home and abroad, and to bring the second edition up to date, a fresh chapter has been added, dealing with this method of treatment, together with other subjects—*e.g.* sludge digestion. With a view to increasing the usefulness of the second edition, the information previously given has been amplified and extended where it appeared to be necessary.

The great war naturally altered all previously accepted figures of cost relating to sewage treatment, and even at the present time (1925), prices are by no means stabilised. In cases where figures of cost are given in this book, and there can be no ambiguity as to the date to which they refer, pre-war figures have been retained, as they form a useful landmark.

In all post-war data regarding costs, the year to which they refer is given.

The author has endeavoured to meet the valuable suggestions of the reviewers of the first edition, and he trusts that the new matter may render the book of greater service to the reader.

G. BERTRAM KERSHAW

9, VICTORIA STREET,
WESTMINSTER, S.W.
January, 1925.

CONTENTS

LIST OF ILLUSTRATIONS

CHAPTER I

INTRODUCTION

Early sewers intended solely for surface water. The early sewers in towns were intended for use as surface water sewers only, their use as foul water sewers being prohibited. Later, however, after the introduction of water closets, about 1810, they were utilised to take the overflow from cesspools in addition to surface water whilst continuing to discharge into rivers or streams as formerly. Further, the pollution of rivers became legalised by the Towns Improvement Clauses Act of 1847.

As a natural sequence of events, certain rivers in thickly populated districts not unnaturally became foul, and complaints followed. As a result of the investigations and reports of various Royal Commissions appointed from time to time to deal with the subject, the Public Health Act of 1875 came into force, and the discharge of sewage into rivers and streams was prohibited.

To go back a few years prior to the year 1870, with the exception of a few towns which dealt with their sewage by land treatment, sewage purification, as understood at the present day, may be said to have been practically non-existent, and instances of sewage disposal not over numerous.

The Rivers Pollution Commission, 1868. The Rivers Pollution Commission appointed in 1868, marked the advent of fresh activity in matters relating to sewage treatment, and as a result of this Commission's reports, the purification of sewage by land treatment was put on a sounder basis.

Acting upon the findings of the 1868 Commission, the Local Government Board insisted that land should form the final part of the treatment adopted for sewage purification.

The practice, however, of invariable insistence on the use of land (whether light sandy loam, or dense boulder clay) for sewage purification led to difficulties in many cases, and tentative experiments were made in the direction of artificial processes, having for their ultimate aim the attainment of such a degree of purity in the effluent as would justify dispensing with land in cases where it was either unsuitable or its price prohibitive.

About the year 1896, several of these artificial processes had been adopted, either wholly or in part, by various local authorities, and applications were made to the Local Government Board by many authorities for loans to construct artificial plants.

The Rivers Pollution Commission of 1868 had already put forward reliable chemical data as to land treatment, and it fell to the lot of the Sewage Disposal Commission appointed in 1898 to place the artificial processes of sewage treatment on a scientific basis, whilst land treatment of sewage was also dealt with, special regard being given to the bacteriological point of view, as this side of the question had not been discussed by the 1868 Commission.

In former days it gradually came to be recognised that it was inconvenient and unhealthy to retain waste filth in the house or on the premises, and so it was promptly turned into the nearest ditch, stream, or river.

Modern ideas of sanitation do not, however, admit of the passing on of waste products to people dwelling further down the river, unless local conditions as regards volume of river, velocity, etc., are such as to ensure the adequate oxidation of the polluting matter before a fresh pollution occurs. In the case of certain inland towns, these conditions sometimes exist, but they are somewhat rare ; and in the vast majority of cases, the authorities concerned have very wisely gone to some expense in providing sewage disposal or purification schemes by which effluents of varying degrees of purity are obtained ; and at the present day it is somewhat exceptional to find even a small town without sewers and sewage disposal or purification works.

As regards large villages, there are difficulties in way of sewers and sewage purification, owing to the initial cost of such undertakings, the low rateable value of such districts, and the consequent heavy rate involved, together with the fact that long lengths of sewers are often needed to connect up comparatively few houses.

It is frequently found to be the case that the cesspool system answers fairly well for villages (when the cesspools are watertight, and rain and bath water are excluded) if they are properly supervised. Then a public water supply is installed, and the cesspool system naturally goes to pieces. Cesspools in connection with an unrestricted water supply, and receiving bath and rain water, are worse than useless.

It would, therefore, seem eminently desirable that when a practically unlimited water supply is brought into a village, it should be thoroughly well understood that sooner or later it means sewers, and in the vast majority of cases a purification works. This must not be taken to mean that a public water supply is a thing to be avoided, but that water supply, sewerage and sewage purification should go hand in hand.

Mortality statistics sometimes misleading. Of recent years there has been a gradual awakening of the public to the fact that insanitary surroundings are to be regarded as a menace to health ; although even at the present day, villages can be found with wretched sanitation, whose inhabitants proudly point to the fact that their death rate is one of the lowest for the rural districts of the county.

All that can be said of such cases is that so far they have been remarkably lucky in escaping. With regard to mortality statistics generally, it may be remarked that no statistical table yet devised gives what is really needed, *viz.* the general standard of health in a particular district. For example, the population of a district may be for a time in a poor state of health, or " sore throat " may be recurrently prevalent ; but unless the persons affected actually die, this general state of bad health is not brought out in the statistics for the period.

Again, continued bad health, ascribed to insanitary surroundings, often means that those who are able to do so, leave the district. Further, an outbreak, say, of typhoid fever, though very soon over, is apt to discount indefinitely a reputation for healthiness previously acquired by the district, though that condition of healthiness has, since the fever outbreak, been fully maintained.

It needs to be remembered that, in a rural district, the majority of the workers are in the open air during the greater part of the day, and this doubtless acts as a set-off against an insanitary home life. Moreover, it is probably quite possible to become more or less inured to insanitary conditions, but the visitor, who is not immune, often suffers.

In some instances, indifference of local authorities to sanitary improvements is put forward as an excuse by individuals, who are often themselves the chief stumbling blocks to reform. Granted that occasionally the authority is at fault : a community generally gets the type of council it deserves. The remedy is to see that those who are elected to positions of trust are men who will do their duty. When this is the case, the hope expressed by the Archbishop of York at the Congress of the Royal Sanitary Institute, held in that city in 1912, may be realised :—" There is now, I hope no need of the trenchant eloquence of that noble-hearted pioneer of sanitary science, Charles Kingsley, to insist that it is not religion, but something more nearly approaching blasphemy, to say that an outbreak of disease is God's will being done, when patently it is man's duty which is being left undone."

CHAPTER II

CONSERVANCY METHODS, COMPOSITION OF SEWAGES, ETC.

By " conservancy " is meant the conserving or keeping of refuse matter in privies, pails, earth closets, etc., for its periodical removal.

The system is not one to be recommended when other methods are economically practicable, although with certain methods, on a small scale, given cleanliness and attention, palpable nuisance may be absent, or at any rate minimised. Unfortunately, flies of many kinds haunt refuse matter, and risk of infection from enteric fever by their agency is a very grave matter.

It has without exception been found to be the case where water closets have superseded conservancy systems, that the rate of mortality has become very noticeably lower as a result.

Dr Parsons, in his evidence before the Sewage Disposal Commission, gave the following statistics with reference to the average annual number of cases of enteric fever in Nottingham : *viz.*

1 in every 45 houses provided with midden privies.
1   ,,   217   ,,   ,,   pail closets.
1   ,,   376   ,,   ,,   waste water closets.
1   ,,   861   ,,   ,,   water closets.

Such figures as these speak for themselves.

All conservancy methods are expensive as regards maintenance and working cost if properly carried out.

Privies. Privies may be dismissed very shortly ; they are as a general rule insanitary ; in hot weather they attract hosts of flies of various kinds, and should not be tolerated.

A system which has for its aim and object the accumulation of several weeks' filth in the immediate neighbourhood of houses, stands self-condemned.

Pail closets. The ordinary form of pail closet, *i.e.* where no earth is employed, is not much better than the privy, except that the emptying of the pail *must* be more frequent than the emptying of the privy.

Pail closets where earth is properly used as an absorbent and deodorant—and in what follows, the term " pail closet " must be taken to refer to the pail closet used in conjunction with earth—stand on a different footing altogether.

A large and strong galvanised iron or zinc pail, costing 2s. or 2s. 6d., or a tub formed from a small cask cut in halves, well charred and tarred and provided with a drop handle makes a suitable receptacle, and when an ample supply of fresh soil is available, and applied after using the closet, this system may be made to answer well enough in a district where the cottages are scattered, always provided that proper supervision is forthcoming to ensure regular emptying of the pails.

Very much depends upon the extent of garden land attached to the houses or cottages, and also upon the type of tenant, and unfortunately many cottages in villages possess no gardens at all. An intelligent labourer, possessing a small garden, will attend to the emptying and digging in of the contents of the pails in quite a satisfactory manner. Moreover, such a man will, usually for a small consideration, attend to premises where the tenants, by reason of age or other disabilities, are unable to do the work themselves.

There are, however, nearly always certain premises in every village where the tenants are not intelligent, and where the sanitary conditions are correspondingly unsatisfactory : consequently, one finds many villages or portions of villages where the work is done by contract in a more or less desultory manner.

The pail closet system where earth is employed is especially useful in rural areas immediately outside a special drainage district, where the lie of the land and other matters would render its treatment as a contributory place inadvisable. In some districts the normal level of the subsoil water lies within a few feet of the surface of the ground, and in such cases pail closets are to be preferred to cesspools, which, under these conditions, are seldom made watertight.

The main points to be kept in mind in dealing with pail closets, may be summed up as follows.

(1) See that a box containing an ample supply of fresh[1] garden soil[2] is available in the closet and a shovel for handling it.

---

[1] Ashes *can* be used if no garden soil is available, sand is useless , baked brick earth is said to be good, also peat dust. It is not essential that the soil should be absolutely dry when used, although it should be so when used with the automatic earth closets. So long as the soil does not " cling " together when squeezed in the hand it will not be too damp, and if stored in a garden shed for a week or so in a layer about three or four inches deep it will be sufficiently dry for use.

[2] It would seem advisable not to use the same soil over again without baking and exposure to the weather, to become repeopled with suitable microbes.

(2) See that at least a shovelful of soil is thrown into the pail *before* use as well as after.

(3) See that the pail is in its proper position under the seat, and this is easily done by making a recess for the bottom of the pail about one inch deep. The floor of the closet should, of course, be formed of impervious material and preferably of concrete, brought to a smooth surface, or rendered (plastered) with a mixture of portland cement and sand in the proportion of 1 to 1.

(4) See that the pail is *frequently* emptied—daily in hot weather.

(5) See that the pail is rapped quite empty, scraped inside when needed, and *well* dusted internally with fine soil before replacing.

(6) See that flies are rigidly excluded from the pail when in position in the closet : (*a*) by a movable cover to the seat, and (*b*) by other suitable means as regards vent, door and window.

(7) See that a small metal plate is fixed to the underside of the seat to deflect the urine to the centre of the pail.

Disposal of solids from pail closets. Next as regards the disposal of the contents of the pail in cases where good garden land is available : the quantity of garden land necessary for this purpose is given on p. 18. The faeces should be lightly covered with earth in a very shallow trench—say, 3 to 4 inches deep. The faeces and urine are now disposed of, but there still remains the " washup " water, and water used for washing clothes, together with a small quantity of urine. This liquid should be disposed of on a separate area of garden land to that in which the solid matter is trenched. It may be said that the manufacture of the various liquids is sometimes spread over a matter of a couple of hours daily, and that it would mean many journeys to the garden. That need present no serious difficulty ; a pail under the sink pipe will obviate this. If it is raining there are usually intervals when it rains less heavily, and advantage can be taken of these. The liquid should not be dumped down day after day on the same spot, but systematically distributed, beginning at one end of the plot and using a fresh area daily until the whole plot has been treated, when the process can be repeated. It is the waste water from household operations which causes difficulty in treatment, especially when the garden land is clay. In such cases, if there is no other outlet, the soil can be lightened with fine ashes and road grit to the great benefit of the garden from the gardener's point of view.

Another method of dealing with slop water, etc., by means of rough filtration and absorption will be found in the sections dealing with Dr Poore's system.

Laundry waste. When, as is often the case, certain cottages take in much laundry work from larger houses in the neighbourhood, a great difficulty is often experienced in disposing of the laundry water satisfactorily in the absence of a large garden with suitable soil and subsoil.

Sometimes, however, the cottages where this work is done lie fairly close together, and in such cases, the laundry and slop water from a series of cottages could in most cases be drained to a common storage tank from which it could be pumped at intervals into an iron tumbler cart (covered) and finally distributed upon land. The question of who should pay for the cost of pumping, etc., would arise, but it would not be a large matter, as solids should not enter the pipes, which could be formed of iron tubing.

Cesspools. Cesspools came into general use after water closets had been introduced and their discharge to surface water drains prohibited, the discharge from the water closets being conveyed by a drain to the cesspool.

The earth pail system just described, is of no use where w.c.'s are used : in the latter case if ditches and watercourses are to be kept clean, it is a question—in the absence of sewers— of cesspools or nothing, except, of course, in the case of large isolated houses, which may have their own private sewage plant ; and even in quite small villages, where the pail system is in general use, it is usual to find one or two houses provided with w.c.'s, the water flushing them being pumped daily to a cistern at the top of the house by means of a force pump.

In such cases the well from which drinking water is obtained is generally not too far off from the cesspool, and it is of vital importance that this should be constructed in an absolutely watertight fashion, and bath and drain water excluded.

It is not in the interests of public health to have a leaky cesspool 10 feet distant from the drinking water well, and to find that when the surface water level of the well is lowered— say, 3 inches by pumping—that there is also a fall of about three inches in the water level of the cesspool : yet such cases occur. In the first place, the cesspool must be absolutely watertight, and this is not impracticable. If sewer manholes can be constructed in a watertight manner in a water-bearing gravel, there is no reason why cesspools should not be made equally watertight, even if this increases the cost.

There are persons who say that where there are no wells, cesspools should be purposely made leaky—(and they are frequently made so after having been passed by the sanitary authorities)—so that the liquid can percolate away into the subsoil, since no cost in emptying them is involved. Now with regard to this point, it may be that in the case of isolated houses on the outskirts of a village standing on a suitable geological formation, such leaky cesspools may do little or no harm, but a good deal depends upon the depth below the surface in the cesspool at which leakage takes place, and in most soils it may be taken that the purification of the cesspool leakage will be very slight for some considerable zone from the cesspool, and this zone must in course of time become saturated with filth in the absence of underground water containing an adequate supply of dissolved oxygen to assist in its purification. Further, the absence of wells---failing a rainwater drinking supply—sometimes means a copious public water supply, and there is risk, even if somewhat remote, of polluted water being drawn in to the water mains during breakages, alterations, etc. Again, if there is a public water supply to the village close by, it may be taken for granted that in the more thickly populated parts, the subsoil is in a chronic state of pollution from leaking cesspools, and it is unfortunately a common experience that the owners of large isolated houses possessing leaky cesspools, whilst professing to be extremely

concerned about the insanitary state of the cottages in their
village, not infrequently do their utmost to frustrate any
scheme for bettering the conditions under which the poorer
inhabitants live, which is likely to cause a material increase
in the rates.

In large villages, *where there is ample garden land attached
to each house,* however small the house, and where the water
supply is small, watertight cesspools can be made to answer
fairly well when properly attended to, but even in small villages
with a water supply derived wholly from wells, the trouble,
already mentioned under the heading of pail closets, arises
when laundry work is taken in by cottagers, and large volumes
of water are used for this purpose.

Where the public water supply is a large one for a rural
district—say 15 to 20 gallons per head per day—and bath
water, sink water, and water used for flushing w.c.'s, etc.,
are admitted to a watertight cesspool, it must be obvious that
either (1) heavy expenditure will be incurred in emptying a
properly constructed cesspool at frequent intervals, or (2) that
steps will very soon be taken to evade this burden by rendering
the cesspool leaky, or constructing surreptitious overflows,
should the subsoil be of a nature to favour such evasion.

A simple case will illustrate the futility of using cesspools
when they receive all bath and rain water.

A large cesspool contains, say, 2000 gallons. Assume a
small house with a bath (the chief offender so far as the cesspool is concerned) and two water closets, and occupied by four
persons.

> Say the w.c.'s are used four times daily with a two gallon
> flush each time = 8 gallons × 365 = 2920 gallons.
> Washing up, etc., say, 6 gallons × 365 = 2190 gallons.
> One bath daily, say, 40 gallons × 365 = 14600 gallons.
>   Total   ..   19710 gallons.

On this basis—a fairly low one—the above cesspool would
require emptying (disregarding rainwater) every five weeks or
so, and taking the cost of emptying at 25s. a time, the total
annual cost would come to about £12. Cesspools are utterly

unsuited to villages and houses having an unrestricted water supply. It is needless to add, that in such cases, far more is spent annually in an inefficient and potentially dangerous system, than would be required to pay the annual instalments of principal and interest on a sewerage and sewage purification scheme. Moreover, with cesspools, the bulk of the cost of emptying falls on the poorer classes of the community, who are least able to afford it. The writer has heard it urged on behalf of cesspools that the opening up of the polluted ground necessary for a sewerage system would cause an epidemic : if this be so, why are not epidemics rife all over the kingdom when such works are constantly in progress in a polluted soil and subsoil ? Apparently, so long as the cesspools leak into the subsoil surrounding them, all is regarded as satisfactory, but it may well be questioned whether it is not preferable to have visible a danger signal in the shape of the liquid from a cesspool overflowing into a street or ditch in broad daylight, than to have this systematically going on out of sight in the subsoil.

Sometimes, where cesspools are not leaky, it is possible to arrange for the contents to be drawn off periodically into an airtight iron tank cart, and the contents distributed on fields, preferably arable, or in other circumstances it may be advisable to connect several cesspools to one central tank. This method, however, is not unlikely to cause trouble if the village should ever come to be sewered, as it might be contended that the pipes connecting the cesspools had become a sewer within the meaning of the definition in Section 4 of the Public Health Act, 1875.

Character of cesspool liquid. The ordinary liquid from a watertight cesspool is a very strong over-septicised oily-looking, yellowish-coloured liquid, generally possessing a disgusting smell, and it is hopeless to expect to be able to purify such a liquid on small indifferently constructed filters, without first rate preliminary treatment involving chemical precipitation with lime. It may be noted in passing that the mere act of connecting up the overflows from several leaky cesspools and attempting to deal with the overflow liquid is practically futile ; the leaky cesspools remain, in a possibly more insidious form than previously.

Disposal of liquid from cesspools. Concerning the disposal of liquid from cesspools, it must be borne in mind that this is a most offensive liquid to deal with, and requires considerable care or a nuisance results.

A not uncommon procedure is to distribute it in the raw state over pasture land, but applied in this way, without any dilution, it is very apt to burn the grass and to be more harmful than beneficial. Careful distribution upon arable land or freshly dug garden soil appears to be the best method of dealing with it : rain and contact with the air and soil soon purify the liquid, and the land can be cropped in about a month's time.

Deodorants. As regards deodorants, while the liquid is being distributed, a solution of bleaching powder if mixed with the liquid will practically deodorise it, or lime can be applied in a similar manner, or bleaching powder or lime may be dusted over the surface of the ground which has been sewaged.

A method of dealing with cesspool liquid, which has its advantages in the case of a small garden, is to dig trenches similar to those used for celery, but much shallower ; the cesspool liquid is then run into the trench, given a light sprinkling of fine soil, and then very lightly covered with a layer of fresh soil.

If even this plan is likely to cause trouble by reason of closely adjoining houses, a covering of boards over the trench in the shape of an inverted V will tend to prevent smell, particularly if the liquid can be conveyed from the cesspool to the trench direct by pumping through a length of 2-inch or 2½-inch hose. Excellent pumps for ordinary cesspool work are those of the diaphragm type.

Crops suited to manured ground. With regard to the crops which thrive upon cesspool liquid and also pail closet matter, any of the ordinary vegetables (except potatoes), *e.g.*, cabbages, cauliflowers, and brussels sprouts, do best of any as the first crop from freshly manured ground, and as a rule any other crop flourishes well as a second crop off the same ground. As to the period which should elapse before the ground is ready for cultivation, much depends upon the weather : in fine dry weather the ground will be ready in about a month's time : in wet, or in frosty weather, the period will be longer, possibly extending to six weeks or two months. Fruit trees and bush fruit, such as gooseberries, currants, and raspberries, do very well on doses of liquid manure, especially if applied at intervals when the fruit is commencing to swell. In the case of pail closet stuff, a trench should be dug round the tree about 3 inches deep, 12 inches away from the stem, and a dressing of manure applied, the excavated soil being replaced. Slops can be poured over the trench about once a week in hot weather. One of the commonest errors is that of supposing that the manure should be deeply trenched in ; as a matter of fact, the more lightly this is done the better, if it is out of the reach of flies. A trench 2 inches to 3 inches deep is ample, and the contents of a pail may be spread over a length of 12 or 15 feet of trench : the earth should be immediately turned back into the trench before the flies have time to visit it. When one trench is full, another can be started alongside the old one.

It may be observed in passing that with leaky cesspools in a gravel soil where the level of the subsoil water varies, it is difficult to get at the true cost of emptying them, since in hot dry weather, when the ground water level is low, the contents of the cesspool leaks into the surrounding subsoil, whereas the converse takes place when the ground water level is high ; instances frequently occur where cesspools may be pumped out one night, and be full of subsoil water the following night.

Cost of emptying cesspools. In his evidence before the Royal Commission on Sewage Disposal, Dr Parsons gave some interesting details regarding the cost of emptying cesspools. At Caterham in 1900, for example, the cost worked out at 12s. for each cesspool emptied, or 1d. for every 11·7 gallons removed, whilst in another case where the cesspool was leaky the cost of emptying was 1d. per 2½ gallons removed. At the same place in 1901, the total cost was £832 for a population of 9486 inhabitants. In one case when the cesspool was emptied by pneumatic cart, the cost came out at 5s. per load.

In Staines Rural District, emptying of cesspools by pump and hose cost 5s. 6d. for a cesspool of 300 gallons : 3s. 6d.

per load for one of 750 gallons, the load being 300 gallons, and
1s. 9d. per load for one of 3000 gallons. The cost of emptying
a 1000 gallon cesspool quarterly worked out at £2 per annum.
A cesspool of only one load capacity, i.e., 300 gallons, cost
£3. 6s. per annum.

At another place by a pumping system, the cost was from
one-eighth to one-tenth of a penny per gallon.

At yet another place, emptying 172 cesspools cost £265 a
year. In the case of a large village near London with which
the writer is acquainted, having a population of barely 1000,
the annual cost of dealing with the cesspools exceeds £300 in
ordinary seasons, and approaches £400 in wet seasons, i.e., a
sum sufficient to pay annual loan charges on a scheme of
sewage disposal costing £7000 ! !

The method of building up a cesspool with 14-inch
" stretcher " brickwork in ground apt to become water-logged,
shown in Fig. 1, may be found useful; the writer has used it for

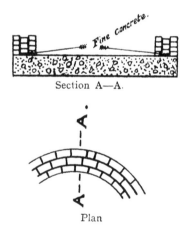

Section A—A.

Plan

Fig. 1.   Stretcher brickwork for cesspools.

rectangular sewer manholes in water-logged subsoils with every
success. For circular work in plan, specially made bricks would
be needed, and these can be obtained to any radius.

Earth closets. The "earth" pail closet perhaps falls
under this heading, but the above title is intended to apply to

the various automatic arrangements by which earth is discharged automatically into a pan, often by means of a rocking seat or a " chucker."

Nearly all these automatic contrivances seem to go wrong sooner or later, generally at the worst possible moment, and either half a hundredweight of soil comes down in a rush filling the pail, or a few particles of soil trickle down.

With the type of closet where the soil is supplied by a shovel from a bin, the case is altogether different, and with a little practice it is possible to distribute the soil evenly over the contents of the pail in much the same manner as a fireman on a locomotive spreads the fuel evenly over the firebars.

Although the law can enforce a supply of water for a water closet, there appears to be no means of enforcing the provision of an adequate supply of earth or for earth pail closets, and an earth closet without earth is no better than a privy[1].

For a village, and for general cottage use, the writer prefers the " earth " pail closet.

In large villages, where there are rows of cottages, there is sometimes a public scavenging service, and as a rule this effects an improvement in sanitary matters; it is, however, somewhat expensive, and for that reason it is often difficult to persuade local people to contract for the work, owing to the ill-feeling caused by an increased rate amongst their neighbours.

Mortality caused by disease during war. The difference caused by sanitation where large bodies of men—such as armies—are temporarily congregated together in bad climates, far away from sewerage systems and purification works, and where they must necessarily be provided for by temporary methods, is well brought out by an instance taken from a recent war. Statistics are perhaps apt to be somewhat misleading unless the full details are known, but it may not be amiss to point out here that in the Russo-Japanese war, the Japanese lost only 250 men from disease as against 100 killed by the enemy.

[1] Where a scavenging service exists, there should be no difficulty in the scavenging carts bringing a supply of earth to those who have no gardens.

Dr Poore's System. The late Dr G. V. Poore took a deep interest in village sanitation, and his methods as carried out at Andover are well known to sanitarians.

In the Milroy lectures[1], 1899, Dr Poore, speaking of the sanitation of camps, gives a very clear description of his mode of operations, and they may be quoted as follows :—

" I have always advocated the burial of faeces[2] in shallow furrows rather than in deep trenches, and, in this country at least, where alone I have had experience, I am convinced that this is the only reasonable course to pursue. If properly done, all offence to eyes or nose is thus ended and the faeces cease to attract either flies or rats. The faeces can be covered continuously as soon as they are dropped, and there is no need of having malodorous open trenches partially filled which are waiting to be completely filled before being covered up."

  ＊ ＊ ＊ ＊ ＊

" If a plot of ground 50 yards long and 50 yards wide— slightly more than half an acre—be allotted for the disposal of faeces, this should be marked off into, say, 16 strips, each about 8 feet wide and 50 yards long, with a narrow path of about 18 inches between each strip to allow for watering and cultivation. The line of the furrows must be accurately marked by a cord and reel in the ordinary way, and the digger must move continuously backwards in order to avoid trampling on the freshly dug ground. The making of the furrows should commence at the point furthest from the latrines, and it should gradually come nearer to them. The earth removed from the first furrow should be wheeled down near the latrines, where it will be ultimately wanted to cover the last furrow which is dug. The capacity of the furrow or little trench will depend upon the size of the spade. I find that, working in ordinary garden soil with a spade having a blade 9 inches long and 7 inches wide (the furrow being consequently 9 inches deep and 7 inches wide), eight stable-bucketsful of soil, each holding

---

[1] Republished in *The earth in relation to the preservation and destruction of contagia*, by Dr G. V. Poore. Longmans, Green & Co. London, 1902.

[2] The domestic cat, given a garden, is one of the best of sanitarians (Author).

2½ gallons, or about 22 lbs. weight of earth, were removed. This amounts to 2½ bushels of soil, weighing 176 lbs., or the measure of the capacity of a trenchlet 8 feet long. This trench must be filled with excreta, and great care must be taken that nothing except faeces and paper and the accompanying urine is placed in it. If broken crockery or old tins are accidentally mixed with the excreta, they must be removed.

" The trench being filled with faeces, mark out a digging line at a distance equal to the width of the spade (7 inches) behind the edge of the first trench and then cover the faeces in the first trench by the earth removed in making the second. Owing to the draining away of urine and moisture, and their great compressibility, it will be found that the excreta undergo a considerable diminution of bulk when tipped into the trench. When the earth of the second trench has been removed and shovelled on to the top of the first trench, it will be found that there is a general raising of the level of the ground, and the second trench will be found to have a cross section which is rather triangular than rectangular, owing to the oblique direction of its front wall, which is composed of a sloping bank of friable earth. The surface of the ground must be left crumbly, smooth, and perfectly neat, like a well-prepared garden bed. No particle of faeces or paper must be left uncovered. There will be no offence to eyes or nose, no putrefaction is possible, and the faeces are beyond the reach of dipterous insects, and if there has been no delay in the collection and burial of the faeces they cannot have been used for oviposition to any great extent, so that the soil will not become infested with ' grubs.'

" How many men will provide the quantity of faeces which can be placed in a trench 8 feet long from which 176 lbs. weight of earth have been removed ? The answer to this question is governed by bulk rather than by weight. If faeces and earth were equal in bulk for equal weights, and if we allow a quarter of a pound of faeces for each man—for the urine soaks away and *qua* bulk may be neglected—then the answer would be 176 × 4 = 704. If the faeces are weight for weight four times as bulky as the earth, the answer is 176. In any case it seems safe to say that a trench 8 feet long, 9 inches deep,

and 7 inches wide will suffice to take the faeces of 100 men.
This estimate entirely accords with my experience gained in
my garden at Andover, where the faecal accumulations of 20
cottages have been disposed of daily in the manner indicated
for 18 years, and when it takes at least five years to cover an
acre of ground in this way. Those who have not had experience in this method are apt to have exaggerated views as to
the amount of land required. If a trench 8 feet long and 7
inches wide is sufficient for the disposal of the daily quota of
excreta from 100 men, then ten such trenches occupying an
area of 8 feet by 70 inches—say 6 feet—is enough for 1000
men, and one strip of ground 50 yards long and 8 feet wide
would serve for a regiment of 1000 men for 25 days, and the
16 strips would serve for 400 days—let us say half an acre per
annum per 1000 men. The actual area necessary will depend
to some extent upon the nature of the soil and the care and
skill of the scavenger, but in no case can the area required be
a bar to the process—certainly not on the veldt or on Salisbury
Plain. It need not be insisted on that a scavenger must be
incessantly at work. The excreta should be taken up as soon
as dropped and be placed in a covered pail, and the pail when
full should be emptied into the furrow and covered up. In
this way effluvia are stopped and oviposition by diptera is
rendered impossible. Further, this method of disposing of
faeces necessitates no increase of the impedimenta of an army ;
no lime or chemicals are needed, and no apparatus beyond a
spade and a set of garden tools.

" The ground beneath which the faeces are deposited should,
when the work is done, have the appearance of a well-prepared
garden bed and it will need little attention until it is covered
with herbage of some kind. The only question remaining to
be decided is as to what that herbage should be. There can
be no camp without water-supply, and in every camp one of
the sanitary problems is the disposal of waste water. Some
of this waste water should be used in time of drought for
laying dust, and encouraging fertility in that small area of
ground beneath the well-tilled surface of which the faeces are
safely bestowed. Then, the higher the temperature, the quicker

will the ground bring forth green leaves to freshen the air. Whether the crop be grass, cabbage, cereals, onions, mustard and cress, lettuces, spinach, or what not must depend upon circumstances. I think the seed sown in such ground should always be those of culinary vegetables which may prove a real blessing if the camp is long occupied."

The above system as described for camps by Dr Poore will answer equally well for cottages in rural districts providing good supervision—so often lacking—is obtainable.

Disposal of slops. Later on in his book, Dr Poore gives an account of " an experiment in sanitation " carried out at a cottage near Andover, and it may well be quoted here since it has reference to that bugbear of rural communities, namely, slopwater.

" The disposal of slopwater is always an important consideration in cottage management. Usually this means slopwater plus roof water, but in this cottage the roof water has been provided for. The amount of slops, allowance being made for evaporation in cooking, and washing and drinking, must always be considerably less than the water consumed. Economy in the use of water lessens the slop difficulty.

"In this instance the slops are strained and filtered, and allowed to flow away in a ' filtration gutter,' to be presently described. The arrangements are on the south side of the cottage, well exposed to the sun, so as to favour evaporation.

" The sink is just below the window of the scullery, and the waste pipe, without trap of any kind, passes through the wall and terminates in a free end about 18 inches from the wall and 2 feet 6 inches above the level of the ground. The waste pipe empties itself into a strainer and filter, which are placed about 15 inches from the cottage wall, so as to avoid the risk of splash or back soakings or accumulations of " dirt " and insects between the wall and the filter. The strainer is placed on the top of the filter, and the filter discharges its water to a filtration gutter.

... " The strainer consists of a basket with a wisp of straw in it. This arrests all but the finest particles, and is the best fat-trap I know—the only one in fact which does its work efficiently and without offence. The straw may be changed as often as necessary—every day, once a week, once a month, according to the amount of accumulations, which will largely depend upon the thriftiness and knowledge of the cook. The contents of the strainer may be given to the chickens, put on the manure heap, or burnt. A new handful of straw is then put in and the strainer replaced. The changing of the straw has the advantage of giving a new direction to the water. Any old basket of suitable size which will hold the straw answers the purpose of a strainer. After months of use it will get greasy and rotten, and may then be burnt and be replaced by a new one. From the strainer the slops flow into the filter, which is simply a galvanised iron vessel, with an outlet at the bottom and filled with broken clinker varying in size from peas at the bottom to walnuts at the top. This filter effects a further purification of the slops, and acts partly mechanically and partly by virtue of the growth of bacteria, on the surface of the broken clinker. The filter...has been specially constructed, and is duplicated, and the waste pipe of the sink is provided with a reversible nozzle so that either half of the filter can be used. For a cottage, however, this is not necessary, and an old galvanised iron bucket with a hole in the bottom will be found to answer every purpose.

" The filtration gutter consists of strong cast-iron guttering, perforated with conical holes, having the small ends upwards so that they cannot get jammed. This guttering, which is 9 inches wide and in lengths of 6 feet, is laid upon loose porous rubble or gravel placed in a trench.

" A trench 18 inches wide and 18 inches deep was first dug from the filter due south, care being taken that the bottom of the trench should slope away from the cottage, in order that water should not flow back towards the foundation of the building. The lengths of guttering are then laid on a level with the top of the trench, the level being maintained by means of bricks-on-edge, built up without mortar in little columns of four from the bottom of the trench, each column, except the first and last serving to support the ends of adjacent lengths of guttering. It being ascertained that the level of the guttering is true, with the slightest possible slope downward from the filter, the trench is finally filled with loose rubble of any kind—builders' rubbish, burnt clay, lumps of chalk, gravel, clinker, coke, whatever may be most readily obtained.

...."Care should be taken that the packing be accurately done at the junctions of the lengths of guttering, in order to give support and firmness to the brick supports. When finished, the filtration gutter looks as though it had been simply laid on the ground, there being, of course, no indication of the rubble-filled trench beneath it. The iron guttering is sufficiently strong to permit a wheel barrow or cart to pass over it, and there is no objection to taking the gutter across a path. The sides of the trench should be planted or the trench may be dug in a shrubbery or plantation.

...."The straw in the basket has been changed about once a fortnight. The filter has never been changed ; we have never seen the slops run further than the end of the first length of guttering, and when the slops are not running the gutter and its neighbourhood look perfectly dry. There is absolutely no smell, no offence to eye or nose. The length of gutter provided is 24 feet (four lengths) but the water has never been seen to travel more than 6 feet...."

Initial cost of process for treating slop water. "The guttering has been made for me by Messrs Tasker, of the Waterloo iron works, Andover, and costs 1s. 6d. per foot run, and the special duplicated slop filter was supplied by the same firm at a cost of 27s. 6d.

"The total cost, therefore, of draining this cottage was as under :

	£	s.	d.
Labour for digging trench, etc.	0	2	6
Basket	0	0	9
Filter	1	7	6
Four lengths of filtration gutter (24 feet in all)	1	16	0
48 old bricks, clinkers, etc., say	0	1	0
	£3	7	9

"But if an old basket or an old galvanised pail be employed, and if two lengths of guttering be used instead of four, then the above bill will be reduced by £2. 6s. 3d., leaving £1. 1s. 6d. on the total cost for providing drainage for the cottage. Not only does the filtration gutter allow the slop-water to run away, but it stops back dead leaves which otherwise would soon choke the porous rubble in the trench.

"I may say that I advise nothing but open guttering to be used for slop-water, be it perforated or otherwise. Wherever this putrescible mixture flows in the dark, the faint smell of drains is soon perceptible. Where all is open, those little accidents which will proverbially happen are seen at once."

The foregoing quotations show very clearly the mode of operations used by Dr Poore in disposing of excreta and slop-water. The writer visited Andover in 1901, and can fully endorse all Dr Poore's claims for his system. It must, however, be borne in mind that in Dr Poore's case, excellent supervision was forthcoming, and the tenants of the cottages referred to were all under one landlord, himself a man of science.

Utilisation of rainwater for domestic purposes. It may not be out of place at this point to refer briefly to rainwater collected from the roofs of cottages and outbuildings as a drinking water supply for places where water is scarce. It seems strange that this source of water supply is not more frequently utilised in England. In Bermuda, the only water supply is obtained from the rainfall falling on roofs and specially constructed "catches," from which it flows into large tanks cut out of the limestone and rendered with Portland cement. All roofs of dwellinghouses have an inclined fillet of cement running round them to collect the rain falling on them at one point. Unfortunately, the water is seldom filtered. Fig. 2 shows a plan and section of a rainwater tank constructed by excavation in rock, the walls and floors being rendered.

In many instances, rainwater could be advantageously collected from the roofs of houses in this country, and after having passed through a Doulton[1] candle filter, it could be

---

[1] All filters on the "candle" principle require the candles to be removed, cleaned, and sterilised periodically.

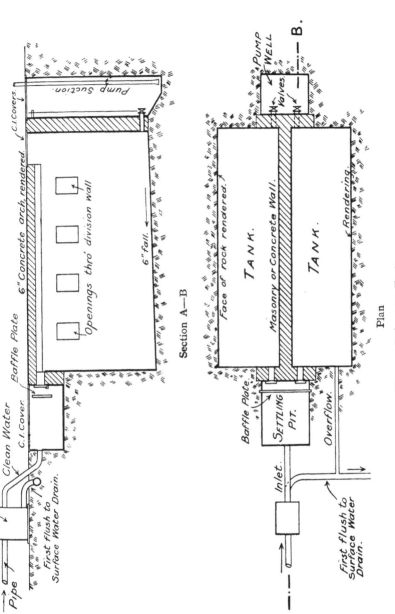

Section A—B

Rainwater
Pipe

Clean Water

Baffle Plate

6" Concrete arch, rendered.

C.I.Covers.

Pump Suction.

C.I.Cover.

First flush to
Surface Water Drain.

Openings thro' division wall

6" Fall.

Plan

Face of rock rendered.

T A N K.

Masonry or Concrete Wall.

T A N K.

Rendering.

PUMP
WELL

Valves

B.

Baffle Plate.

SETTLING
PIT.

Overflow.

Inlet.

First flush to
Surface Water
Drain.

A.

Fig. 2. Rainwater Tank.

used for potable purposes, care being taken to use suitable piping (not lead) owing to the solvent action of soft rainwater.

The following table[1] gives the run-off of rain from a roof having an area of 100 square feet with varying degrees of rainfall.

TABLE I.—*Showing daily yield of water from 100 square feet of roof with varying rainfall.*

Mean Rainfall	Loss from evaporation	Requisite capacity of tank	Mean daily yield of water	Mean daily yield wettest year	Mean daily yield driest year
inches	per cent	cubic ft.	gallons	gallons	gallons
20	25	52	2·1	3·3	1·6
25	20	67	2·8	3·7	1·9
30	20	72	3·4	4·7	2·2
35	20	77	3·9	5·5	2·5
40	15	83	4·8	6·1	3·6
45	15	85	5·5	7·1	4·3

Thus with a roof area of 1000 square feet the mean daily yield in a district having an annual rainfall of 25 inches would be equivalent to 2·8 × 10 = 28 gallons.

Rainwater separators. As the first washings from roofs generally contain soot, dust, bird droppings, decayed leaves, etc., it is advisable to turn to waste the first washings off the roof, before running the rainwater to the storage tank. To effect this, automatic contrivances termed Rainwater Separators have been devised, that form known as the " Roberts " Separator, made by Rogers of Haslemere, being perhaps as well known as any.

These separators are guaranteed to take a rainfall at the rate of 2 inches per hour, and to work with a rainfall of $\frac{1}{2}$ inch per 24 hours on the areas given in the table below. In tropical countries where the rainfall sometimes exceeds 2 inches per hour, and in smoky cities, large separators are needed.

It should be remembered that the separator must correspond to the size of the roof if it is to work properly.

---

[1] Taken from *Quantity Surveyors' Diary and Tables* (Metchim & Sons, Princes Street, London, S.W.).

TABLE II.—*Giving particulars of rainwater separators.*

No.	Area of roof in square feet		Distance between the levels of inlet and outlet pipes		Free to any Railway Station in Great Britain
	In the country	In the city or tropics	Pure outlet	Foul outlet	£ s. d.
1	600 to 1000	—	4½ ins.	11 ins.	3 0 0
3	1000 to 3000	700 to 2000	6 ,,	13 ,,	4 10 0
5	3000 to 5000	2000 to 4000	7 ,,	13½ ,,	6 0 0
7	5000 to 7000	4000 to 6000	8 ,,	15 ,,	7 10 0
9	7000 to 9000	6000 to 8000	9 ,,	15½ ,,	9 0 0
11	9000 to 11000	8000 to 10000	10 ,,	16 ,,	10 10 0

Each further increase of 2000 square feet in area of roof adds 30s. to the cost. The makers observe that the separators need no attention except washing out at intervals of about three months in the country and one month in town.

With regard to the construction, size, and position of the storage tank, this should be constructed of cement concrete, or brickwork in cement with access manholes and placed underground for reasons of temperature. According to the makers of the separators it should be capable of holding a rainfall of about 4 inches, or say, 1 cubic foot for each three superficial feet of roof, so that for a roof having an area of about 2000 square feet, the storage tank should hold 666 cubic feet or about 4150 gallons ; a larger capacity is desirable, however, if it can be obtained, but much depends upon what purposes the water is used for. In the case of most houses a tank holding 100 days' supply would be " drought-proof." The water before being used for drinking purposes should be passed through an efficient filter.

There is no question that many rural districts might make far more use of rainwater for domestic purposes than is now the case.

Alternative methods of sewage disposal for villages. Before leaving the subject of village sewage disposal, it may be useful to consider a few cases which are commonly met with in practice. As a rule it will be found that there are some three or four alternative plans of dealing with the sewage of villages, and it is not necessary in many cases that the same system should be in use throughout the village ; various modifications may be necessary according to local conditions.

The most suitable methods would appear to be as given below.

Nature of water supply	Suggested system of disposal
Water supply very small	Earth pail system or watertight cesspools
Water supply moderate	Earth pail system or watertight cesspools
Water supply large	Sewerage system and purification works

Take first of all the case of a small country village with a non-migratory population of 150 to 200 persons, and a water supply obtained from a solitary pump. Most of the houses will be cottages occupied by labourers, two or three houses occupied by shopkeepers, and a few larger houses occupied by, possibly, the doctor, farmers, and others.

The larger houses will probably be provided with cesspools and large gardens, and there should be little or no trouble experienced in dealing with the waste liquid and solid matter produced. Coming to the smaller houses and cottages : as a general rule, the small householder can obtain the services of some of the cottagers in attending to the emptying of pail closets, as the cottagers are anxious to get this on their own gardens or allotment ground ; but here a difficulty arises, namely the disposal of slop-water, if, as is sometimes the case, there are no gardens attached to the houses.

This means, in the majority of cases, a cesspool for slop-water, in or near the back yard, or, if several cottages are drained to one cesspool, in some convenient central position. A small parish iron tank cart would not cost a great deal of money, and might be placed at the disposal of persons requiring it for a nominal sum each time, and the contents disposed of on land in the neighbourhood. This would get over the difficulty of the shopkeeper and also of the cottager who has no garden for slop-water. There would still remain the disposal of solids from the pail closets of the cottages possessing no garden, and as a general rule the farmer who employs the labourer will be found ready to take the refuse.

The alternative way of getting rid of the slop-water is to let it flow by means of a drain to the ditch at the side of the road, often causing a nuisance in hot weather : further, there may not be a ditch, or it may be too far off to drain to, or the ground may fall the wrong way, and in cases where there are no gardens it is difficult to see how the slops can be disposed of without a small cesspool. Even supposing the tenant to possess an allotment, he is not likely to be able to cart the slops there every two or three days.

Taking the case of a village possessing a moderate water supply, such as might be obtained by wells dug in gardens. In such a case it is of vital importance, if any cesspools are used for slop-water, that they should be watertight, for very obvious reasons, and the utmost care exercised in disposing of the solids on the garden land. Either earth pail closets or Dr Poore's system might suitably be considered, in conjunction with cesspools for slops, where no gardens exist. In this case there is perhaps less likelihood of several cottages being without gardens, but on the other hand, the cottages having none, will usually be found to be let at the lowest rentals, and therefore generally let—but by no means always—to an undesirable type of tenant. In such cases it is questionable whether it would not be better to let the cottages remain unlet ; but, unfortunately, even insanitary cottages in rural districts are too valuable to the owners to let them remain unlet, and in such instances the parish cart previously suggested would seem to be the only solution of the problem.

In every case, as has already been pointed out, one of the chief difficulties experienced in a village is lack of efficient administration.

The third case—*i.e.*, where the water supply is large—only admits of one solution ; unless it is in the happy position of lying on the banks of a river of sufficient volume to take the sewage of the community without treatment other than removal of the grosser solids ; and that solution undoubtedly is a sewerage system and purification works.

Cost of small sewage disposal works. It is the sewerage which entails the greater part of the cost ; the purification works, as Dr Handford in his evidence before the Sewage Disposal Commission has shown, need not necessarily be costly. The particulars cited by Dr Handford are given below, and he observes that the works are efficient.

TABLE III.—*Giving particulars of village sewage works. Particulars of four sewage disposal works in the Basford Rural Sanitary District in the County of Nottinghamshire*[1].

Name of Outfall	Estimated Population	Description of Works	Approximate cost
			£
Beaufit Lane ..	220	Septic tank, revolving sprinklers, two series of bacteria beds	250
Plainspot ..	220	do. do.	250
Jubilee Pye Hill	200 (Provision for 400)	do. do.	500
Watnall ..	200	Septic tank, two filters. Sewage distributed over two bacteria beds through galvanised iron pipes fed by tippers.	150

Possibly the suggestion in the Eighth Report of the Sewage Disposal Commission, published in 1912, may give a stimulus to village sewage disposal. The sentences referred to run as follows :

" We think, therefore, that the Rivers Boards might be well advised to turn their attention first to securing compliance with the standard by the larger towns whose works were as yet inefficient. The smaller communities might meanwhile employ this period of grace either in making provision for a scheme of sewerage and sewage disposal which would be adequate for their increasing requirements, or, if their population were stationary or diminishing, in adopting some system of dry conservancy which would materially lessen the amount of pollution which entered the river."

Flies. Considerable attention has been devoted of late years to the part played by flies in conveying and disseminating infection, and the subject is an important one where conservancy systems are concerned, since the majority of these methods unquestionably tend to attract flies of many species.

The subject of flies as carriers of disease is fully dealt with by Dr G. S. Graham Smith in his book on *Flies in relation to disease (non-bloodsucking flies)*, Cambridge Public Health Series, and the reader is referred to it for detailed information.

---

[1] The district referred to by Dr Handford is a mining one, and the population are chiefly colliers.

Composition and strength of sewages. In the Fifth Report of the Sewage Disposal Commission, page 11, paragraph 13, the following definition is given of sewage. " Sewage generally may be said to consist of a mixture of saline matter in solution, and nitrogenous and carbonaceous organic matter in solution and suspension, together with a certain amount of grit and mineral matter."

The composition of sewages may for present purposes perhaps be best discussed under the headings of :—

(1) Domestic Sewages.

(2) Sewages which contain trade refuse.

Domestic sewages. Taking domestic sewages first ; in plain language, domestic sewage as it enters the house drains in dry weather consists mainly of dirty water derived from various household operations, containing, amongst other things, faeces, urine, paper, soapsuds, bath water, hair and fibre, soap, matches, candle ends, and various other articles ; after this mixture has passed into the sewers it often receives drainage from urinals, stables, pigsties, etc.; further, it usually becomes mingled with a certain—or rather an uncertain—volume of subsoil water which gains admission to the sewers. If the sewerage system is what is known as combined (*i.e.*, when all street and roof water enters the sewers), it will also, in dry weather, receive washings from streets when they are watered, containing grit, horse dung, oily and tarry matters. During rainfall, soot, leaves, dust, excreta of birds, etc., will be washed to the sewers from roofs of houses, *via* the house drains, and the sewers will also receive from the road gullies organic and inorganic matter washed from backyards, gardens, and street surfaces. If the sewerage system is partially separate, only the rainwater from back roofs of houses and backyards should reach the foul water sewers.

It will be recognised that the chief constituents of domestic sewage in dry weather are common to most towns, and there would appear to be no reason why the amount of refuse matter produced by individuals in different towns should vary very materially : the water supply per head of the population, however, with which the sewage matter is diluted, varies considerably in various towns, and exercises a very great influence on the quality or " strength " of the sewage as it is termed : in fact, so important a factor is it, that were it not for the question of subsoil water, the strength of a domestic sewage could be arrived at quite nearly enough for purposes of sewage purification by employing the water supply (taken as gallons per head per 24 hours) as the scale of strength. Thus, a sewage derived from a water supply of 30 gallons per head per 24 hours, would, other things being equal, be half the strength of one resulting from a water supply of 15 gallons per head.

The great variability of the quantity of water consumed per head per day in various towns can be seen in the following table :

TABLE IV.—ʃ ɔwing water supply per head in various towns.

Name of to		Water supply per head per day	Name of town		Water supply per head per day
Durban	..	2	Brisbane	..	34
Madriʳ	..	3·3	Paris	..	36
Tries'	..	4·4	Aberdeen	..	38
Hoɲ ῀ong	..	6	Belfast	..	39
Ve ɉ	..	8	Christiana	..	40
L ɹre	..	10	Hamburg	..	46
ʄ ʋerley	..	10	Adelaide	..	50
ɔchdale	..	18	Baltimore	..	54
∧ndover	..	20	Boston	..	74
Exeter	..	25	Toronto	..	82
Hendon	..	30	New York	..	114
Liverpool	..	32	Washington	..	145
Munich	..	33	Chicago	..	200
London	..	33-·36			

It by no means follows that the total water supply of a town reaches the sewers : part is used for watering streets and gardens, whilst there is a certain amount lost in steam from kitchen boilers, or in some cases water used for filling locomotive tenders is taken out of the district.

In some towns where the water supply is limited, slop-water closets are in use, the household slops being employed to flush the closets, and in such cases the sewage is generally strong, since the water used for flushing is already fouled.

Hourly variations in strength of sewages. It is found, as might be anticipated, that domestic sewages vary in strength throughout the day, being usually strongest in the case of a small town about 10 a.m., and weakest in the early morning, usually from about 3 a.m. to 6 a.m.

The habits of people in towns are generally more or less regular, with the result that the variations in strength of sewage, in the absence of rain, are more or less regular.

For example, in a town where a number of houses are provided with baths, there will generally be a large discharge of fairly clear water to the sewers between the hours of 7 a.m. and 8 a.m. from certain districts, followed later on by flushes from water closets, slop-water, and water from washing-up operations, whilst from other districts in the same town where possibly water is used sparingly, a stronger sewage will be entering the sewers ; from about 12 p.m. to 2.30 p.m., there will be a further rush of dirty water to the sewers containing grease and bits of fat derived from cooking and washing up, whilst from 4 p.m. to 6 p.m. a further pronounced flow of waste water occurs. The length and gradients of the sewers, as will be seen presently, tend to equalise these variations, and the larger the town the greater the equalisation, but the larger variations can usually be detected. From what has been said, it will be seen that domestic sewage, even in dry weather, is a liquid of extremely variable composition ; it is doubly so during heavy rainfall, when the foul matters are washed from roofs and streets into the sewers.

Strength of sewages. It does not come within the province of this book to touch more than briefly upon chemical points, but the following facts should be known by those who are called upon to design sewage purification works.

It was formerly very usual to measure the strength of a particular sewage by the number of gallons per head of sewage arriving at the works, or by the chlorine content, but the chlorine method gave unreliable results where certain trade wastes were present, whilst subsoil water vitiated the former method.

One particular sewage may be strong as regards free ammonia, another in trade wastes which absorb oxygen from permanganate rapidly, and yet another in suspended matter or albuminoid ammonia.

The Sewage Disposal Commission, in their Fifth Report, recommend the dissolved oxygen absorption test, saying "...where, however, a more exact measure of strength is needed, we are inclined to think not only on theoretical grounds, but also as the result of experience, that this can at present be best obtained by ascertaining the amount of dissolved oxygen taken up during the complete, or practically complete, oxidation of the organic and ammoniacal matter in the sewage.

" The purification of sewage is to a large extent a process of indirect oxidation through the agency of bacteria, and one of the chief things required to be known about any particular sewage is how much oxygen is required for its complete oxidation. The rate at which the sewage will take up oxygen is also a factor of importance, in that it furnishes information as to the character of the organic matters."

*   *   *   *   *

" The amount of oxygen which a sewage can take up is, however, only an approximate measure, for purposes of purification, of its strength, as some constituents of sewage are oxidised by filters or land more readily than others, and the proportion which they bear to the total organic matter varies largely in different cases.

" To determine the amount of oxygen which a sewage requires for its oxidation, a definite quantity of the sewage is allowed to remain in contact with a known excess of oxygen until it is completely oxidised, and the oxygen remaining over is then measured."

As a result of numerous experiments, Dr McGowan found that 100,000 parts by weight of an average sewage took up about 100 parts by weight of dissolved oxygen from water in two months or more, by which time practically all the oxidisable matter present had become oxidised, an average septic tank liquor about 80 parts, and an average precipitation liquor about 60 parts.

The test just alluded to has the disadvantage that a long time is required to oxidise the organic matter completely, and Dr McGowan, therefore, made a large number of observations to see whether the dissolved oxygen absorption test bore a more or less constant ratio to other rapid tests.

As a result of these investigations, figures were obtained which showed that the amount of dissolved oxygen which a sewage would take up during oxidation (*i.e.* its strength) could be arrived at fairly closely by a formula based on the figure for oxygen absorbed in four hours, together with the figures for ammoniacal + organic nitrogen[1].

The No. 1 formulæ were as follows :—

For sewages
    (ammoniacal + organic N.) × 4·5 + (oxygen absorbed in 4 hours × 6·5)
For septic tank liquors
    (ammoniacal + organic N.) × 4·5 + (oxygen absorbed in 4 hours × 6·5)
For precipitation liquors
    (ammoniacal + organic N.) × 4·5 + (oxygen absorbed in 4 hours × 6·)

Turning again to the Commission's Fifth Report, and referring to the table facing page 202, it will be found that figures of analysis showing the chief characteristics of strong, average, and weak sewages are as given in the following table:

Table V.—*Showing composition of various sewages.*

Water supply, etc.	Strength of sewage	Ammoniacal nitrogen	Oxygen absorbed[2] in 4 hrs.	Suspended solids
Strong or very strong sewage — Parts per 100,000				
Slopwater town—10–15 gallons per head. Partially separate system of sewers	200–230	6·0	25	40
do. do.	175–200	7·5	20	40
W.c. town—25–30 gallons per head. Separate system of sewers	160–170	9·0	17	40
Sewages of about average strength				
W.c. town—30 gallons per head. Some subsoil water in sewage	100	4·0	10–12	28–30
Weak sewages				
W.c. or slopwater town—25–30 gallons per head. Much subsoil water in sewage	60	2·5	7–8	20

[1] *Sewage Disposal Commission*, Appendix IV to Fifth Report, p. 1, *et seq.*

[2] Oxygen absorbed in 4 hours means, oxygen absorbed in 4 hours at 27° C. (80° F.) from an eighth-normal solution of permanganate of potash (3·94 grams per litre) rendered acid with dilute sulphuric acid.

Strong, average, and weak domestic sewages. A few typical analyses of strong, average, and weak domestic sewage taken from Appendix III to the Fifth Report may now be given.

TABLE VI.—*Giving typical analyses of strong, average, and weak domestic sewages.*

	Parts per 100,000			
	Caterham Barracks (very strong sewage)	Little Drayton (strong sewage)	Oswestry (average sewage)	Exeter (St Leonards) (weak sewage)
Ammoniacal Nitrogen	13·41	7·57	3·53	2·49
Albuminoid ,,	1·75	1·41	0·91	0·55
Total organic ,,	3·87	2·76	2·25	1·39
Oxidised ,,	—	0·00	trace	—
Total ,,	17·53	10·33	5·85	3·89
Oxygen absorbed at 27° C. (80° F.) in 4 hours	17·99	24·44	11·27	6·53
Chlorine	13·57	11·40	9·16	6·58
Solids in suspension..	42·10	23·90	29·40	26·70

In the case of Little Drayton, the figures given above are the average of three sets of hourly samples, at Oswestry four sets, at Caterham Barracks four sets, and at Exeter (St Leonards) three sets.

Broadly, the ammoniacal nitrogen or " free " ammonia is derived from the fermentation of the urine, the albuminoid ammonia coming from organic matter of animal origin.

The total organic nitrogen is also derived from animal organic matter, and the figures include the " albuminoid " ammonia.

The total organic nitrogen represents a separate determination of the whole nitrogen.

The oxidised nitrogen figures represent nitric with a little nitrous nitrogen, derived mainly from the oxidation of the ammonia of the liquor. Its presence in a weak sewage or during the early hours of the morning is an indication that there is subsoil leakage to the sewers.

The oxygen absorbed may be taken approximately as a measure of the oxidisable carbonaceous matter present.

The chlorine is derived almost entirely from urine (except when there is any manufacturing refuse present).

The solids in suspension are derived from various sources which will be described in the chapter dealing with sludge.

It may be remarked here, however, that the term " solids " does not only mean large lumps of faeces, but includes quite fine matter, almost imperceptible to the eye when in suspension.

Sewages containing trade wastes. In most towns of fair size certain trades or manufactures exist, producing various liquid and semi-solid waste products which are often disposed of by turning them into the sewers, where these exist. Some of these trades produce very polluting liquids, and when present in the sewage in large quantities, they sometimes render its treatment a matter of some difficulty, especially as the waste is often turned into the sewers in flushes and not equably.

The principal trade wastes met with in this country are given in the chapter on trade wastes, and they need not be enumerated here.

Possibly waste from breweries is more frequently met with in small towns than any other, and when its ratio to the volume of sewage is at all large, it is often a source of trouble, causing great nuisance if the sewage is allowed to become at all septic.

Composition of sewage from some American cities. Since some references are made to American practice in sewage disposal and purification, it may be useful to give, for purposes of comparison, some figures of analysis showing the composition of sewages from some American cities.

The following table is compiled from a table given by Mr Langdon Pearse in *The Sewage Disposal Problem in the United States and abroad* [1] (p. 571).

TABLE VII.—*Showing comparative analysis of crude sewage of various American cities.*

			Parts per 100,000			
	Boston 1905–1907	Columbus 1904–1905	Waterbury 1905–1906	Gloversville 1908–1909	Worcester 1908	Chicago 1909–1910
Free ammonia	1·14	1·10	·78	1·20	2·22	·88
Organic nitrogen	·91	·90	1·48	2·30	—	·76
Nitrites	·000	·009	·014	·038	—	·011
Nitrates	·004	·020	·152	·088	—	·035
Oxygen consumed	5·6[a]	5·1[a]	4·6[a]	9·5[a]	11·7	3·8
Chlorine	—	6·5	4·8	15·8	5·7	4·0
Suspended matter	13·5	20·9	16·5	40·6	25·8	14·1
Fats	—	2·5	2·6	4·8	—	2·3

[a] Sample is boiled five minutes.

It will be observed from the above figures that, generally speaking, American sewages are very much weaker than the sewages in England.

Issued by the Sanitary District of Chicago, 1911.

The taking of samples. It might be thought that this is quite a simple matter, and that a random or chance sample taken at any time and with no particular precautions is sufficient to give reliable indication on analysis of what kind of effluent a particular plant is turning out. If the character of sewage were fairly uniform, as for example in the case of most water supplies, this belief would, to a certain extent, hold good, but it has been shown that sewage is a most variable liquid as regards character and strength, and it therefore follows that unless the sampling is carried out in a most careful manner, and spread over a proper period, the results obtained from single chance samples at infrequent intervals of time may yield most misleading data. There are, of course, times when a chance sample will give all the information required, as for example when it is required to ascertain whether a filter has commenced to produce nitrates, but in the majority of cases what are known as average samples of sewage or effluent should be taken, and the manner of taking these will be described presently. Before going any further, it may be well to note that effluents as well as sewages vary considerably, not only from day to day, but also throughout every hour of the 24 hours, albeit these hourly differences may not in some cases be large.

With land effluents, the strongest effluent sometimes does not occur until, say, from 6 p.m. onwards, the time depending largely upon the nature of the soil and subsoil, rate of treatment per acre, whether the land has been recently sewaged, etc. When the land is underdrained, it is a good plan to dry off a particular plot until the underdrains run dry ; this will show that there is no subsoil water mixed with the effluent— although this can sometimes be obtained approximately from the chlorine figures—sewage can then be applied to the plot and samples can be taken at intervals from the underdrains until well after the normal flow has been reached. Another method of ensuring the obtaining of "corresponding" samples is to add fluorescin to the sewage as it flows on to the land, and to note when it appears in the effluent. Fluorescin is a dark reddish powder, costing about 10s. per 1 lb. tin. A very small quantity of this powder mixed with water, and a stick or two of caustic potash will colour a very large volume of sewage or water a most brilliant green.

By "corresponding" samples is meant, two or more samples of practically the same liquid taken at various stages of its purification; thus, supposing three samples in all are taken of (1) a sewage, (2) a tank liquor, and (3) a filter effluent, and assuming that where a sewage sample was taken, some fluorescin was poured into the sewage entering the tank; then, if a sample of tank liquor is taken when the green colour begins to show strongly over the tank sill, this will be a corresponding sample to the sewage sample; *i.e.* it will be practically the same body of liquid as was sampled for sewage, but it will have undergone tank treatment in the meantime. Consequently, it is possible by comparing the two samples after analysis to see what degree of settlement is produced by the tank process.

Again, if a sample of the filter effluent is taken from the filter, after showing a strong green colour, this will also be a corresponding sample both to the tank liquor, and also to the original sewage.

It is most important in taking samples of effluent, and also of sewage, that suspended matter lying on the floor of a chamber, or invert of effluent channel or pipe, shall not be stirred up and included with the sample, otherwise the sample is valueless. A case once occurred where pollution causing damage to cattle was alleged, and where samples were taken above the alleged point of pollution, at the point itself and also below it. At the point of pollution a small boy was sent in to stir up the sediment whilst this particular sample was taken! Unfortunately there does not appear to have been any undue anxiety to stir up the mud at the point where the sample was taken *above* the point of pollution. Such a sample is, of course, quite worthless—in one case only water was sampled and in the next sample, water plus river bed was taken, the sediment consisting of possibly months of deposit of vegetable matter. Similarly, if sediment lying at the bottom of a sampling chamber is included, it should be properly mixed with the whole of the effluent from which it was derived,—probably a few hundred thousand gallons, and then the sample might be taken!

The proper course to adopt in the case cited would have been to have dealt with the liquid and solids separately, and by means of carefully sampling and subsampling, to have taken proper samples of mud at all three points.

Another point to be remembered in sampling is, that the bottles used should be scrupulously clean, of white glass, and glass stoppered, and the stoppers should be carefully ground in with fine " wash " emery to ensure a tight fit.

What are known as Corbin or half-Winchester bottles are almost universally used for holding samples, and as a rule they are amply large for all purposes of analysis. Should a specially large sample be required, however, Winchester quarts can be used. The bottle should be filled quietly to overflowing, and the stopper gently worked into place. It can then be secured by passing a piece of stout unbleached calico over the stopper, and tying it round the neck with string, just under the raised ring of glass on the neck of the bottle.

To take average samples of sewage, tank liquor, and effluent, involves a good deal of labour (three men being required to take samples every hour, night and day), and some apparatus. As a general rule a 24 hours' sample consists of a sample made up of 24 separate samples drawn hourly throughout the 24 hours, the hourly quantity of sewage or effluent used for the final mixed sample being proportionate to the rate of flow for that particular hour. This naturally means gauging of the sewage, tank, and effluent flows throughout the period of sampling. If the final 24 hours' sample was composed of 24 hourly samples, taken in equal quantities each hour, it would not represent the *average* quality of the sewage, etc., liquors, since the volume of this varies from hour to hour throughout the day. If the whole operation of taking average samples is described it will possibly make things clear.

In the first place, a gauge and weir must be set up to record the flow of sewage (or whatever it is desired to sample) on a chart automatically : when the gauge and weir have been fixed and are in working order samples can be taken at any time, but it is usual to commence sampling at, say, 9 a.m., in order to get the sample to the laboratory as quickly as possible.

About 30 to 36 wide-mouthed glass stoppered bottles holding
12 to 16 ounces each are required for the hourly samples, and
a large mixing bottle holding, say, 1 to 1½ gallons for the final
sample. If bacterial samples are desired, two or three sterilised glass stoppered bottles will also be needed, each holding,
say, 75 to 100 c.c.

Assuming the automatic gauge to be started at 9 a.m.;
at 9.30 a.m., one of the small hourly sample bottles is filled
with the liquid to be sampled, the stopper gently replaced,
and the bottle labelled thus, "Sewage, 9.30 a.m."; the same
process takes place at 10.30 a.m. and so on throughout the 24
hours, the last sample of the first 24 hours finishing at 8.30 a.m.
the next morning. The chart on the drum of the automatic
gauge is removed at 9 a.m. and a fresh one substituted whilst
the heights traced by the pen are worked out for each hour
and written in as gallons per hour. The date is also marked
on the chart. There now remains the taking of a certain
amount of liquid from each of the 24 small hourly sample
bottles, proportionate to the rate of flow shown for each hour
on the chart, and its transference to the large mixing bottle.

The removal of the desired quantity of liquid from the
smaller bottles can be quickly effected by turning the small
bottle over two or three times to mix up any sediment, and
pouring it into a long measuring glass graduated in cubic
centimetres.

It is convenient in most cases to mark off one or two places
from the number of gallons shown for each hour on the chart,
to make this fit in with the capacity of the hourly sample
bottle ; or, if the flow is a small one, each hourly figure can be
multiplied by a constant throughout to obtain the desired
quantity of liquid ; so long as the hourly flows are either
divided or multiplied throughout by the same figure, the
result will be the same. When all the proportional amounts
have been taken from the hourly bottles and placed in the
large mixing bottle, its contents should be well but quietly
mixed, and the ordinary sample bottle filled, stoppered, and
tied down, packed and sent off to the laboratory. The bottle
for bacterial analysis is filled from the large mixing bottle.

It is well to have all the hourly sample bottles arranged in one line of 24, and to work from one end to the other, noting on the chart the times of weakest morning sewage, time of influx of any trade effluent, and the like : and it is also frequently advisable, when the approximate time of weakest sewage flow is known, to take a sample of this to ascertain whether it contains nitrates, since this is an indication of subsoil water in the sewers.

The whole of the operation of working out the chart and sampling takes from one and a half to two hours according to circumstances, and whilst the making up of the final sample is in progress the gauge is recording on a fresh chart, and samples can be taken in the spare bottles.

The working out of the charts takes some little time until one or two have been done, especially if the flow of sewage is irregular, when the hours must be divided up by several ordinates and the average flow between each ordinate worked out. The writer has designed a slide rule for gauging in connection with the taking of average samples, rectangular weirs being used ; it is shown in Fig. 3. A pencil line or point is

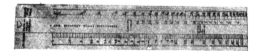

Fig. 3. Slide Rule for calculating flow of sewage or water.

made on the chart at the average height, and the height from the base line is scaled off on the edge of the rule ; the slide in the rule is marked width of weir, and the right hand side is marked height over weir in inches (and fractions of an inch). If the line on the slide corresponding to width of weir used is made to coincide with the line giving height of liquid over weir in inches as scaled off, the arrow on the slide will show the volume of flow passing over the weir in gallons or cube feet per minute. The rule is adapted to the weir gauging tables given in Santo Crimp's Tables, but any coefficient desired can be employed by drawing a fresh arrowhead with a fine hard pencil.

As regards conditions suitable for gauging with a rectangular weir. The weir sill itself should be about one-third the full width of the channel in which it is placed, and the section of liquid falling over the weir should not exceed about one-fifth of the cross section of the liquid in the channel immediately above the weir, appreciable velocity of approach being avoided thereby. Further, the weir should not be " drowned " but should have a free overfall, and the gauge should be set sufficiently far above it to be uninfluenced by curvature of surface. The weir plate itself may be suitably made of rolled brass, with bevelled sill and screwed to the gauge-board or dam. The float of the gauge should be protected from string, rags, etc. by being enclosed in a cylinder of perforated zinc. In some cases it may be necessary to provide a small sluice door in the weir dam to admit of sludge being flushed through occasionally.

If an automatic gauge cannot be obtained, measurements can be taken with a thin steel rule from a point level with the crest of the sill and a few feet upstream ; this, however, involves much additional labour as readings should be taken at least every ten minutes throughout the 24 hours

It may be useful to suggest when average samples should be taken so as to obtain a good idea of the strength of the sewage in dry weather, since small places cannot afford to pay for large numbers of analyses, and they must be limited in number.

Supposing that the samples are to extend over a period of four days, Monday to Friday inclusive :

As a general rule, about two or three dry days should precede the sampling, but if, say, ·01 to ·05 inch of rain falls during the two or three days or during the sampling period, it will not, if of ordinary intensity, affect the sewage flow appreciably, especially if the sewerage system is a partially separate one, but much must be left to the judgment of those in charge of the sampling ; for example, a rainfall of ·10 inch spread over the 24 hours with dry dusty surfaces may not affect the sewage flow at all, whilst a fall of ·05 inch in 10 minutes on a wet surface will possibly cause a large run-off to the sewers ; it all depends upon the intensity of the rainfall and the condition of the surfaces upon which it falls.

Generally speaking, three to four days of average sampling (*i.e.* three to four 24-hour samples) will show fairly definitely the nature of the sewage, but in some cases it may be advisable to extend the sampling to seven days.

It would doubtless be well to have seven absolutely dry days prior to the sampling, and to carry the sampling over seven dry days in every case, but the average number of rainy days in the British Isles is somewhere about 190 in the year, and in most districts 14 consecutive dry days could scarcely be relied upon.

If calculations for volume of filtering material, etc. are based upon dry weather analysis of the sewage, they will certainly be upon the right side, but in many cases, not only the sewage flow but its character alters at different seasons of the year, owing to influx of subsoil, water, etc., and in such cases it may often be advisable to have average samples taken in summer, autumn, and winter.

Bacteria in relation to sewage purification. In a few words, bacteria or microbes may be described as being excessively minute organisms only visible with a high power microscope, and many of them with an infinite capacity for applying themselves to the work of breaking down the organic matter upon which they subsist. Pasteur classified bacteria under the following headings : (1) aerobic bacteria, or microbes requiring oxygen, (2) anaerobic bacteria or bacteria living practically without oxygen, and (3) facultative bacteria or those living either with or without oxygen. Some of these are known as pathogenic or disease producing bacteria as distinguished from the harmless or non-pathogenic bacteria.

Most of the bacterial life found in sewage is derived from the faeces and urine of human beings, and one cubic centimetre of ordinary sewage may contain many millions of microbes. It will therefore be seen that sewage contains in itself the active agents required for its purification, in the bacteria which break down the complex organic matter present in the sewage to simpler substances. Chemical and physical actions also come into play in breaking down the substances found in sewage, together with the higher forms of life, such as larvae, worms, and insects of various species, and finally, in most cases algae and water plants.

The final process of sewage purification in which the nitrogen is converted into nitrites and finally into nitrates is carried out by nitrifying bacteria.

To sum up, sewage purification is the outcome of the activities of bacteria mainly, but assisted by chemical and physical actions and the purifying agencies of various algae and water plants.

Degree of purification should be adjusted to local conditions. All purification is relative, and since local circumstances differ widely as regards different towns and rivers, it follows that a lesser degree of purification may suffice in one case, whilst a much higher degree of purification may be demanded by another case.

This was in the minds of the Sewage Disposal Commission when they wrote (Fifth Report, page 9):

" The two main questions, therefore, to be considered in the case of a town proposing to adopt a system of sewage purification are, first, what degree of purification is required in the circumstances of that town, and of the river or stream into which its liquid refuse is to be discharged."

BIBLIOGRAPHY.

Barnett, Major K. B. *Handbook on Military Sanitation for Regimental Officers.* Forster, Groom and Co., Ltd., Charing Cross, S.W. 1912.
Graham-Smith, G. S. *Flies and Disease, non blood-sucking flies* (2nd edition). Cambridge Public Health Series. Cambridge University Press. 1914.
Kershaw, G. B. *Modern Methods of Sewage Disposal,* Chapter III. Chas. Griffin and Co., Ltd., London. 1911.
Poore, G. V., M.D. " Flies and the Science of Scavenging," *Lancet,* May 18th, 1901.
——. *The earth in relation to the preservation and destruction of Contagia.* Longmans, Green and Co., London.
Royal Commission on Sewage Disposal. Fifth Report, 1908. Appendix IV to Fifth Report. Eighth Report, 1912.
Minutes of Evidence. Q. 32955 to Q. 33443.
Appendix III. Fifth Report.

CHAPTER III

SEWERAGE SYSTEMS, VARIATIONS IN SEWAGE FLOW, STORM WATER, ETC.

It is not generally appreciated how very largely the sewerage system in use in a particular town influences the average character of the sewage throughout the year, *i.e.* all weathers included, and it may therefore be well to discuss at some length the various systems in use at the present day.

The two main systems are :
(1)　The combined system ;
(2)　The partially separate system ;
while, in a few cases, the entirely separate system is in use.

The combined system. In this system, all rainwater— mainly derived from street surfaces, pavements and roofs of houses, is received into the foul water sewers.

There are several serious disadvantages attending the use of a combined system of sewers, whilst it also possesses certain advantages in special cases. The main disadvantage is that in times of heavy rainfall very large volumes of storm water enter the sewers, and all surface water and storm water, with the exception of that passing away by the storm overflows, must be conveyed to the works. In many cases where the general contour of the land is steep, it would be quite impracticable, on the ground of expense alone, to attempt to convey the whole volume of storm water and sewage to the purification works without relief storm overflows (discussed later in this chapter), or, supposing it to be practicable, to treat it satisfactorily when it arrived there.

Further, sewers with a carrying capacity sufficient to carry off all sewage and storm water from a hilly district without frequent storm overflows, would probably need a great deal of flushing in dry weather, and difficulties would be liable to arise with the ventilation of the sewers.

When the depth of liquid in the sewers varies say from one quarter to seven-eighths of the diameter of the sewers, the result of such extreme fluctuations is to leave a large surface of slimy deposit on the sewers and manhole benchings above the line reached by dry weather flow variations, and this coating, owing to gradual fermentation and putrefaction, is apt to cause nuisance from smell from vents and open manhole covers ; in many cases, too, where a large volume of storm water is received into the sewers, some of them become surcharged, the dirty water rising up in the manholes, and leaving a foul coating on the manhole walls ; and cases have occurred in fairly recent schemes where, when the sewers are flowing under pressure, certain of the manholes have been below the line of the hydraulic gradient, and manhole covers have been lifted off as a result.

In the combined system the street gullies are connected to the foul water sewers, and in rural and suburban districts, where gravel and macadam roads occur, grit and small gravel are washed into the gullies, and very often out of them into the sewers—since gullies are seldom systematically attended to in a rural district—the result being that the grit and gravel become coated with gelatinous growths, silt, etc. and gradually entangle pieces of paper and fibre, resulting in decreased velocity and discharge, and possible ultimate blockage.

The question of detritus reaching the disposal works by way of the sewers is fully discussed in the chapter upon sludge (p. 121).

When the gullies are connected to the foul water sewers, if the gully traps should become unsealed in dry weather—a not infrequent occurrence—sewer gas will escape through them.

It is often said that the scouring-out effect of rain storms on a combined system of sewers is beneficial ; no doubt it is beneficial when it occurs, but in hot dry weather—such for instance as the summers of 1911 and 1914—no system of sewers can be regarded as satisfactory which depends upon adventitious rainfall for flushing-out purposes. Further, after a long spell of dry weather, large masses of filth are suddenly washed down to the purification works as the result of rain, causing trouble to the man in charge and frequently injury to filters. Where the sewers, by reason of unavoidably slack gradients need flushing, this is best provided for by suitable flush tanks, due regard being had to the size and gradient of the sewer it is desired to flush.

Another objection to the combined system arises when the sewage is pumped, the large volumes of storm water requiring pumping and adding very greatly to the cost.

The greatest difficulty of all, possibly, occurs at the purification works, where, in the course of perhaps less than an hour, without much warning, the manager may be called upon to deal with perhaps twelve times the ordinary flow of sewage for the particular time of day.

Even supposing stand-by tanks to be provided, in some instances it is impossible to empty these by gravitation, and it means pumping the tanks empty after every storm, besides disposing of the sludge, a great part of which is derived from the road surfaces ; possibly the road tarring system now in general use will help to keep this grit and silt on the roads, but there can be no doubt that the rate of run-off to the sewers will be much faster than with macadam roads, and the liquid will contain much more impurity. It is a common experience too, that in continued wet weather, the surfaces of roads that have been tarred work up into a regular slurry an inch or so deep.

It will be obvious, where so many factors have to be taken into consideration, that any accurate estimate of the extra amount of liquid due to rainfall liable to be received at the disposal works during the year with a combined system of sewers is out of the question, but at a rough approximation it will probably not be less than a 50 % increase on the dry weather flow.

In large cities, it may often be advisable to retain a combined system of sewers for the densely populated, and often insanitary areas, whilst providing the partially separate system for the suburbs of the city, and also for all new streets.

The partially separate system of sewers. With the partially separate system, rain falling upon the front portions of the roofs of houses, pavements, and street surfaces, often passes, as in the combined system, into the street gullies, but the gullies are connected up to lines of separate surface water sewers, which discharge into the nearest watercourse or river or sea, as the case may be. At the same time a short length of rainwater drain is sometimes necessary when the houses stand back some distance from the road.

The chief objections are the increased initial outlay involved by its adoption, and the consequent opposition by frontagers on the roads to be sewered.

When the water from backyards and roofs of houses is also separated from the sewage, two sets of house drains are needed for each house, one line for the sewage proper and one line for the rainwater, whilst a double set of sewers will require supervision and maintenance.

It is often said that with two sets of house drains, there is danger of sewage or sink wastes being connected up to the rainwater drain. In this connection, the writer has made a practice with new work, of having each cement joint on the rainwater pipes lightly stamped while green with the letters " R.W." This can easily be done when the pipes are being laid, and a rainwater drain can then be recognised as soon as the pipe socket is laid bare, thus leaving no excuse for mistakes.

With the partially separate system of sewers, smaller sewers can be used, and the violent fluctuations in flow common to the combined system will be smoothed down, but it must be remembered that the average character of the sewage over a particular year will be stronger in rainy weather than would be the case if all the rainfall were admitted to the sewers ; on the other hand, the total volume will be smaller, and very much less detritus will reach the sewage works, less sludge in consequence being produced. It is probable that future improvements in the separate system of sewers, may go far towards eliminating the sludge difficulty so far as mineral matter is concerned, by excluding it from the sewers as rigidly as possible.

Generally speaking, it may be said that modern practice in sewerage tends to the provision of the partially separate system of sewers wherever feasible, particularly in pumping schemes where it is specially necessary to reduce the volume of sewage to be lifted to the lowest possible limit.

A very great advantage of the partially separate system is that in many cases storm overflows can be considerably reduced in number, as compared with the number which would be advisable for a combined system, and in a few exceptional cases it may be possible entirely to dispense with them.

The entirely separate system. In this system the whole of the rainwater is supposed to be excluded from the sewers, but this rarely occurs in practice, and in continued rainy weather the sewage flow is generally increased to a greater or lesser extent.

At Reading and Hampton, Middlesex, the separate system is in use, but increases in sewage flow due to rainfall occur notwithstanding—at Hampton an increase of some 10 % on the year's sewage flow.

It will be seen from what has already been said that the particular sewerage system provided must depend on the local requirements of the special case under review, and that in many cases a modification of the systems just described may be the best to adopt.

Velocity in sewers. The question of what the character of the sewage will be when it reaches the purification works, will depend, other things being equal, upon the time it remains in the sewers, and this will in turn depend upon the size and contour of the district sewered, and in particular upon the velocity of flow in the sewers.

It is a very common thing even now-a-days to find sewers of far too large a diameter employed for slack gradients, under the impression that the velocity of flow is increased thereby. If the hydraulic mean depth of the sewage flowing in the sewer were increased thereby this would be so, but it is not : it is diminished ; *e.g.* supposing a 6-inch sewer with a gradient of one in 110 gives a velocity flowing full (or half-full) of 177 feet per minute, and a 9-inch sewer with a similar gradient is substituted, the velocity in the 9-inch sewer flowing half-full will certainly give a velocity of 232 feet per minute, but the volume of sewage flowing in the 6-inch sewer—say half-full—

will not anything like half fill the 9-inch sewer of similar gradient. To do this, the volume of sewage would have to be considerably increased.

Quite recently, the writer had to replace some old sewers and house drains; one of the latter, used to drain a small detached house, was a 9-inch drain ! The drain itself was choked with solid matter, all but a waterway of about three square inches kept open through the solid matter.

It is now quite a usual thing to employ sewers of 6-inches and 7 inches diameter, whereas not many years ago it was deemed inadvisable to employ a sewer of less than 9 inches in diameter.

There are now many tables giving velocity and discharge of sewers in diagrammatic form, the best known perhaps being Crossthwaites' tables[1], the Alexander diagram[2], tables by T. C. Ekin[3], and tables and diagrams by Crimp and Bruges[4].

Variations in sewage flow. Variations in sewage flow may be classified under the following headings :

(*a*)   Annual variations.

(*b*)   Seasonal   ,,

(*c*)   Daily   ,,

(*d*)   Hourly   ,,

Annual variations. These may be caused by several factors, *e.g.* increase or decrease in yearly rainfall, increase in population, in impervious area and in water supply, advent of new industries, the periodical rise and fall of the subsoil water in the ground in which the sewers are laid. It may be said that all sewers should be watertight and therefore insusceptible to the influence of any subsoil water, but the joints of stoneware pipes however well made when the sewers are put in, will not last for ever, owing to expansion and contraction, slight settlements, etc., and sooner or later hair cracks form at the cement joints, and in course of time these enlarge and allow water outside the sewers to enter. Again, in soft waterlogged soils, a certain degree of flotation may take place. In some

[1] E. and F. N. Spon, London.
[2] H. P. Woodhouse and Co., Pelsall, Walsall.
[3] Constable and Co., London.   [4] Biggs and Son, London.

localities the effects of the autumn and winter rains are not reflected in the flow of streams until the following spring.

It seems doubtful whether the periodical influx of a moderate volume of subsoil water would materially interfere with the treatment of the sewage by, say, percolating filters, since, although the rate of treatment per cube yard would increase, the strength of the sewage would be less than normal, and thus the two factors would tend to balance one another.

Seasonal variations. These are mainly caused by seasonal increase in population, by variations in the seasonal distribution of the rainfall, also by the varying subsoil leakage to the sewers at different times of the year, and they occur more or less regularly year after year ; they may, however, sometimes be due to difference in water supply per head in summer and winter, or in certain cases to the presence of trade wastes from certain industries—such as the whisky distilling industry—where the work is only carried on for a portion of the year. It follows, therefore, that if for special purposes it is desired to obtain full information as to the character of the sewage for the year, any samples which may be drawn for purposes of analysis should embrace, if possible, a period in summer, winter, and early spring.

At seaside towns, the sewage flow alters in character and volume during the season when the influx of visitors is greatest, and with inland watering places the same thing occurs.

Daily variations. These are due to several causes, the chief—apart from rainfall—being the result of (in the case of domestic sewages) the influx of laundry waste to the sewers on certain days, usually Mondays and Tuesdays, and in the case of sewages containing trade refuse, to the fact that the waste liquids from various industries are generally turned into the sewers on particular days.

It will be found that variations in flow on different days of the week due to the above causes may be considerable ; as a general rule sewage flow is least on Sundays.

Hourly variations. The flow of sewage is never constant, varying from hour to hour, and these hourly differences in flow are known as hourly variations (see Fig. 4), their cause being

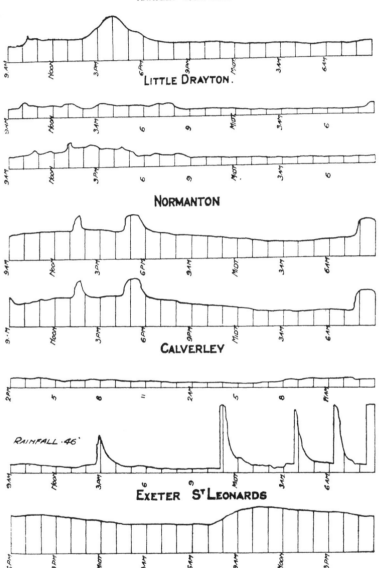

Fig. 4. Diagrams showing hourly variations in sewage flow.

mainly due to regular habits of the population served by the
sewers. As a general rule, the maximum sewage flow occurs
from 9 to 10 a.m. in the case of small works, to 11 a.m. to noon
or even later in the case of larger works where the district
sewered is an extensive one, but much depends upon the
gradients of the sewers, and the length of the outfall sewer.
When much subsoil water reaches the sewers, its effect is to
smooth down the hourly variations.

Minimum hourly flow usually occurs in the early morning,
say from 1 a.m. to 5 a.m. In cases where the sewage is pumped,
the hourly variations in dry weather are smoothed down,
especially when the sewage flow is not large and is stored in
a suction tank for some hours before being pumped.

Were subsoil and tap leakage to the sewers non-existent,
there would be little or no sewage flow after 1 a.m. in the
morning in the case of very small towns. When the early
morning flow of sewage is high it may be taken for granted
that there is a considerable volume of subsoil water entering
the sewers.

Hourly proportions of sewage flow. Since hourly
variations in sewage flow occur in dry weather at about the
same hours on the same week-days—on Sundays they are
usually later—it will be of interest to see what proportion
they bear to the total sewage flow for the 24 hours.

The proportions will vary somewhat in nearly every instance
but, broadly speaking, it may be said that during the hour of
maximum flow, as much as 8 % of the total flow for the day
may be delivered at the purification works, that is to say, if
the total flow per 24 hours is 100,000 gallons, 8000 gallons or
about one-twelfth of the total daily flow may be received at
the works in one hour, and this is known as the maximum
hourly flow. The minimum hourly flow is generally considerably below one-half of the maximum, or about 2 % to 3 %.

The average hourly flow is arrived at by dividing the total
flow per 24 hours by 24, and it bears, roughly speaking, a
ratio to the maximum hourly flow of from 1 : 1·5 to 1 : 2·5,
but in the case of small works the difference may be very
much greater.

Rainfall and sewage flow. If it were not for the fluctuations caused in sewage flow by rainfall, sewage purification would be a much simpler matter than at present, and the sludge difficulty would not reach such alarming proportions.

Duration and intensity of rainfall. These are of the utmost importance in relation to sewage flow and the provision of storm overflows.

By duration of rainfall is meant the number of hours during which rainfall occurs, and by intensity is meant the rate at which it falls during a certain unit of time. For example, an equable rainfall of ·50 inch spread over five hours is said to have an intensity or rate of fall of ·10 inch per hour. The intensity of rainfall is often very variable as regards distribution ; even in the case of a particular shower, the intensity or rate of fall may differ considerably in different parts of the same district affected by the rainfall.

From ·05 inch to ·06 inch per hour is a very usual rate of rainfall in the London district.

How important the average intensity of rainfall is, may be seen when it is considered that the sewers have to be designed with adequate carrying capacities to deal with a certain proportion of the rainfall, and a rainfall of ·50 inch in say two hours is a very different matter from ·50 inch spread over the 24 hours. A sewerage system which may be amply sufficient to cope with the latter rate, may be quite incapable of carrying off the surface water resulting from the former, such as might occur as the result of a heavy thunderstorm, and it is at such times, when the intensity of the rainfall is high and the duration short, that the sewers are apt to become unduly burdened, and flooding of low-lying streets and basements occurs. It may be noted that in rainy years the intensity of the rainfall is generally lower than in normal years.

Run-off from rainfall. Only a certain proportion of the rain which falls in a particular district will reach the surface water or foul water sewers. Some of it will become absorbed, some utilised and some evaporated, whilst some will flow away by sources other than the sewers.

The nature and character of the surface on which the rain

falls will modify the run-off of surface water ; for example, tarred roads and asphalt, paved and slated surfaces will in the case of sharp showers contribute a .arge run-off, especially if these surfaces were moist before the shower. Macadam roads and garden soil on the other hand absorb a great deal of moisture before they become saturated and any run-off occurs. Again, with a high temperature and drying wind, the effect produced on the flow in the sewers may be insignificant even with a fairly heavy shower, if of short duration : a certain quantity of rain has to fall and saturate the surface on which it falls before any surface water can run off.

Again, when the water begins to flow from the various surfaces, some time must elapse before it reaches the sewers, this being mainly dependent upon the average surface slope of the district draining to the sewers.

As regards the actual annual proportion of the rainfall reaching the sewers, records are not numerous, but in the case of Croydon (where there is a partially separate system of sewers), Mr Baldwin Latham found that during 1880 to 1881, 38·92 % of the actual rainfall reached the sewers. Again, at Rhyl, in North Wales, during the year 1901, 52·92 % of the rainfall reached the sewers.

As a very rough guide, with a combined system of sewers, about one-half to five-eighths of a sharp shower (say ·25 inch in half-an-hour) may find its way to the sewers. A sudden thaw and warm rain occurring abruptly after a sharp frost and snow, often produce a rush of water to the sewers equal in volume to that produced by a heavy thunderstorm.

The question of dealing with the excessive volumes of surface water reaching the sewers at certain times leads to the subject of storm overflows. It is quite impracticable in most sewerage schemes within reasonable limits of expenditure, to provide sewers capable of dealing with all the volumes of storm water which may reach them under certain conditions, and relief must therefore be provided at certain points in the sewers by means of specially constructed outlets known as storm overflows.

Storm overflows. Storm overflows may be divided into two classes :

(1)   Local overflows.

(2)   Main overflows.

The object of local storm overflows is to relieve the tributary sewers before they become surcharged, otherwise, an enormous outfall sewer would be requisite, quite out of proportion to dry weather requirements.

Main storm overflows may be described as being overflows placed on the main outfall sewer or sewers, so that the volume of liquid reaching the purification works shall not exceed a given volume—usually expressed in terms of the dry weather flow ; thus, with an average dry weather flow of sewage of 30,000 gallons per hour, the storm overflow may perhaps come into action when the flow in the sewer exceeds, say, six times the average hourly dry weather flow, or 180,000 gallons. The Sewage Disposal Commission in their Fifth Report state that they consider that in most cases full treatment of three times the dry weather flow will be sufficient, so that when the sewage flow exceeds this rate, the balance will pass through the stand-by tanks and thence to the river or stream.

It must be borne in mind that even with the partially separate system of sewers, an appreciable proportion of the run-off due to rainfall will go to the foul water sewers, and therefore storm overflows are often advisable and frequently essential in districts where the built-upon areas have a steep fall to the sewers.

Various kinds of storm overflow. The ordinary type of storm overflow, but constructed with a long weir, is shown in Fig. 5, and consists of a manhole on a line of sewer containing a weir whose sill is placed at the required calculated level to come into operation when the depth of sewage in the sewer reaches this level. It is open to the objection that if 4 inches of storm water are passing over the sill, the depth of liquid flowing in the sewer will also be about 4 inches in excess of the depth needed to secure the requisite discharge, hence, if the storm overflow sill is set to allow six times the dry weather flow to pass down the sewer, a volume considerably in excess of this will actually pass, the excess volume increasing with the depth of liquid passing over the sill. A long weir lessens this disadvantage, but means increased cost in the construction of the storm overflow manhole.

A better type of storm overflow in some ways is shown in Fig. 6, where a thin horizontal iron plate placed at the level of the overflow sill with vertical deflecting plate, diverts the excess water (which would otherwise pass down the sewer) to the storm overflow pipe or culvert. With this type of overflow it is possible to approximate fairly closely to the desired discharge through the sewer, but even with this type a slight excess will pass down the outfall sewer. Attention is required after storms to remove rags, etc., from the plate, and therefore it is not so well suited to rural districts where supervision is apt to be casual.

It may be observed in passing, that it is not practicable to construct an overflow to come into operation at a mathematically exact number of dilutions, nor, indeed, would there be any object in doing so, assuming it to be feasible. Sewage varies greatly in strength during storms, and a dilution of six times the dry weather flow may at certain times be more polluting than a dilution of say three times the normal flow.

Another type of overflow, suitable for surface water sewers, is shown in Fig. 7.

By this method, the first washings from streets and roads flow to the foul water sewer ; when, however, the flow of surface water in the sewer increases, and therefore the velocity, the water jumps the opening and passes away to the nearest watercourse or river.

All storm overflows should be visited after storms, and rags, paper, and the like removed from the sills. The use of screens and scumboards to cover overflow sills is not generally advisable : in the former case they generally become blocked during the first few minutes of storm, whilst in the latter case the " draw " caused by the liquid overflowing the sill will carry most of the solids with it, even if there is a scumboard.

It must be borne in mind that the discharges from overflows are intermittent and not continuous, and the effect produced on the river or stream into which they discharge is not so deleterious as a *constant* dribble of polluting liquid, *i.e.* the

DIFFERENT TYPES OF STORM OVERFLOW

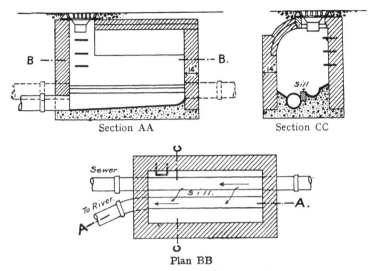

Section AA

Section CC

Plan BB

Fig. 5. Ordinary type of storm overflow.

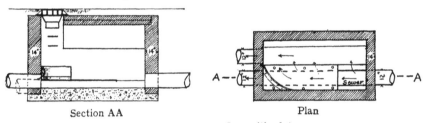

Section AA

Plan

Fig. 6. Storm overflow with plate.

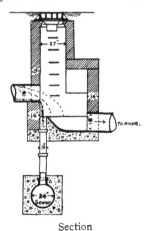

Section

Fig. 7. Leaping weir overflow.

stream has time to recuperate as a rule ; and it is frequently, but not always, in flood at the time of receiving storm overflow discharges. It is the suspended matter from storm overflows which causes the real mischief.

As to the number of times a particular storm overflow comes into operation, a good deal will depend upon the time of day when the storm occurs. If, for instance, the rain comes at about the time of maximum sewage flow, the storm overflow will come into action sooner than if the rain occurred in the early morning when the sewage flow is at its minimum.

The average number of " rainy " days in the British Isles is about 190, but included in this figure are many days on which the rainfall would be quite insufficient to cause any increase in sewage flow, let alone bringing storm overflows into operation.

The question of how much the sewage should be diluted before permitting discharge by overflows is of the utmost importance where the whole of the sewage flow is pumped. In many cases the sewage flow proper is normally diluted with an equal volume of subsoil water, a weak sewage sometimes resulting even in dry weather, and the question at once arises, are such places to be required to dilute to an equal extent as places producing a strong sewage. It does not seem to be of much value to say that there should not be this excessive subsoil leakage ; the facts have to be taken as they are, and it must be remembered that were the subsoil water eliminated a stronger sewage would result, and, as a probable sequence, a worse effluent.

One point in connection with storm overflows seems to stand out prominently, namely, that it would appear to be preferable in many cases to have in new schemes a separate or partially separate system of sewers with very few overflows, and these only coming into action on rare occasions, rather than to have a combined system of sewers, and overflows discharging at frequent intervals. In the first case, the bulk of the liquid discharged to the watercourse or river would not be mingled with a polluting sewage containing possibly typhoid or other objectionable germs, whereas, with the combined system this must be of fairly frequent occurrence. The presence of storm overflows would seem to render sterilisation of sewage effluents worse than useless, when in wet weather discharges from storm overflows may be passing untreated into the same river which receives the sterilised effluent.

BIBLIOGRAPHY.

Crimp, W. Santo. *Sewage Disposal Works.* Charles Griffin and Co., Ltd., Exeter Street, London.

Kershaw, G. B. *Modern Methods of Sewage Purification*, Chapters V, VI, VII, and VIII. Charles Griffin and Co., Ltd., Exeter Street, London. 1911.

Royal Commission on Sewage Disposal. Fifth Report. Appendices I and III to Fifth Report. Fourth Report, vol. IV.

CHAPTER IV

REMOVAL OF SUSPENDED MATTER

Screens and screening. All crude sewages contain suspended matter from coarse floating solids, such as faeces, corks, matches and paper, down to particles almost invisible to the naked eye. Sewages also contain a certain amount of colloidal matter, which is invisible to the eye, and consists of infinitely fine particles, which are neither in true solution nor suspension. When land treatment of sewage was more or less general, the crude sewage generally received only what may be termed rough treatment before passing on to the land, whilst it was seldom even roughly screened unless pumped[1], and in several instances at the present day the crude sewage is distributed on the land direct from the outfall sewer. The advent, however, of artificial filters and contact beds rendered it necessary in most instances that the larger suspended matters should be removed by screening before grit settlement and tank treatment, as a preliminary to treatment either by percolating filters or contact beds, the reason being that clogging of the material rapidly took place when the suspended matter in the

[1] Sewage should be screened when the sludge is pressed.

liquid filtered was high, and medium to fine material was used
It will be pointed out in the chapter on sludge and its disposal
(p. 121) that the general modern tendency of reducing the
solids in the tank liquor to a figure as low as possible before
passing it on to filters or contact beds, results in the production of a large quantity of sludge.

Faeces excluded from most sewage analyses. An average
English sewage contains about 35 parts of suspended matter
per 100,000, but it is doubtful whether this is not a low
estimate, except in the case of stale sewages where the solids
are well broken up before reaching the works. Lumps of faecal
matter are always numerous at certain times of the day in a
fresh sewage, but in most samplings they do not figure in the
analysis since they are too large to pass the neck of a half-
Winchester bottle : still, such matters have to be disposed of
either by screening or tank treatment, before the sewage can
be filtered efficiently, and, if thoroughly broken up and mixed
with the sewage, so as to pass into the sample bottle, it would
seem highly probable that not only the strength of that sewage
would be greater, but, that the quantity of suspended solids
per unit volume of the sewage would also show a higher figure
upon analysis.

**Sewage discharged without tank treatment should be
screened.** In England, screening as previously stated is
usually regarded as a preliminary to facilitate further treatment, or to protect pumps when the sewage is lifted. This no
doubt is due to the fact that in most instances the English
rivers and streams are small in volume, and, save in somewhat
exceptional cases, unsuited to the burden of receiving crude or
screened sewage. In the *Eighth Report of the Sewage Disposal
Commission* however dilution is countenanced whenever the
ratio of the volume of the river to the volume of sewage discharged into it exceeds 500 to 1. In such cases, however, the
sewage should, if practicable, be screened, to prevent likelihood
of solids travelling long distances down stream, or causing
offence to the eye locally.

In Germany, where the rivers are for the most part of large
volume, screening has been almost brought to a fine art, and

it is regarded in many instances as a final process of treatment for the sewage of large towns.

Forms of screen. In the English practice, the simplest form of screen met with is of the fixed bar type, set leaning at an angle with the sewage flow, and cleared either by hand, or, in the case of large works, by automatic contrivances. A bar screen and screening chamber is shown in Fig. 8.

The bar type of screen is open to the objection that unless it is regularly cleaned it is apt to choke up; and further in

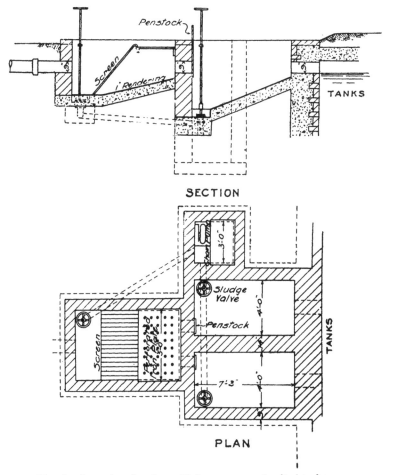

Fig. 8. Screening chamber with bar screen and grit chambers.

clearing the screen some of the screenings are almost unavoidably forced through the bars.

In the design of screens, an adequate transverse area should be presented to the sewage flow, and a sufficient depth of the bars should be submerged.

When the ordinary type of centrifugal pump is used for lifting the sewage after screening, the screens should be efficient and carefully looked after. With other types of pump, too, small pieces of hard matter are apt to prevent the valves from closing properly, causing thereby a large amount of slip.

The angle at which the screen leans away from the sewage flow should be such as would facilitate the removal of the screenings, and, in most cases, an angle of about 45° will be suitable. In the case of a screen raked by automatic rakes the angle at which the screen or screens lean away from the sewage flow should be increased, otherwise a portion of the screenings will keep falling back into the screen chamber, and eventually become broken up. As a rough guide, about $1\frac{1}{2}$ square feet of submerged screen should be provided per 1000 persons draining to the works, but much will depend upon the size of the works and the character of the sewage, *i.e.* whether it contains such trade wastes as woolscouring liquors, and whether it is fresh or stale on arrival at the purification works.

Bar screens, unless regularly attended to, effect comparatively little useful work, except in pump or filter press protection where the sewage is subsequently pumped or the sludge pressed.

Cage screens are used at some sewage works ; they should be in duplicate, so that when one screen is raised for clearing purposes, the other can be lowered to take its place.

Automatic screens. Another form of screen (Smith's Carshalton screen) which works automatically consists of an endless band of woven wire meshes, moving at an angle with the sewage flow, the motive power being obtained from a small water wheel driven by the flow of sewage; the solids in the sewage pass against the wire mesh and are gradually drawn clear of the sewage to the top of the screen and over it, when they fall into a trough in which an Archimedean screw revolves, transferring the screenings to the end of the trough, where they fall into a wheelbarrow.

An ingenious revolving screen, designed by Mr Baldwin Latham, is in use on the Croydon outfall sewer at Brimstone Barn. This screen resembles a large iron sieve revolving in a vertical plane, the sewage flow providing the motive power. The sewage passes through the sieve, the solids being intercepted by the wire meshes, and pushed out of the sieve into a trough by means of a revolving screw. Other good types of moving screen are the Reinsch-Wurl, in use at Dresden, Windschild's drum screen, Brunnottes' screen, and Jennings' Chicago screen.

The Weand rotary screen has been used in various cities in America. Briefly described, it consists of a cylindrical frame covered with wire cloth with various sized meshes according to the sewage it is designed for (usually 35 to 40 meshes per lineal inch), this cloth being superimposed on copper wire netting of 1·5 inch mesh as a support. A steel worm attached to the interior of the frame conveys the solids clear of the machine to a receptacle underneath.

The crude sewage enters the screen near its axis and falls from a platform at right angles to the flow in the sewer. Travelling jets of water playing outside the top portion of the screen wash any adherent matter off.

The screen revolves at a speed of from 8 to 12 revolutions per minute, and requires 3 to 5 H.P. motors for driving purposes.

Quantity of screenings produced. Unless the screens are very fine and the sewage fresh, the matter removed by them will be found to be comparatively small.

Colonel Harding and Mr Harrison carried out experiments in screening at Leeds[1], and it was found that even when using fine screens, the screened out matter, on drying, represented under 10 % of the suspended matters present in the sewage.

The quantity of screenings produced per million gallons of sewage screened will depend mainly upon the condition of the sewage when it reaches the works, i.e. whether fresh or the reverse, together with the kind of screen and the spaces between the meshes or bars.

In particular cases the figures may range from 2 cwt. to 18 cwt. per million gallons of sewage screened.

At the Stratford-on-Avon sewage works, Mr H. D Bell, the chemist in charge, gives the following figures showing the quantity of garbage removed from the screens[2] for the years 1908–12.

[1] City of Leeds, *Report on Experiments in Sewage Disposal*, June, 1905, by Col. T. W. Harding and Mr W. H. Harrison. Jowett and Sowry, Leeds.

[2] Borough of Stratford-on-Avon, *Second, third, fourth, and fifth Annual Reports on the Sewage Disposal Works*, by H. D. Bell. Stratford-on-Avon.

TABLE VIII. *Showing quantity of screenings produced yearly at Stratford-on-Avon Sewage Works.*

Year	Total sewage flow during the year (gallons)	Tons of garbage	Tons per million gallons	Cost of removal of garbage per million gallons	per ton	Rainfall for the year
1908–9	126,375,570	100·5	·79	1s. 3d.	1s. 7d.	21·06″
1909–10	134,458,070	103·5	·77	1s. 1d.	1s. 3½d.	26·95″
1910–11	136,241,480	99·	·73	5·9d.	8·1d.	25·17″
1911–12	127,294,700	*114·	*·89	10·7d.	11·9d.	22·24″

* Including removal of sand from pump well.

The Stratford-on-Avon sewage is a strong one, and contains much brewery waste.

Fuller states[1] that in America it has been found that medium-sized bar screens (openings ·5 inch to ·75 inch) remove from about ·5 to 10 cubic feet per million gallons, the majority of results showing a removal of from 4 to 8 cubic feet per million gallons.

At Plainfield, using inclined bar screens with spaces of ·5 inch, the quantity of screenings removed per million gallons averages about 5·7 cubic feet, weighing when removed about 46 lbs. per cubic foot and containing about 84 % of water, the cost of screening being about 2s. per million gallons of sewage screened.

The same authority states that " at Brockton, Mass., the wet screenings amount to about 50 cubic feet per million gallons of the strong local sewage."

In comparing these American results with English practice, it must be remembered that American sewages are on the whole far weaker than the English, and that in consequence the quantity of screenings removed *per million gallons* is low by reason of the dilution.

Removal and drainage of screenings. Screenings should be frequently removed from bar screens by the attendant, allowed to drain, and then set aside for removal: the finer the screens, the greater will be the attention required.

A small embanked bay formed of earth, or, if the circumstances warrant it, of concrete, underdrained and with open jointed land tiles discharging back to the sewer or pump well, is advisable for receiving screenings prior to removal (see Fig. 9). The underdrains should be covered with about 6 inches of small cinders to allow the moisture to percolate freely to the underdrains, or, if a concrete floor is used, malthouse tiles can be employed.

[1] *Sewage Disposal*, G. W. Fuller. McGraw-Hill Book Company, New York and London. 1912.

As each relay of screenings is deposited in the bay, they should receive a sprinkling of lime, or a light covering of ashes or peat dust.

If practicable, the bay used for holding screenings should be protected from rain by a light roof of corrugated iron, and in some cases, notably in the vicinity of houses, a closed shed should be provided for the screenings, both to obviate risk of smell and to shut out flies.

In the case of small works, the screenings and grit from the grit chambers are often placed in the same bay, and the grit disposed of together with the screenings.

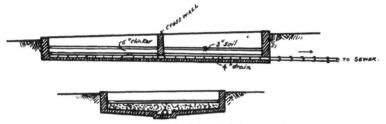

Fig. 9. Sections of draining bed for screenings.

Disposal of screenings. Screenings should be removed as frequently as possible (daily in hot weather), from the pumping station or outfall works as the case may be, and at once disposed of. In some cases it is convenient to set aside a small area of land where these can be dug into the soil ; if the area in question is a sewage farm area, and fruit trees are grown there, screenings form an excellent manure, trenched in about 2 feet from and round the trees.

In some cases nurserymen and farmers will remove the screenings, but even when they will do this, they will only as a rule fetch them during certain months of the year, and even then at irregular intervals, and steps should be taken for their proper disposal throughout the year.

In some cases, where a destructor adjoins the sewage works, arrangements can be made for burning them, and if this is practicable the greater the proportion of cinders mixed with the screenings, the better. In any case care should be taken not to expose the screenings to the visits of flies and other insects, and in some circumstances a " dusting " of bleaching powder over each relay of screenings will act as a deterrent to insects.

Detritus tanks or grit chambers. Although screens will remove the grosser solids floating in the sewage, they do not, unless of exceptionally fine mesh, affect the heavy particles of grit such as travel along the invert of the sewer. If it is desired to remove this matter it must be removed either by tank treatment, or prior to this by means of grit chambers (detritus tanks).

When settling tanks are used in series, the first tank always contains the greatest proportion of mineral matter, derived from roads, and when pressing is adopted, the sludge from the first tank in the series is usually much easier to press than that removed from the other tanks in the series, since the high percentage of coarse mineral matter allows the moisture of the sludge to drain away more rapidly : in such a case grit chambers would not be needed.

In the English practice wide variations are to be found respecting the ratio of the detritus tanks to sewage flow as regards capacity.

Apart from variations in the amount and character of the suspended matter present in different sewages, the velocity of discharge from the outfall sewer due to its gradient is a variable factor, and from 1 a.m. to 6 a.m. the suspended matter in the sewage is often quite 80 % less than normal.

Working capacity of grit chambers. Theoretically, the velocity of the flow through the detritus tanks should be regulated to allow the heavy mineral matter time to settle, whilst allowing the putrescible matters to pass on to the settling tanks.

From $\frac{1}{100}$th to $\frac{1}{200}$th part of the total dry weather flow of sewage per 24 hours is perhaps a usual capacity provided.

All detritus tanks should be constructed in duplicate, one tank being kept empty in reserve for sudden increases in flow due to storms.

American practice with regard to grit chambers. Turning to American practice with regard to the interception of heavy mineral detritus in grit tanks, Fuller quotes from a paper by Eddy and Fales[1] containing comments on grit chambers in use at Worcester, Mass. The grit chambers referred to were in duplicate, each 10 feet wide, 40 feet long, and holding a depth of about 9 feet of sewage and silt.

It was found that with the ordinary flow of sewage up to 15 million gallons per 24 hours, the organic matter settled was excessive if both chambers were in use at the same time. During storm times, when the flow was above 15 million gallons, it was found necessary to use both chambers at the same time to collect the bulk of the sand and gravel. The following table gives some statistics regarding the Worcester grit chambers.

TABLE IX. *Giving particulars of grit chambers at Worcester, Mass.*

	Customary use of chambers	Two chambers in use at rates below 15 million gallons
Deposit per million gallons of sewage passed through chambers	·16 cubic yard	·52 cubic yard.
Cost of cleaning chambers and hauling refuse 1000 feet	3s. 2d. per cubic yard	3s. 9d. per cubic yard.
Cost of cleaning chambers and hauling refuse 1000 feet (per million gallons of sewage passed through basin) ..	6d.	2s.
Dry solid matter contained in refuse ..	50 %	30 %
Volatile (loss on ignition) matter contained in refuse	35 %	50 %
Organic nitrogen in dry solid matter ..	·75 %	1· %
Weight of refuse as removed from chambers	67·2 pounds per cubic foot	—

Later figures (1910) from the same works give ·11 cubic yard of deposit removed from the grit chambers per million gallons. The velocity of flow through one chamber when all the sewage flow was being passed through it was, roughly speaking, about 3 inches per second, or a rate of flow through of about 2·66 minutes.

German practice regarding grit chambers.

Some grit chamber velocities given by Schmeitzner[2] are :

Aachen	3·4 feet per minute.
Weisbaden	100 ,, ,,
Elberfeld Barmen ..	10 ,, ,,

A rate of 1 foot per second has been selected for the new Hamburg works.

Tank treatment. Since tank treatment of sewage in one form or another forms a most important part of modern sewage purification it will be discussed at some length.

---

[1] *Journal of the Association of Engineering Societies*, vol. XXXVII. p. 67. 1906.

[2] *Clarification of Sewage*, by Dr Ing. Rudolf Schmeitzner, translated by A. Elliott Kimberley, 1910. Engineering News Publishing Company, New York, and Constable and Company, Ltd., London.

Objects of tank treatment. Even after passing through grit chambers, there still remains a very large amount of suspended matter in the sewage liquor, depending largely upon the extent to which the sewage is broken up before it reaches the sewage works, and when it is desired to remove a certain percentage of this, resort must be had to further methods of preliminary treatment devised to reduce to a greater or lesser extent the suspended matters present.

With most artificial processes, it is customary to remove the suspended solids as far as it is economically practicable. Unfortunately, the greater the quantity of matter removed from the sewage the greater is the bulk of sludge to be disposed of ; but, in most cases at all events, it is cheaper to remove the sludge from the tanks than to allow it to pass into filters or contact beds, and to remove it later on by washing operations.

The extent to which the removal of suspended matter is carried out should depend upon the purification process (if any) which follows, and the means adopted to effect this removal usually consist of some form of tank treatment. A diagrammatic section is given in Fig. 10 of a common form of rectangular settling tank used in this country.

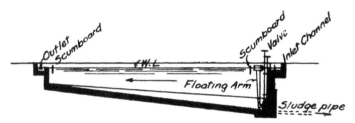

Fig. 10. Diagrammatic section of rectangular settling tanks.

Conditions vary in almost every case, and there is no one type of tank treatment universally applicable to every sewage met with.

Various methods of tank treatment. The various methods of tank treatment may be broadly classified as follows :

I. *Settling or Sedimentation Tanks.*

1. Simple settlement without chemicals, (*a*) continuous flow settling tanks, (*b*) quiescent settling tanks.

II. *Chemical Precipitation Tanks.*

2. Chemical precipitation in (*a*) continuous flow precipitation tanks, (*b*) quiescent precipitation tanks.

III.

3 Septic tank treatment (including other forms of tank treatment).

Although septic tank treatment possibly comes under the first heading, it will be more convenient to consider it under a separate heading, together with other special forms of tank.

Before going further it may be well to describe in a few words the main types of tank treatment enumerated above, subsequently dealing with each method of tank treatment more fully.

I. *Settling Tanks.*

(*a*) **Continuous flow settling tanks.** With this method the sewage passes continuously through one or more settling tanks, the suspended matter falling to the floor of the tanks, to be dealt with subsequently under the name of " sludge." The flow of sewage through the tank is only interrupted when the tank is temporarily thrown out of work, for the purpose of removing the suspended matter or sludge.

(*b*) **Quiescent settling tanks.** In this method sewage is run into one or more of a series of tanks until they are full ; the flow of sewage is then diverted into other tanks, whilst the contents of the full tanks are allowed to remain quiescent for two to three hours, when the tank liquor is drawn off and the tanks are ready to be refilled with sewage, and so on throughout the whole series of tanks, when the operation is repeated. The sludge is removed periodically after the supernatant liquid is decanted.

II. *Chemical Precipitation.*

(*a*) **Continuous flow precipitation tanks.** This plan of tank treatment resembles continuous flow settlement except that chemicals are employed to assist the settlement of the suspended matter.

(*b*) **Quiescent precipitation.** This process is the same as quiescent settlement, except that, as in the last mentioned method of treatment, chemicals are added, and for precisely similar reasons.

III.

Septic tank treatment. In this process the flow of the sewage through the tank or tanks is slow, and the contents of the tank become putrid or septic (so-called), the main object in most cases being the reduction of the sludge to as small a bulk as practicable.

4. **Various methods of tank treatment.** There are several of these, and some of them will be described later on when the more usual methods have been dealt with.

Returning to the five main types of tank treatment.

I. *Settling or Sedimentation Tanks.*

Settlement of suspended solids. The rate at which solids settle in a still liquid depends mainly upon their specific gravity, shape and size, upon the quantity of matter present, and the density of the liquid ; further, if the liquid being dealt with is a fermentable one, such as sewage, it very often depends also upon a most variable factor, *i.e.* the absence or presence of gas bubbles rising from accumulations of sediment or sludge on the tank floor. Hence, settling tanks should be cleaned out sufficiently frequently to prevent these conditions arising.

Grit, such as that derived from roads, settles rapidly ; very fine silt, such as the finer particles of china clay, may remain suspended for weeks in a still liquid.

The passage of gas bubbles through the liquid in the tank produces eddies, similar to those produced by the inequalities of a river bed, and these, in nature, play a most important part in lifting the finer suspended matter which is just about to settle, the current of the river then transporting it still further, until an opportunity of settlement on the river bed occurs. The particles themselves tend naturally to settle, but when the upward force produced by the eddies balances or is greater than the resistance of the particles they remain in suspension.

Temperature has a marked influence on the rates of settlement of fine particles; again, the presence of much finely divided matter in a liquid acts almost as if it were in solution and raises its specific gravity ; with fine particles, too, the ratio of their surface area to their weight increases rapidly the finer they are.

The rate of fall of fairly large particles such as grit and coarse sand is said to vary roughly as the square root of their diameter, and the more nearly they approach spheres in form, the more rapidly do they settle.

Aggregation or flocculation of small particles occurs, and chemicals are added to induce this action and to hasten settlement. The larger particles, which settle very rapidly, are usually retained by the grit chambers already described.

The primary object of all tanks is to remove a certain percentage of these suspended matters, and this is brought about either by complete stagnation, or by causing the sewage to flow slowly, with or without the addition of chemicals, through one or more tanks, sometimes rectangular in form and sometimes circular, the suspended matter being deposited on the floors of the tanks, and removed from time to time as sludge.

To bring about a satisfactory degree of settlement, several factors need to be borne in mind in the design and use of tanks, and they may be conveniently considered under the following headings, *viz.* :

Rate of settlement of suspended solids.	Ratio of length to width.
	Longitudinal floor slope.
Capacity.	Sludge sumps.
Shape.	Outlets.
Velocity of " flow-through."	Scumboards.
Currents.	Baffling walls.
Inlets.	Number of units.
Depth.	Working of tanks in series and
Cross section.	in parallel.

It should be observed that most of the points dealt with under the foregoing headings apply to many forms of tank other than continuous flow settlement.

Rate of settlement of suspended solids[1]. In 1899 Bock and Schwartz showed that settling tanks respectively 162 feet and 243 feet long, and worked with a velocity of ⅛ to ⅓ inch per second, deposited 55·7 % of the suspended matter from the day sewage in the 162 foot tank, and 61·5 % in the longer tank. On increasing the velocity to ⅓ inch per second, the figures for the longer tank were only reduced to 57 %.

The sewage with which these experiments were carried out deposited 88·8 % of the suspended matter on standing quiescent for 24 hours, 11·2 % consisting of fine particles which would not settle.

Settlement for an hour and a half produced a result practically similar to that obtained in three to four hours, 68·1 % of the suspended matter being deposited.

Imhoff determines the amounts of " settleable " solids by allowing a bottle of sewage to remain quiescent for two hours. The matter still remaining in suspension after this interval, he regards as too fine to belong to sedimentation processes.

It is now generally recognised that the extra amount of suspended matter deposited by a stay in excess of, say, eight to ten hours continuous flow settlement is not proportionate to the large extra outlay needed in tank capacity.

Stuernagel in 1900 carried out experiments at Cologne in a tank 146 feet long, the velocities used during the experiments ranging from ⅛ inch to over 2 inches per second.

The results obtained at Cologne resembled those obtained by Bock and Schwartz.

During the treatment of the day sewage and using a velocity of ¼″ per second, 72·31 % of the suspended matter was deposited. The velocity was then increased five times, the percentage of removal being 69·08 %. This velocity was then doubled, 58·9 % of the solids being then deposited. On allowing the tank liquor obtained at a velocity of ¼″ per second to stand quiescent for 12 hours, a further deposit of 11·7 % resulted.

At Clifton, in Lancashire, a velocity of 1·7 inches per minute reduced the suspended solids from 49 to 24 parts per 100,000 or a 51 % reduction.

At Halton, Yorkshire, a velocity of ·66 inch per minute reduced the suspended solids from 17·7 to 10·7, a reduction of about 40 per cent.

[1] Dunbar, *Principles of Sewage Treatment*, translated by H. T. Calvert. Griffin and Co., Ltd., London. 1908.

At Oswestry, Cheshire, a velocity of 3·40 inches per minute reduced the solids from 28·4 to 13·7, a reduction of about 50 %.

At the Dorking testing station, a velocity of ·31 inch per minute brought about a reduction of solids from 20·8 to 10·1 or a percentage reduction of 50 %.

Capacity of tanks. On the assumption that it is desired to obtain a fair to good tank liquor from a domestic sewage of average strength containing about 35 parts of suspended matter per 100,000, the following table[1] shows the results which would need to be aimed at. (Chemical precipitation and septic tanks are also included in this table.)

TABLE X. *Showing reduction in suspended matter effected by different methods of tank treatment.*

Preliminary Process	Strength of sewage	Strength of tank liquor	Average amount of suspended matter in tank liquor in parts per 100,000
Quiescent precipitation ..	100	50	1 to 4 parts
Continuous flow precipitation	100	60	3 to 6 parts
Quiescent settlement.. ..	100	70	5 to 8 parts
Continuous flow settlement ..	100	80	10 to 15 parts
Septic tanks	100	80	10 to 15 parts

The above figures show results which might be reasonably anticipated when employing rectangular tanks of the capacities stated in the table below, the dry weather flow of sewage per 24 hours being 1,000,000 gallons, and of average strength, it being assumed that in times of storm the tank capacities would be sufficient to deal with a storm flow up to 3,000,000 gallons per 24 hours.

TABLE XI. *Giving total capacities of tank required to treat a daily flow of one million gallons.*

Preliminary process	Stay in tanks (hours)	Total number of tanks	Number of spare tanks	Total capacity of tanks required (gallons)
Continuous flow precipitation	8	8	2	444,440
Continuous flow settlement ..	15	8	2	833,333
Quiescent precipitation ..	2	10	2	1,041,660
Quiescent settlement.. ..	2	10	2	1,041,660
Septic tanks	24	6	1	1,200,000

[1] See *Fifth Report*, Sewage Disposal Commission, p. 41.

It should be carefully borne in mind that the above capacities include spare tanks for bringing into use when some of the tanks are out of action for sludging operations.

Continuous flow settlement experiments carried out at Dorking with a tank having a capacity of 2000 gallons and a ten hours flow through, reduced the suspended solids from 21·50 to 9·39 parts per 100,000. (Average of 21 estimations extending from November 1905 to June 1906.)

Shape of settling tanks. Apart from the liquid-holding capacity of settling tanks, it should be noted that in the case of continuous flow tanks, the shape of the tank largely influences the rate of flow through them. Thus, with two tanks, each holding a 24 hours flow, but one of them (*a*) 60 feet long and the other (*b*) 40 feet long, the rate of flow through the tanks per minute will be (*a*) $\dfrac{60 \text{ feet} \times 12 \text{ inches}}{1440}$ and (*b*) $\dfrac{40 \text{ feet} \times 12 \text{ inches}}{1440}$ or a velocity of $\frac{1}{2}$ inch per minute and $\frac{1}{3}$ inch per minute respectively.

The main points to be borne in mind in the design of settling tanks, are (1) the bringing down of the desired amount of suspended matter as rapidly as possible, and (2) the facilitating of sludging operations.

Circular tanks of the Dortmund type are frequently used where the subsoil is not waterlogged and space is valuable. The Dortmund tank will be noticed later.

Velocity or rate of flow through settling tanks. This is generally stated in inches per minute, the assumption being made that the flow is a constant one throughout the 24 hours and the flow the same throughout the whole section of the tank; but it may be observed that this assumption is very far from being correct, since the flow of the sewage (unless it is pumped) is rarely constant for more than a few consecutive minutes, consequently the rate of flow through the tank also varies, being at a maximum at about mid-day—when the sewage is strongest—and least in the early hours of the morning, when the sewage in dry weather contains a minimum quantity of suspended matter. Again, storms may double or quadruple the rate of flow through the tanks, unless additional units are brought into use.

A most important point in connection with the rate of flow through tanks should be mentioned here, namely, that supposing two similar tanks to be dealing with the same sewage, but one having a rate of flow through the tank of say 50 % in excess of the other, a unit volume of the sludge deposited at the higher velocity will contain very much more heavy solid matter than a unit volume of sludge obtained at the lower rate.

Steuernagel's experiments. This point is well exemplified in Steuernagel's experiments cited by Dunbar in his book on *Principles of sewage treatment*[1].

Steuernagel obtained the following figures from his experiments, taking a day's observation in each case.

TABLE XII. *Showing sludge produced per* 1000 *gallons of sewage, at different velocities.*

Velocity (Inches per second)	Sludge (gallons)	Analysis of sludge	
		Moisture (per cent.)	Dry matter (per cent.)
$\frac{1}{6}$	4·040	95·57	4·43
$\frac{5}{6}$	2·474	92·87	7·13
$1\frac{2}{3}$	1·838	91·34	8·66

Further, the sludge produced at the higher velocity was easier to deal with than that obtained by employing a lower rate of flow through, presumably owing to the greater percentage of grit which it would contain.

Currents in settling tanks. Experiments on this matter have been carried out by Schmidt at Oppeln, and they showed that, as has been noticed in many cases in England, the sewage during the cooler months of the year being warmer flowed at the surface of the tanks.

This is very noticeable in English manufacturing districts in cold weather, when the various trade effluents are treated in settling tanks. Some of these liquors are discharged at a high temperature, and make a short cut through the tank at the surface, in many cases taking only a few minutes to pass out. This can very easily be tested by pouring dye into the inflowing effluent.

Temperature also exercises a very material effect on the rate at which suspended solids come to rest in water, and for this reason quiescent settling tanks are to be preferred where the local conditions are such as to justify putting them down.

[1] Griffin and Co., Ltd., London.

Inlet channels. These should be designed to effect as even a distribution of the sewage as possible over the cross sectional area of the tank. With a large sewage flow the best form of inlet for continuous flow tanks is undoubtedly a sill extending the whole width of the tank and a similar outlet. By this method of construction eddies are reduced to a minimum and practically the whole area of the tank is utilised.

A very usual method of constructing inlets for tanks consists in providing one or more inlets to each tank regulated by sluices. Where this construction is used for continuous flow tanks the ratio of length to width should be high. It will be found that eddies are set up in the corners of the inlet end of the tanks, and therefore, as far as the velocity of the flow through the tank is concerned, these corners might be filled in without affecting it.

A feature of the continuous flow tanks at Rochdale is that the outlets as well as the inlets of the tanks are provided with adjustable weir penstocks, by closing which the capacity of the tanks can be materially increased, the tank liquor flowing over the penstock weir when the increased tank capacity is in use. This design is due to Mr S. S. Platt, M.Inst.C.E. the Borough Engineer.

Depth of settling tanks. As a general rule, with the ordinary types of continuous flow rectangular tanks, it is not an advantage to construct them much deeper than an average depth of, say 6 feet, and it is doubtful whether the advantages obtained by constructing them as shallow as 3 feet average depth, are not more than neutralised by the extra cost necessary to provide the requisite total tank capacity, and increased risk of nuisance from exposed sludge when the tank liquor is drawn off to allow of sludging. It must be borne in mind that with the common form of rectangular tank, the deeper the tank the longer a given particle of suspended matter will be in falling to the floor of the tank, and, if the tank be too deep, it may be carried over the tank sill. If the available space for tanks is limited, it will probably be better, if the ground is good, to provide deep tanks of the Dortmund or Imhoff type, since the sludging operations are thereby facilitated, as the sludge can be removed periodically without emptying the tank, which is often necessary with the shallow rectangular form, unless special sludge sumps are provided ; again, sludge withdrawn frequently from shallow tanks often carries a high percentage of moisture with it.

Cross section of settling tanks. The cross sections of most of the earlier constructed settling tanks in England were rectangular in form ; in many cases the angles where the longitudinal walls meet the floors, both in quiescent and in continuous flow settling tanks, might be rounded in form with advantage, to facilitate the sludging processes, and it is now usual in many cases to provide a central sludge channel in the floors, which slope to this channel from each of the walls.

If the slope of floor is intended to cause the sludge to flow by gravity to the channel, a considerable fall will be needed, and hence it is inadvisable to construct tanks of too great a width, as much fall will be lost in connection with the sludge drain.

With quiescent settling tanks the sludge generally settles fairly evenly over the entire floor in a thin film, and when, as is usually the case, these tanks are cleared out after the first[1], second, or third filling, the sludge is not as a rule sufficient to form a surface slope of its own, and squeegees must be used.

When continuous flow tanks are used in series they are sometimes constructed with different cross sections, the smallest section occurring at the inlet end of the first tank, the greatest section being at the outlet of the last tank. This arrangement has the effect of reducing the rate of flow through each tank successively.

Such an arrangement of tanks is in operation at Viersen, and is stated by Schmeitzner to have a high efficiency, removing 82 % of the suspended solids.

By constructing tanks wedge-shaped in plan, it is practicable to preserve a uniform cross-sectional area and velocity throughout the tanks.

Ratio of length to width. As previously mentioned, the formation of the sewage inlets to the tank exercises a great

[1] If the sludge is not removed frequently from quiescent settling tanks, there is danger of it being stirred up when the tank is re-filled.

influence on the rate of flow through the tank, but where several sluice gate inlets to each tank are provided it will generally be found advisable to have a ratio of length to width of at least three to one in order to eliminate as far as possible the effect of entrance eddies, and to admit of the settlement of some of the finer particles.

Longitudinal slope of floors of settling tanks. In all modern settling tanks, a longitudinal fall is given to the floors towards the sludge sump, to facilitate sludging operations, and also to admit of a certain amount of sludge accumulating in the deeper end of the tank without materially interfering with the rate of " flow through " between the intervals of cleaning.

The amount of fall necessary to enable a " free " sludge to gravitate naturally to the sludge sump is, roughly speaking, about 1 : 30. In some instances glazed tiles have been used to line the floors of the tanks to cause the sludge to slip towards the sump freely. In many cases the fall available is insufficient to allow a longitudinal fall of, say 1 : 30, and in such cases squeegees are used or a hose is applied to cause the sludge to flow, or some tank liquor siphoned off from an adjoining tank which is full. With some larger tank installations movable scrapers on wheels run along lines laid on the floors of the tanks, pushing the sludge before them. It follows that with a longitudinal slope, the cross-sectional area of the tank must be constantly diminishing towards the outlet, and that consequently the velocity of flow through the tank is increasing. This objection can be lessened, as has already been pointed out, by designing the cross section of the tank so as to meet this point, but there are so many other factors to be considered such as storm flows, etc., that it seems an unnecessary refinement

Sludge sumps. The position of the sludge sump in continuous flow tanks is generally advantageously placed at the inlet end of the tanks, where the greatest quantity of heavy gritty sludge is likely to collect. When the sump is rectangular in plan, the four sides should slope sharply to the sludge outlet pipe, with a slope of say 1 to 1.

In many instances with small rectangular tanks the sludge can be removed while the tank is in use, if a small portion is removed at frequent intervals; if, however, the sludge is allowed to accumulate for a week or so, it is a common experience to find that when the sludge valve is opened, only a small portion of the sludge in the immediate vicinity of the sludge outlet comes away, leaving a cavity resembling an inverted pyramid with the apex over the sludge outlet. This is of frequent occurrence with the usual form of septic tank

Sludge drains. The gradient at which the sludge drain will act satisfactorily depends upon the nature of the sludge to be conveyed by it. With tanks used on the quiescent system, where they are cleaned out after every second filling or so, the sludge will generally be of a watery nature (say 95 % moisture) and the gradient of the sludge drain can be 1 in 100 or even less where an ample area of land is available for the sludge, since in such a case small flushes of sewage can be employed to flush the drain after each sludging. (The specific gravities of sludge are said to vary between 1·02 and 1·06. Ordinary 90 % moisture sewage sludge weighs about 10·6 lbs. per gallon.)

For the sludges containing less moisture, say 90 %, the gradient of the sludge drain will probably have to be steepened to 1 in 50, and for sludges containing under 90 % moisture, the gradient should be still steeper.

Outlets of settling tanks. Without question, one of the best forms of outlet is the weir or sill extending the entire width of the tank, and as the floating solids should have been removed before the sewage reaches the outlet, there is no risk of their accumulation on the outlet sill during periods of slack flow. When the tanks are built out of the ground, drop outlet pipes can be provided in the outlet channel communicating with a carrier at a lower level if land treatment is used, or to a pipe supplying filters or contract beds as the case may be. If the tanks are also used on the quiescent plan, the outlet from the floating draw-off arms will communicate with the carrier or pipe at about the same level as the drop pipes. The main reason for having the outlet end of the tanks at the shallow end opposite to the inlet, is to avoid the narrowest cross section in the tank being still further reduced by accumulating sludge, as would otherwise be the case.

In some tanks the outlets are arranged in the form of movable hand sluices, whilst in other cases floating draw-off arms are relied on. A further method of withdrawing tank liquor is by means of telescopic draw-off pipes.

Scumboards. All continuous flow tanks should be provided with scumboards. These not only arrest floating matters but tend to still the surface eddies formed in the tanks. As a rule two scumboards are provided to each tank, one at the inlet and the other at the outlet. Scumboards may be either fixed or movable.

With continuous flow tanks, where the liquid is drawn off for sludging purposes by a floating draw-off arm, it is advisable to have one of the scumboards made to slide in grooves in the tank side walls, so that, as the water level in the tank sinks, the scumboard falls with it, and protects the floating arms from such matters as corks, match sticks, etc. With quiescent settling tanks floating scumboards in the form of a box without top or bottom can be used to surround the floating arm, but some floating arms draw off the tank liquor at some distance below the water's surface, and scarcely require scumboards. Care should be taken to place the scumboards near the inlet of the tanks at a sufficient distance from the end wall to prevent the flow of sewage carrying floating matters under the scumboard; as a general rule a distance of about 3 feet will effect this object.

As regards the depth below the water level in the tank to which the board should dip, a submerged depth of from 9 to 18 inches has been found to answer well. The outlet scumboard should not be placed nearer the outlet wall than about 3 to 4 inches to avoid any " dragging-up " action caused by increased velocity of flow-through during storms. Scumboards are essential in the case of septic tanks where a heavy blanket or scum is apt to form, and for septic tanks with long weir sills, cleaned out at frequent intervals, 2 feet is not too much to allow for the depth of the submerged portion.

Baffling walls. These consist of cross walls, one or

more in number, built across each tank at intervals, the top of the walls lying below the water level of the tanks.

As a general rule baffle walls should not come nearer the water level in the tank than about $\frac{1}{4}$ to $\frac{1}{3}$ the total water depth in the tank at that particular point.

In cases where it is desired to retain the heavy gritty sludge at the lower end of the tank, a baffling wall is a useful adjunct where very large quantities of sludge have to be manipulated.

Number of tank units. It is not advisable to have less than two tanks in the smallest installation, and three is a much better number for satisfactory working. If, where there are only two tanks, a storm coincides with the sludging of one of the tanks, much suspended matter will be washed out of the tank in use. A third tank would get over the difficulty.

In the case of a larger installation, very much depends upon how the sewage flow arrives at the works, and the tank units should be arranged accordingly. Few things are more annoying to a sewage works manager than to have one solitary tank— often much too large—in which to give the sewage preliminary treatment.

Fig. 11 shows a plan and section of the new continuous flow settling tanks recently constructed at the Cambridge sewage farm, where the fall between the existing tanks and the ground level was very small. The tanks are five in number with a total combined capacity of 1,200,000 gallons.

With the ordinary sewage flow the sewage passes from the grit chambers into a long shallow channel, whence it is fed into the five new tanks, each of which is provided with four inlets, two being generally in use at any one time.

During heavy sewage flows, the sewage overflows into the old tank; the rate of flow through the new tanks is, therefore, not unduly increased in times of rainfall.

Each of the new tanks is divided into two compartments, the sludge deposited in the smaller compartment being removed weekly without emptying the whole tank. The larger compartments are only sludged once a month. Both the old and new tanks discharge the sludge into the same channel near the grit chambers.

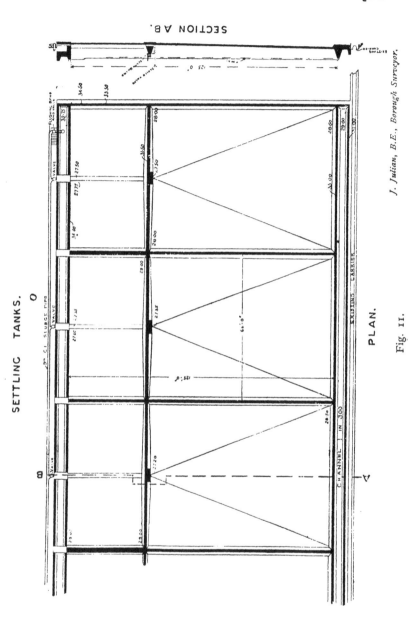

BOROUGH OF CAMBRIDGE.

SETTLING TANKS.

SCALE.

SECTION A B.

PLAN.

J. Julian, B.E., Borough Surveyor.

Fig. 11.

The sludge can be removed from the small compartment in half an hour, and from a large compartment in about $2\frac{1}{2}$ hours.

The writer is indebted to Mr J. Julian, B.E., Borough Surveyor of Cambridge, for the foregoing plan and particulars.

Working of tanks in series and in parallel. With both chemical precipitation and simple settlement, when the flow of sewage is passed through two or more tanks one after the other, they are said to be used in series ; when the sewage is run through two or more tanks simultaneously, they are said to be worked in parallel.

If kept sludged frequently, tanks worked in series are useful during storms. Quiescent settling tanks are almost universally worked in parallel. With ordinary rectangular tanks, other things being equal, the lowest rate of flow through is brought about when the tanks are worked in parallel.

A good deal depends upon facilities for getting rid of the sludge or the reverse, as to whether it will be economical to run the tanks in series. If this is done, the first tank will receive the heaviest sludge, containing the smallest percentage of water, whilst the sludge from the last tank will be excessively watery : again, if the last tank of the series is allowed to run too long without sludging, there is danger of gas bubbles rising and carrying suspended matter over the sill thus frustrating one of the chief advantages of working tanks in series.

Quiescent settling tanks. With quiescent settling tanks, if it is required to withdraw a maximum amount of suspended matter from the sewage, the tanks must be sludged frequently. Experiments carried out at Leeds[1] and Sheffield showed that good settlement could be obtained by quiescent settlement in from two to three hours.

Some sewages, however, which receive certain wastes, e.g. brewery, tannery or woolscouring wastes, contain matters which are extremely difficult to treat without causing smell, and in such cases chemical precipitation would probably give better results.

One of the main drawbacks to quiescent settling tanks is to be found in the fact that in gravitation schemes they require

---

[1] *Fifth Report*, Appendix I. Evidence of Mr W. H. Harrison.

considerable fall when used as a preliminary process, unless
pumping is to be resorted to : again, considerable attention is
necessary for filling and emptying and sludging the tanks, and,
if the sewage is a variable one containing trade refuse, it may
so happen that instead of its being equalised with the rest of
the sewage, one particular tank may be filled with virtually
nothing but trade waste liquor.

As regards the production of sludge by this method, it is
somewhat greater as a rule than that produced by septic tanks
or continuous flow settlement, whilst the sludge, owing to the
frequent drawing-off, contains more water. On the other hand,
the tank liquor will contain a minimum of suspended solids,
whilst a very great advantage is the absence of eddies and
velocities, and the influence of varying temperature during the
period of quiescence ; moreover, the actual quantity of sewage
passed through the tanks can easily be recorded, and this is
desirable.

, **General.**   There is a good deal to be said in favour of continuous flow settlement, the main point, perhaps, being that
very little fall is lost as regards the outflow from the tanks, the
tank liquor leaving the tank at a level but little below that at
which it enters.   Again, the initial cost is not large, and little
attendance is needed, whilst the volume of sludge produced is
not excessively large, and variations in the strength of the
sewage are equalised.   On the other hand, it must be noted
that the sludge will contain a large percentage of water—at
least 90 %, and, in hot weather, possibly 95 %, since the tanks
must then be frequently emptied.

Probably continuous flow tanks are as well suited as any
for the preliminary treatment of the sewage of small places
where the sewage gravitates to the disposal works.

In cases where the whole sewage flow is pumped to the tanks
in a few hours by centrifugal pumps, it is often very convenient
to have the tanks designed so as to be capable of being used
either on the continuous flow or quiescent plan : if this method
is followed, the tanks can be filled in succession during the
morning pumping spell, being run off when the pumps have
stopped and the sewage is collecting in the pump well ; the

tanks can be left at night ready to work on the continuous flow plan, should there be likelihood of storms occurring, necessitating night pumping.

Fig. 12 gives a plan and section of the tanks at the Hatfield sewage farm, which are worked in this manner.

If some such method is not adopted, *i.e.* to ensure quiescent settlement, where centrifugal pumps are used at small works, it will often be found that the sewage is rushed through the tanks so quickly as to preclude any chance of proper settlement.

If the tanks are designed to be used interchangeably on the continuous flow or quiescent settlement plan, a portion of the tanks, in the absence of a rapid fall, will have to be built out of the ground, otherwise in the case of land treatment a considerable area of land near the tanks will be out of use.

In dealing with some sewages it may be advisable to use precipitants during the hot weather, reverting to sedimentation during the winter months; it is usually a simple matter to provide in the design of the tanks for precipitation, if this should be needed.

Nuisance from settling tanks. If the tanks are kept clean and not run for too long periods without sludging, there should be very little smell from them, if domestic sewage is being treated. Where brewery or tannery liquids are present in the sewage, smell may arise during the ordinary working of the tanks. During sludging of the tanks, local smell is apt to arise in hot weather.

II. *Chemical Precipitation Tanks.*

There has been a tendency of late years to look upon chemical precipitation as being out-of-date. This view, however, was by no means held by the Sewage Disposal Commission, and, whilst it would be unreasonable to expect chemical precipitation to produce a tank liquor suitable for discharge in large volumes into a river or stream of small volume, there can be no question that it frequently forms a very valuable preliminary to modern filtration processes, especially where the absence of smell is desirable. The main disadvantage is the fact that the volume of sludge produced is large, and in many cases difficulty is experienced in getting rid of this.

Chemical precipitation is specially suited to sewages containing such trade liquors as those derived from breweries and tanneries, where a nuisance would be apt to arise with other methods of tank treatment. With ordinary domestic sewages it is also useful, where it is essential to produce a tank liquor with a minimum of suspended solids, as, for example, where the tank liquor is to be treated upon very fine filters.

It is possible with two hours' quiescent chemical precipitation to produce a tank liquor containing an average of from two to four parts of solids per 100,000, whilst with eight to ten hours' continuous flow precipitation, the tank liquor may contain from three to six parts per 100,000.

Various precipitants used. Many chemicals have been used such as lime, alumino-ferric, ferrous sulphate, sulphuric acid, ferrozone, ferric sulphate, etc. The chemicals in most general use, at the present day, are lime and alumino-ferric, or lime and alumino-ferric used in conjunction. Alumino-ferric is manufactured in blocks, and has the advantage of not requiring mixing machinery ; lime, on the other hand, is usually added as milk of lime, and requires mixing machinery.

At Chorley in Lancashire, alumino-ferric has for some years been manufactured at the sewage works by treating bauxite with sulphuric acid.

At Kingston, a very effective precipitation method is that known as the " A.B.C. process," the original ingredients added to the sewage being alum, blood and clay ; these substances have been somewhat modified of late years ; it should be noted that at Kingston the sludge is dried, powdered and sold as manure under the name of Native Guano, so that the additional solids produced by the precipitants are rather an advantage.

It has been found that chemicals are most effective when added in the form of a solution, but this presents some difficulty, as the quantity of solution should vary according to the strength and volume of the sewage arriving at the works. Alumino-ferric blocks are useful in this respect, since if they are placed in the inlet channel to the tanks, the sewage flow when it increases will dissolve proportionately more of the block. It will usually be found the most economical chemical for small works unless brewery refuse is present, when lime is better owing to its deodorizing effect. As a general rule it is convenient to add the chemicals to the sewage where it enters the inlet channel to the tanks, and it is advantageous to enlarge the channel and place slate baffles in it, for the purpose of ensuring a thorough mixture of the precipitant with the sewage. As a general rule it will be found advisable to add a fairly large dose of the chemical, if satisfactory results are to be obtained.

When two separate chemicals are used in conjunction, it has been found beneficial to add one chemical a little in advance of the other—for example—when using copperas and lime, it is best to add the copperas after the lime.

At Burton-on-Trent some years ago a very large dose of lime (from 50 to 60 grains per gallon) was used to prevent nuisance from the brewery waste present in the sewage in preponderating quantity. A large dose of lime is still used.

At Bradford and Rochdale sulphuric acid is used as a precipitant by reason of the large quantity of wool scouring refuse.

Merits of various precipitants. Many experiments have been carried out in this country and abroad concerning the value of various precipitants.

Mr Hazen in experiments[1] carried out on a weak sewage at Lawrence, U.S.A. with lime, lime and ferrous sulphate, ferric sulphate and aluminium sulphate, observes :

" Using equal values (*i.e.* as regards price) of the different precipitants, applied under the most favourable conditions for each, upon the same sewage, the best results were obtained with ferric sulphate. Nearly as good results were obtained with copperas and lime used together, while lime and alum each gave somewhat inferior effluents. The range of these results was, however, comparatively narrow, and it may be added that with a sewage of a different character, or with variations in the price of chemicals, it would be advantageous to use copper—as with lime, or even alum. When lime is used, there is always so much lime left in solution that it is doubtful if its use would ever be found satisfactory except in the case of acid sewage "

[1] *Experiments upon the chemical precipitation of sewage.* State Board of Health, Massachusetts. 1890.

At Birmingham, milk of lime was used as a precipitant for many years until it was abandoned in 1901. Lime was added at the rate of 12 grains per gallon[1]. The effect of the lime process is shown in the following figures.

TABLE XIII. *Showing effect of lime process at Birmingham in* 1900.

	Parts per 100,000	
Year 1900	Dissolved Solids	Suspended Solids
Crude sewage	129·1	67·6
Preliminary tank liquor ..	138·0	16·3
Final tank liquor	133·2	4·2*

* The Birmingham sewage contains considerable quantities of iron salts, so that the above results cannot be ascribed entirely to the lime.

It will be observed that the solids *in solution* are increased by the use of the lime.

Mr J. Bolton stated in his evidence before the Sewage Disposal Commission that the best precipitant tried at Heywood was alumino-ferric. With 8 grains per gallon of this precipitant a purification of 62 % was effected at a cost of £1. 7s. 6d. per million gallons of sewage treated.

At Huddersfield, Mr Campbell employed lime and copperas for seven years with good results, a purification of 54 % being obtained at a cost of about 17s. 11d. per million gallons.

It must be carefully borne in mind that the cost of the preliminary process cannot well be considered apart from the subsequent process ; for example, a rather costly precipitation process may enable the resulting tank liquor to be filtered at a much greater rate than a tank liquor produced at a cheaper rate but containing more suspended solids, and therefore only capable of being treated at a much lower rate per cube yard of filtering material, medium to fine filtering material being assumed in either case.

The following table taken from the *Fifth Report* of the Sewage Disposal Commission gives various particulars regarding precipitation of sewage (mainly domestic) at various places.

---

[1] Sewage Disposal Commission, *Fifth Report*, p. 34.

Place	Precipitant	Quantity of precipitant added (in grains per gallon), based on the dry weather flow	Dry weather flow of sewage (treated by the precipitation process) Gallons	Character of Sewage	Cost of precipitant per million gallons — Based on dry weather flow (£ s. d.)	Cost of precipitant per million gallons — Based on average daily flow (£ s. d.)	Year
Withnell	Alumino-ferric	15·7	10,000	Very strong	5 6 0	—	1903
Radcliffe	,,	8·0	800,000	—	—	2 15 0	1902–5
Calverley	Alumino-ferric and ferrozone	17·5	12,000	Very strong	2 10 0	—	1904
Heywood	Alumino-ferric	8 / 8	630,000 / 630,000	Average strength	—	1 7 6 / 1 6 6	—
Guildford	Alumino-ferric	8	300,000	Very strong	2 2 0	1 4 5	1905
Horfield	,,	5	40,000	Average strength	1 10 0	1 17 6	1905
Normanton	,,	6·7	175,000	Very strong	1 5 0	—	1902–5
Hendon	,,	5·5	950,000	Rather strong	—	13 3	1906
Chorley	,,	9	900,000	Average strength	—	12 10	1902
Royton	,,	2·22	367,500	—	—	6 7½	1906
Buxton	Natural iron water, milk of lime	6·7, 6 } 12 to 13 / 13	750,000	—	—	4 6	1906
Dorking	Lime and alumino-ferric	5·6, 3·5 } 9·1	200,000	Average strength	—	15 8	1902–4
Friern Barnet	Lime, alumino-ferric	4, 2 } 6	350,000	—	Lime 5s. 1d. / Alumino ferric 7s. 7½d.	12 8½	—
York	Lime / Alumino-ferric	5·77, 4·33 } 10	3,750,000	Average strength, or perhaps under average	—	10 7	1904–5
Willesden	Lime / Alumino-ferric	3·85, 5·46 } 9·31	1,930,950	—	Lime 1s.5·38d. / Alumino ferric 8s.6·5d.	10 0	—
Ealing	Lime / Alumino-ferric	4, 2 } 6	1,000,000	—	—	6 9	3 years ending Mar. 1906
Leyton	Lime / Hanson's Sulphurous powder	15, 7 } 22	3,000,000	—	—	3 11 0	1905–6
Kingston	Alumino-ferric, blood, charcoal and clay (A.B.C. process)	50	2,750,000	Average strength	—	3 4 0	1902–4
Rochdale	Alumino-ferric / Sulphuric acid	7·3, 4·7 } 12	2,000,000	Very strong	—	1 8 7	1904–5

NOTE. It will be observed in the above table that at nearly all the places where lime is used as a precipitant the cost is relatively low. In regard to this, however, it must be stated that the figures of cost refer to the lime alone, and do not include any charges with respect to the mixing. This might add, we think, from 2s. to 10s. per million gallons according to circumstances.

Nuisance from chemical precipitation tanks. There is generally considerable smell from these tanks when they are being sludged, especially if there is brewery refuse in the tank liquor.   Little smell, as a general rule, arises from precipitation tanks during their working.

III. *Septic Tanks.*

Septic tank treatment came to the front as a result of Mr Cameron's experiments at Exeter, having for their main object the digestion of the organic matter in the sewage.

By this method the sewage is passed slowly through the tanks, and the sludge is only removed at infrequent intervals, being left in the tank to undergo putrefaction and diminution in volume : the tank liquor from a septic tank is generally dark-coloured, and with most sewages is a strongly smelling liquid. It was at one time claimed that septic tanks solved the sludge problem, all the organic matter being digested, whilst all pathogenic microbes were destroyed in the passage through the tank ; further, that septic tank liquor was more amenable to subsequent treatment than other tank liquors.

The digestion of solids is now known to be very considerably less than was originally held to be the case, whilst as regards numbers of bacteria, there is little to choose between the sewage entering the septic tank, and the tank liquor leaving it. Further, experiments at Dorking, Rochdale, Leeds, Sheffield and elsewhere went to show that septic tank liquor was not more easily oxidised by filters than other tank liquors.

Septic tanks, however, apart from the sludge digestion, are sometimes useful for equalising the strength of a variable sewage containing trade refuse.

It is now generally recognised that the chief benefits resulting from the use of septic tanks are the settlement and partial liquefaction of suspended matter in the sewage, together with the equalisation in the strength of the sewage brought about by the long stay in the tanks.

Shape. As regards the shape of septic tanks, the most general form in use in England is the rectangular form, although circular tanks of the Dortmund type are in use. As with all settling tanks, the design should be such as to facilitate the settlement and withdrawal of the suspended matter. Unfortunately, owing to gas bubbles being evolved from sludge lying upon the tank floors and rising up through the liquid, there is a great tendency for large masses of suspended matter to be carried over the tank sills. This may be remedied to some extent with rectangular tanks by providing a cross wall to retain the bulk of the sludge at the inlet end of the tank, the object being to prevent the gas bubbles from rising through the liquid near the outlet sill, where the particles of suspended matter have insufficient time to subside. Another important point in the design of septic tanks is that facilities should exist for removing the sludge which has remained the longest in the tank.

The following table shows the dimensions of several septic tanks in use in England.

TABLE XV. *Showing dimensions of various septic tanks.*

Place	Dimensions
Accrington	{101'–9″ × 59'–8″ × 8'–6″ {101'–9″ × 58'–2″ × 9' 101' × 67'–6″ × 9'
Andover ..	80' × 16'–8″ × 8'–6″
Exeter (Belle Isle) ..	177' × 36' × 6'
,, (St Leonard's) ..	70' × 50' × 7'
Hartley Wintney (1908)	70' × 10' × 7'–9″
York	160' × 40' × 6'–6″
Slaithwaite	20' diam. 21' deep (Dortmund type)
Prestolee	38' × 10' × 7'
Manchester	300' × 100' × 6'
Burnley	80' × 46' × 6'–6″
Barrhead	100' × 18' × 8'
Yeovil	200' × 14' × 6'
Cheltenham	160' × 36' × 7'
Hanley	200' × 75' × 6'

Depth. Since one of the functions of a septic tank is to digest sludge, and sludge digestion takes time, it follows that the accumulation of sludge will in course of time reduce the capacity until an equilibrium more or less has been reached, and much suspended matter comes to be carried out of the tank, the capacity of the tanks should therefore be such as to admit of a certain amount of sludge storage.

As a general rule with rectangular tanks, an average water level depth of six feet or so will be found suitable. If the tanks are much deeper than this, difficulty as regards the withdrawal of the sludge will sometimes arise, if the available fall on the site is limited.

Capacity. The capacity of septic tanks will vary somewhat according to the nature of the sewage to be tanked. It was formerly the custom to make the tank capacity equal to a 24 hours flow of sewage; and, in India, it appears that a three days flow has on occasion been found advantageous.

In this country, from 12 hours to 24 hours is a very usual capacity, but much depends upon the distance the sewage has travelled before entering the tanks, and in many cases where the sewage is pumped and a large suction tank holding possibly from 12 to 24 hours flow provided, an additional stay of say 18 hours in a septic tank would probably result in an over-septicised liquid, and, in the case of a brewery sewage, there would be serious risk of nuisance from the resulting tank liquor.

It may be laid down as a general rule that a septic tank installation should never consist of less than two units.

Inlets. The best form of inlet is a weir extending the whole width of the tank, as recommended for continuous flow settling tanks, as this method causes a minimum of disturbance in the tanks.

Outlets. The outlets should be designed to effect the withdrawal of the tank liquid with as little disturbance as practicable, and this can in most cases be effected by a long weir extending the full width of the tank as in the case of the inlet. The outlet should be protected by a deep scumboard.

One point should be mentioned with regard to weir outlets, namely, liability to smell in hot weather by reason of the surface of liquid exposed; this objection can, however, be overcome by using iron plates or boards fitting in rebates in the outlet channel walls, so that the channel is completely covered in.

Rate of flow through septic tanks. Colonel Harding and Mr Harrison made several experiments upon this point with the Leeds sewage[1], rates of flow through the tanks of 12, 24, 48 and 72 hours being tried with the following results.

TABLE XVI. *Showing effect of different rates of flow through Leeds septic tanks.*

Grains per gallon	1½ hrs flow		24 hrs flow		48 hrs flow		72 hrs flow*	
	Average analysis	Percentage reduction on crude sewage	Average analysis	Percentage reduction on crude sewage	Average analysis	Percentage reduction on crude sewage	Average analysis	Percentage reduction on crude sewage
Total Solids	87·7	—	78·2	—	78·6	—	73·9	—
Suspended solids ..	19·2	52	11·4	71	10·9	73	9·9	76
Free ammonia ..	1·56	22	1·51	24	1·62	19	1·79	37
Albuminoid ammonia	0·54	50	0·45	58	0·38	64	0·34	52
Oxygen absorbed in 4 hours at 80° F. ..	5·21	45	4·84	49	4·30	55	3·59	55

* Experiment at later date with weaker sewage.

Dr Gilbert J. Fowler in his evidence before the Sewage Commission stated that 24 hours stay in the tank was the longest period he would allow.

Messrs Watson and O'Shaughnessy found with the Birmingham sewage that septic treatment for a period of at least 24 hours was distinctly advantageous.

It has been noticed by several observers that if sewage is passed too slowly through a septic tank, " over-septicisation " occurs, with the production of large volumes of sulphuretted hydrogen, and that its subsequent treatment on filters is rendered difficult.

Open and closed septic tanks. It was formerly thought that it was essential to the proper working of septic tanks that they should be covered in, but experiments by reliable investigators at Manchester, Birmingham, Leeds and elsewhere showed that there was no difference between the tank liquors derived respectively from closed and open septic tanks.

[1] City of Leeds, *Report on Experiments in Sewage Disposal*, by Col. T. W. Harding and Mr W. H. Harrison. Leeds, June, 1905.

The main advantages claimed for covered tanks are that

(1)   Smell is avoided,
(2)   The effects of wind, rain and snow are eliminated,
(3)   The temperature is more equable.

As regards the avoidance of smell by roofing in, it is a common experience that it is usually the liquid issuing from the tank which smells rather than the body of the liquid in the tank, which is usually covered with a blanket or scum, and it is during the distribution of the liquid over land or filters that nuisance arises.

A roof certainly protects the liquid in the tanks from effects of weather, but except in the case of tanks adjacent to inhabited buildings, it is not essential.

As regards temperature, a fibrous blanket spreading over the surface of the tank is about the best non-conductor of heat that could be devised.   Further, there can be no question that the permanent covering in of tanks very greatly hampers sludging processes, whilst there is always the risk of explosion through carelessness.   At the Exeter (Belle Isle) works, it has been found almost impossible to remove the sludge effectively from the large covered-in tanks.

Removal of sludge.   If the sludging question alone had to be considered with septic tanks, it would generally be preferable to sludge at infrequent intervals; but there are several objections to this, the chief one being that after a certain time the suspended solids issuing in the tank liquor increase largely, and cleaning out becomes a necessity, whilst the sludge in the tank becomes denser and more difficult to manipulate.

It would therefore appear that some figure should be decided upon as regards the limit of suspended solids permissible in the tank liquor, and when this figure is exceeded the tanks should be cleaned out.   If this is not done, the heavy increase in suspended solids will rapidly choke filters of medium-sized material or land.   With filters of coarse material, it is possible to filter a tank liquor containing, say, 15 to 20 parts of suspended matter.   If such a liquid, however, were treated in contact beds of medium-sized material, trouble from clogging and consequent decreased capacity would very quickly follow.

The nature of the subsequent treatment therefore will to some extent decide how often the tanks should be sludged, *i.e.* with fine material filters any large amount of suspended matter in the liquid treated by them would shorten the life of the filters.

The question next arises, whether it is better to remove all the sludge in one operation, or only to remove partially some of the sludge at more frequent intervals.

As a general rule it will be found that at a small sewage works the tanks are only cleaned out at long intervals of time, regardless of the increase of solids in the tank liquor and the increase of sludge in the tanks. This means that the filters or contact beds are receiving the sludge which should be retained in the tanks.

It must be remembered that if the sludge is left in a septic tank too long, it is often extremely difficult to deal with, since it settles closely together on the tank floor in course of time, and cannot be got to flow unless it is thinned down with tank liquor.

In any case it would seem advisable to remove the oldest and densest sludge from the tanks leaving the more newly formed to digest still further.

Removal of suspended matter from septic tank liquors. Many attempts have been made to effect a reduction of the suspended matter normally present in septic tank liquors, both by layers of fine filtering material, as at Leeds, and by coarse material, as at Guildford and Ilford, whilst at Birmingham Mr Watson has found that tanks on a modified Dortmund system remove about 75 % of the suspended matter present in the Birmingham septic tank liquor.

Experiments carried out at Dorking having the same object in view, showed that by passing septic tank liquor through tanks holding about one quarter of the 24 hours flow of sewage, and adding lime to the liquor at the rate of from 2 to 3 grains per gallon, the suspended matter was reduced from eight to five parts per 100,000 whilst a considerably larger quantity of the liquor could be purified per cube yard of filter, and the offensive character of the septic tank liquor was largely destroyed.

It may be noted that this process was in use at Blackburn for some years, the object there being to assist nitrification on the filters.

Sludge digestion. The amount of sludge digested by septic tanks must depend largely upon the nature of the sewage and of the suspended solids which it contains. Since most of these solids contain from 40–60 % of mineral matter, it follows that in no case can the digestion possibly exceed 60 % at the outside, even supposing that every particle of highly resistant matter were fully digested, which is not the case.

At Huddersfield, Mr Campbell estimated that about 38 % of the solids were digested or gasified.

Mr Harrison gave the figure for Leeds as being about 30 %.

Dr Fowler gives the total at Manchester as being possibly 25 % of the total suspended matter.

At Sheffield, Mr Haworth gave the digestion at 32·9 %, and at Birmingham, Messrs Watson and O'Shaughnessy stated that the figures available indicated a digestion not exceeding 10 % of the suspended matter entering the tanks.

At the experimental station at Lille, Dr Calmette found that 20 % of the total sludge became dissolved.

The above figures, as one would expect, show widely differing results.

The Sewage Disposal Commission, from observations made at Ilford and Exeter, and extending over two years, found that the digestion at Exeter was about 25 %, and at Ilford about 30 %. The septic tanks at both places held about one day's flow of sewage, and the sewages in each case were fairly similar as regards strength.

Passing of storm sewage through septic tanks. So long as the increased rate of flow through the tanks does not produce a scouring action, stirring up the sludge and causing an increase in the suspended matter in the tank liquor, there does not appear to be any reason why increased flows up to say three times the normal rate should not occasionally be passed through septic tanks.

Septic action is probably diminished temporarily by storms, especially if these continue for any length of time, but it has been found that the slight change in the character of the septic tank liquor has not any marked effect upon its subsequent treatment.

It was found at Dorking that the treatment of septic tank liquor and settled sewage on matured percolating filters alternately for 24 hours at a time, did not affect the character of the effluent produced, whilst a like experiment at Leeds gave similar results.

At Rochdale, percolating filters which had previously been treating septic tank liquor for a long time were suddenly dosed with precipitation tank liquor, little or no alteration in the effluent being detected.

The facts afford strong presumptive evidence that the admission of storm water to septic tanks, within reasonable limits, does not in any way prejudice its subsequent treatment upon percolating filters, contact beds or land.

If the detritus tanks are worked in duplicate during heavy rainfall, and are kept properly cleaned out, the heavy road grit brought down by storms will not reach the septic tanks, and if the sludge in the septic tank is kept below a certain limit, say, not more than about one-third of the tank's capacity, scouring out of sludge is not likely to occur, unless the underside of the blanket or scum is of a loose flocculent nature.

As a general rule, three times the mean dry weather flow can be safely passed through septic tanks without detriment, and the same holds good in the case of continuous flow settlement and continuous flow precipitation.

Effect of septic tank gases on Portland cement concrete. Since it appeared possible that septic tank gases might injuriously affect Portland cement concrete or rendering, and little appeared to be then (1903) known about the subject, experiments were carried out by the writer for the Sewage Disposal Commission, with a view to ascertaining whether the gases from closed septic tanks exercised an injurious effect on Portland cement.

The experiments were carried out at three installations, namely, (1) Leeds, (2) Exeter and (3) Knowle.

Six cubes and six briquettes were suspended in wooden

boxes in the gas under the roofs of the tanks at each of the three installations, the exposed[1] surface of the cement in each case lying uppermost.

The period during which the cement was exposed to the action of the gas was about 15 months in each case.

The results, taken as a whole, showed in a fairly conclusive manner that the gases evolved from septic tanks did not, within the period of 15 months, have any deleterious effect upon the Portland cement. It must, however, be borne in mind that the duration of the experiment was short, the dismantling of the septic tanks at Knowle and Leeds preventing a longer experimental period.

Nuisance from septic tanks. Generally speaking, septic tank treatment causes smell, the degree depending a good deal upon the character of the sewage.

If the sewage is a weak one, or if, as at Birmingham or Manchester, the sewage contains iron salts or tarry substances, the smell may be only slight. Where, however, tannery or brewery refuse is present grave nuisance from such smell may arise.

Sulphuretted hydrogen is the chief cause of the smell, together with organic sulphides.

If the outlet channels from the tanks are covered in, the smell from the tanks will be considerably reduced.

Selection of preliminary process. Regarding this question the Sewage Disposal Commission say—Fifth Report, p. 202:

" It has been shown in another section of our Report that, given conditions favourable to each process, there is little difference as regards cost between any of the different forms of tank treatment when the cost of the subsequent filtration is taken into account. For this reason, the selection of the preliminary process should depend mainly upon local circumstances and upon the facilities offered for the disposal of sludge.

If the circumstances were such that considerable quantities of sludge could be easily and effectively disposed of, say, as wet sludge by sending to sea or by trenching in soil, or as

---

[1] One side of each cube and each briquette was left unprotected; the remaining surfaces were protected with pitch.

pressed cake by sale or gift to farmers, it would probably be best and cheapest to adopt a preliminary process which removed as much of the suspended matter as possible from the sewage. If, on the other hand, it were imperative to have as little sludge and as few sludging operations as possible, then septic tanks or continuous flow settling tanks might be cheapest.

The size of the place and the question of smell are also factors of primary importance in the selection of the preliminary process."

Storm water tanks. Whilst treating of the subject of tanks, the question of tanks for treating storm water may be suitably discussed.

The question of the treatment of storm water was somewhat fully dealt with by the Sewage Disposal Commission, and some extracts may be made from their Fifth Report.

The Commissioners say :

" The usual requirements of the Local Government Board in regard to the treatment of storm sewage are that any increase in flow up to three times the normal dry weather rate should be fully dealt with by the ordinary complete plant, and that a certain number of additional dilutions—up to a total of six— should be treated on special storm filters. These requirements should, we think, be modified, they are, in our opinion, not sufficiently elastic ; and, moreover, experience has shown that special storm filters, which are kept as stand-by filters, are not efficient. We find that the injury done to rivers by the dis- charge into them of large volumes of storm sewage chiefly arises from the excessive amount of suspended solids which such sewage contains, and that these solids can be very rapidly removed by settlement. We therefore recommend as a general rule :

(1) That special stand-by tanks (two or more), should be provided at the works and kept empty for the purpose of receiving the excess of storm water which cannot properly be passed through the ordinary tanks. As regards the amount which may properly be passed through the ordinary tanks, our experience shows that in storm times the rate of flow through these tanks may usually be increased up to about

three times the normal dry weather rate without serious disadvantage;

(2) That any overflow at the works should only be made
from these special tanks, and that this overflow should be
arranged so that it will not come into operation until the tanks
are full;

(3) That no special storm filters should be provided,
but that the ordinary filters should be enlarged to the extent
necessary to provide for the filtration of the whole of the sewage,
which, according to the circumstances of the particular place,
requires treatment by filters;

(4) As regards the overflow from the outfall sewer to
the stand-by tanks, the size of the stand-by tanks, the amount
of storm sewage which should be filtered, and the arrangements
generally for dealing with storm sewage at the outfall works,
the Rivers Board, or the County Council in areas in which
no Rivers Boards have been established, should have similar
power to that which we have proposed in regard to overflows
on branch sewers, and the Local Authority should have a
similar right of appeal to the Central Authority."

Further on in the Fifth Report the Commissioners say, with
regard to the size of the stand-by tanks:

" In most cases it will probably suffice to provide stand-
by tanks capable of holding one-quarter of the daily dry
weather flow, and it will not be necessary to provide for *filtering*
more than three times the normal dry weather flow."

It should be noted that the increase of flow through the
ordinary settling or other tanks up to three times the normal
rate is not intended to apply to dry weather flows, but
merely for the time that the storm occurs. It would obviously be unwise to continue working the ordinary tanks
at three times their normal rate, other than for limited
periods. A plan and section of storm water tanks is given
on Fig. 13.

Imhoff or Emscher tank. This form of tank, which at first sight bears
a strong family resemblance to the Travis tank, appears to have been first
installed at Recklinghausen in Germany about 1907, and was the outcome of
work by Dr Imhoff, having for its object the attainment of digestion of sludge

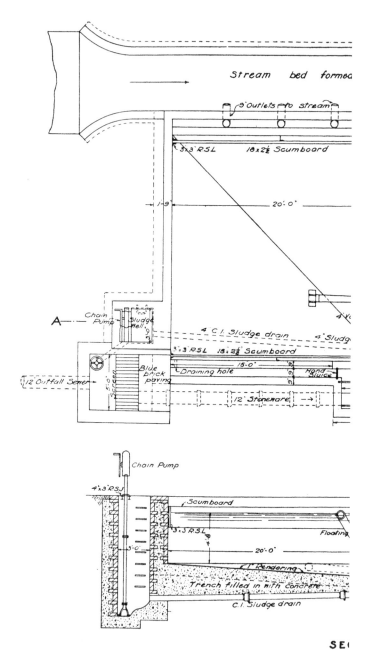

Fig. 13.

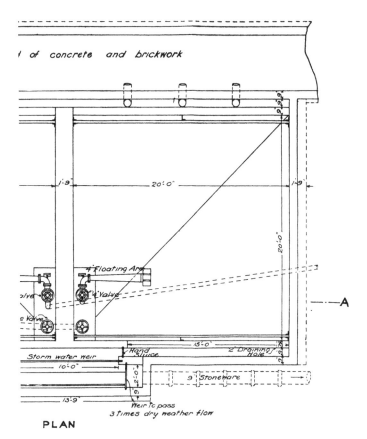

of concrete and brickwork

1'-9" 20'-0" 1'-9"

20'-0"

4" Floating Arm

2" Valve

lve

e Valve

15'-0" 2" Draining Hole

Storm water weir

Hand Sluice

10'-0"

9" Stoneware

13'-9"

Weir to pass
3 times dry weather flow

PLAN

Blue brick coping

Arm

6'-0" 5'-8" 6'-6"

20'-0"

CTION A-A.

Storm water tanks.

in a tank, without allowing the tank liquor itself to become septic, this being effected in a two-storied tank, in the upper portion of which the sewage passes through horizontally in a fresh state, whilst the suspended matter during the passage of the sewage falls through slots in the bottom of the upper or settling chamber into the lower portion or sludge chamber, thus keeping the two processes separate. There is no flow of sewage in the lower, or sludge chamber, and the Imhoff tank thus differs from the Travis tank, in which a certain amount of flow occurs in the lower or sludge chamber. Further, in the Imhoff tank, the slot at the bottom of the settling chamber is overlapped about 3 inches to prevent gas or sludge rising from the lower to the upper compartments, proper vents for the purpose being provided at the sides of the tank.

Through the courtesy of Dr Karl Imhoff the writer is enabled to give on Fig. 14 a plan and section of the Wanne-Nord installation, a medium-sized plant serving 18,000 inhabitants.

This installation is provided with coarse screen, three-divisioned sand arrester, and two settling tanks with horizontal flow over each of the two sludge wells.

The sewage flow is 28,500 gallons per hour, the time allowed for settlement one and a half hours. About $\frac{1}{4}$ lb. of sludge is produced per head of population per day. The sludge well is capable of holding a six-months' supply of sludge.

Imhoff tank sludge is said to contain on an average 75 % of moisture and to dry rapidly when run on to suitably drained lagoons, this being in great measure due to the small gas bubbles imprisoned in the sludge.

The reproduced photographs on Figs. 15–17 refer to the Wanne-Nord installation, and show two views of the tanks, and one view of the sludge lying in the sludge-draining beds.

Many Imhoff tank installations have been constructed in Europe and in America.

The Travis tank. Perhaps the best introduction to this particular mode of tank treatment will be to quote a few passages from *Some Observations on the Principles of Sewage Purification*[1], by Dr W. Owen Travis, in which he deals very clearly with the question of solids in colloidal solution.

Dr Travis says : " It is now generally recognised that the impurities contained in sewage exist in it in the three states of solids in suspension, solids in colloidal solution, and solids in actual or crystalloidal solution, including the volatile solids.

The fact that the two former are to some and even to a large extent interchangeable, is either not as fully understood or perhaps not so freely conceded as it ought to be, considering that the character of the sewage and the methods of elimination of the solids are profoundly modified thereby.

[1] Reprinted from Biggs and Sons' *Contractors' Record and Municipal Engineering*, London, Dec. 13th, 1911.

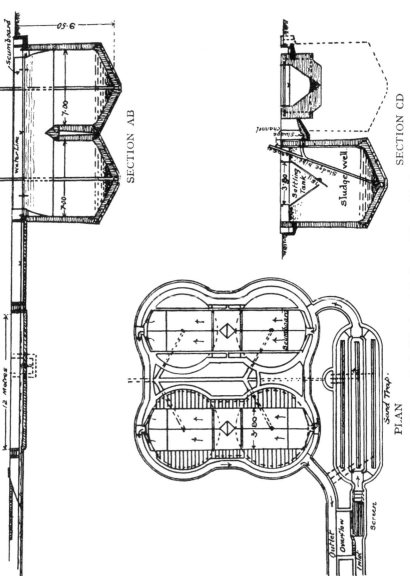

Fig. 14. Imhoff tank installation at Wanne-Nord.

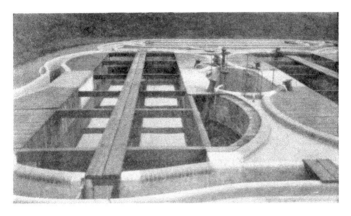

Fig. 15. Imhoff tanks at Wanne-Nord.

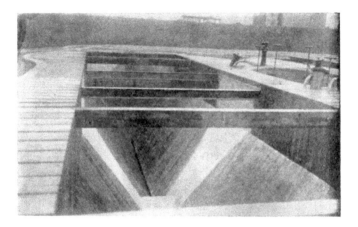

Fig. 16. Imhoff tanks at Wanne-Nord.

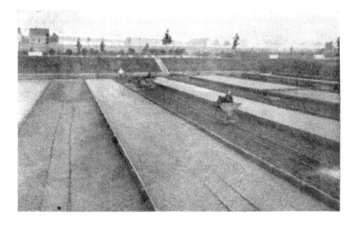

Fig. 17. Sludge draining beds at Wanne-Nord.

The alternate succession from solids in suspension to solids in colloidal solution, and again to solids in suspension—even the further repetition of these phenomena—can be demonstrated, in the same sample of sewage, and can be proved to be the result of purely physical actions.

When a sewage, especially one which has flowed by easy gravitation and which contains moderately gross masses in it, is thoroughly agitated, the solid matters will become finely disintegrated, and a proportion will be thrown into colloidal solution ; the previously clear or translucent liquid will then be found to be opalescent ; and the characteristics of the gravitation sample will have given place to those of one raised by pumping operations. The analyses, before and after, will determine the amount thrown into colloidal solution.

If such a sample be sterilised, and placed on one side in a narrow glass cylinder, the liquid portion will gradually clear, until at the end of from two to four or five weeks it will be found to be transparent. Accompanying this clarification, and proportionate to it, will be noted the formation of particulate solids on the sides and bottom of the glass cylinder. Thus the matter thrown into colloidal solution by mechanical agitation has been re-converted into suspended solids by physical operations.

Further, if the whole sample be again agitated, some proportion of the particulated solids will once more be thrown into colloidal solution ; and will again in due time, redeposit on standing.

Sewages, filtered sewage, tank effluents, and even filter bed effluents, whether sterilised or kept under natural conditions, all exhibit a like series of phenomena ; the solids in the colloidal state become transferred from their condition of solution to that of obvious suspended matter, and the opalescence or translucency, occasioned by the colloidal solution, disappears and gives place to a brilliantly transparent liquid."

     ✻   ✳   ✳   ✳   ✳   ✳   ✻   ✻   ✳   ✳

" The removal of the dissolved and volatile solids from the sewage, and the retention of the withdrawn substances in the immediate environment of the filter or soil particles, can be demonstrated, by sterilisation experiments, to be the effects of physical, in contradistinction to vital operations. In these as well as under natural conditions, the degree of desolution is strictly proportionate to the extent of surface, and to the intimacy and duration of the contact of liquid and surface. An increase in the extent of surface, secured either by deepening the filter, or by diminishing the size of the particles, will result, other things being equal, in the more complete depletion of the impurities from the sewage."

The aims of the Travis hydrolytic tank are to remove more completely the suspended solids, especially those in a finely divided state, and to bring out of solution a proportion of the colloidal matter by presenting large surfaces to the liquid on its passage through the tank.

Below will be found a description of the latest Travis tank installation at Luton ; and on Fig. 18 a plan and section of one of the tanks is shown, which in conjunction with the description, and reproduction of the photograph taken during the construction of the tanks and shown on Fig. 19, will make the mode of working clear.

The installation consists of two tanks which are designed to treat a daily dry weather flow of 1⅓ million gallons of sewage. They are of circular type, are arranged so that they can be worked in series or in parallel, and have a combined liquid capacity of 572,000 gallons.

Each tank consists of a central valve chamber, surrounded by three annular spaces. The two outer spaces are separated by a diaphragm wall, having openings in the bottom, and are subdivided radially into four sections, whilst the inner one is undivided, and forms the fifth section. This section, and all the outer chambers of the other sections, with the exception of the first, are fitted with " colloiders," consisting of wooden frames with 1 inch × 1½ inch vertical slats, placed in series of five, at 9 inch centres in the outer sections, and at 6 inch centres in the inner section. The floor of the tank is constructed in the form of hoppers, with sludge pipes leading into the central chamber.

The sewage issuing from the rising main, enters the regulating well, passes over its weir, and is conducted by three

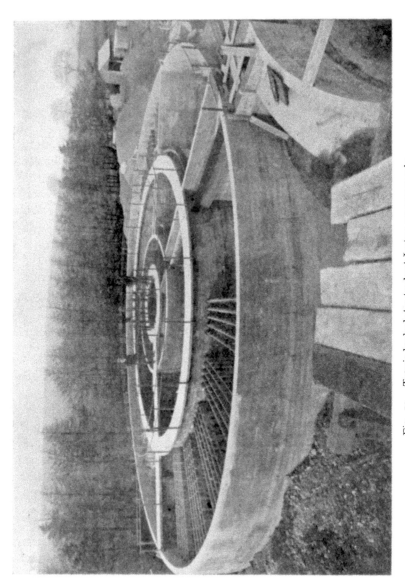

Fig. 19.   Travis hydrolytic tank at Luton sewage works.

down pipes to the foot of the vertical wall of the outer chamber of the first section of the tank. As this chamber communicates with the corresponding inner chamber by openings in the bottom of the diaphragm wall, and as the outflow from both is by weirs which are on the same level, the amount of sewage passing through each is practically in accordance with the relative widths of their respective weirs. The rate of flow is determined by the relative capacities of the chambers to the volume flowing through each. By increasing the capacity of the inner chamber the flow is retarded, and time given for the settlement of the suspended solids. These remarks apply equally to the chambers of the other sections.

The weirs of this section are so arranged that 66·6 per cent. of the sewage passes across the outer chamber to its weir, whilst 33·3 per cent. flows downwards through the openings, carrying with it the heavier suspended solids, which are deposited in the hopper-shaped bottom, the liquid rising upward to its weir.

The separate liquids are carried by a common channel to the downtake of No. 2 Section. In this section the combined liquid passes forward through the outer chamber, between the colloiders, to its weir, over which 70 per cent. flows, whilst 30 per cent. descends through the openings into the inner chamber, carrying the suspended solids, including those which have been arrested by and dropped from the colloiders, which are left in the chamber, whilst the liquid rises upwards to its weir.

The operation is repeated in the third and fourth sections. In the third, 75 per cent. passes through the outer chamber and 25 per cent. through the inner. In the fourth, 80 per cent. flows through the outer chamber directly into the outlet channel from the tank, the remaining 20 per cent. passes through the inner chamber, enters the fifth section, and after traversing it in the opposite direction, amongst the colloiders, is discharged over its weir to join the 80 per cent. volume in the outlet channel.

The deposited sludge is regularly drawn off by operating the valves in the central chamber, from whence it gravitates to a " Shone " ejector, which raises it to trenches in the land, and to sludge drying beds.

The principles of assisting sedimentation by the downward projection of a volume of liquid, and the removal of finely divided suspended and colloidal matter by interposing self-cleansing surfaces in the sewage flow, are peculiar to this type of tank. These principles have been emphasised in the Luton tanks, inasmuch as they are repeated in the several sections.

The Dortmund tank. This form of tank was designed by Herr C. Kniebüher for the sewage works of the town of Dortmund about the year 1883.

It was first of all proposed to use vacuum towers of the Röckner-Rothe type, but owing to the cost of this system, cylinders were sunk in the ground instead. A diagrammatic plan and section of the tank will be found on Fig. 20 which will serve to show the action of the Dortmund tank.

The chemically treated sewage enters the tank through the horizontal inlet pipe, passing down the central vertical cylinder as shown by the arrows ; this central cylinder is about 30 feet deep and at its foot are placed distributing arms or channels radiating from the central cylinder, the object of these being to distribute the incoming sewage evenly throughout the whole transverse area of the tank. The suspended matter in the sewage flocculates in the lower portion of the tank, gradually subsiding to the apex of the tank, whence it is raised through 6-inch sludge pipes and conveyed where desired.

The clarified sewage leaves the tank at the surface, where a network of tank effluent channels is provided connected up to a main outlet. The object of these channels is to secure an even outflow and to obviate any tendency of the tank liquor to carry suspended matter with it, which would probably occur but for this contrivance. It may be mentioned that the sewage of Dortmund contains a very large amount of brewery waste, but faeces do not enter the sewers.

At Dortmund it was found important to keep all floating matters and heavy particles out of the tanks ; further, the sludge required frequent removal.

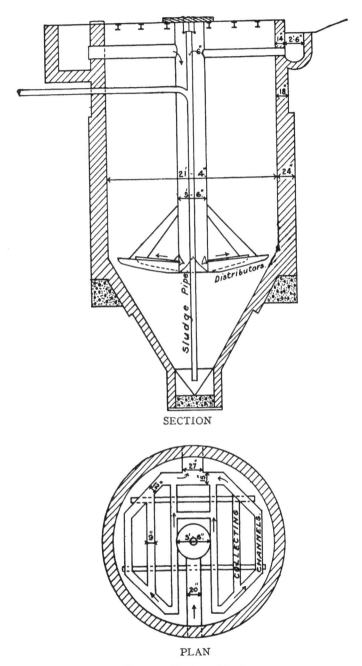

SECTION

PLAN

Fig. 20. Dortmund tank.

There are several modified Dortmund tank installations working in England and the system is well adapted to restricted sites, where the nature of the subsoil is good and not water-logged. The original Dortmund tanks were about 48 feet deep from water level to sludge sump, the diameter being 21 ft. 4 ins., the cost of each tank being about £750.

The Kremer Clarification Process. Three processes carried out by the Sewage Clarification Company of Berlin-Schöneburg[1] are of interest, and may be mentioned here : they are,

(1)   The Kremer process proper.

(2)   The Kremer process combined with separate sludge digestion chambers.

(3)   The Kremer-Schilling grease extraction process.

The Kremer clarification process proper is a sewage clarifying tank, which brings about, through a particular deflection of the current, a mechanical separation of the suspended solids, which are separated according to their specific gravities into two layers.

The inflowing sewage meets with a check, and is deflected by special guide plates, whereby the lighter solids such as grease are directed upwards to the water surface. Here they collect together by adhesion, and form a floating surface layer of grease, whilst the heavier solids freed from grease subside into the sludge cylinder.

In the sludge cylinder the water content of the sludge is diminished from 92 % to 88 %, and in this state it can be forced out and into the sludge pipe by the pressure of the head of water, the narrow cylinder preventing the formation of blowholes in the sludge caused by the sewage. The absence of grease allows the sludge to part with its moisture much more readily than would otherwise be the case.

In this process the sludge is removed before putrefaction sets in.

It may be noted that in bad waterlogged ground, the sludge cylinder offers a distinct advantage over the Dortmund tank, where the body of the tank is carried to a much greater depth.

It is claimed that there is a very high degree of separation rapidly effected as regards fat and suspended solids, that a very small space is occupied by the tanks, whilst first cost and maintenance charges are low, and that the tank liquor is non-putrescent ; further, that extensions of plant are easily made.

The sludge produced is said to have a low percentage of moisture.

If desired, the fresh sludge can be used upon land, since the bulk of the fat, which would otherwise clog the pores of the land, is removed ; or, if it is not intended to dispose of it upon land, it can be run into sludge digestion chambers, whence it is eventually conducted to sludge drying beds.

In the case of large installations, the floating layer of grease is removed by hand by means of a flat perforated shovel ; with small plants, where the grease

---

[1] *Gesellschaft für abwässerklarung*, m.b.h.   " System Kremer."   Berlin-Schöneburg.   Kaiser-Friedrich-str. 9.

cannot be turned to profit[1], it can be made into a compost with a peaty soil, and in this state forms a useful manure for gardens.

The grease is said to contain about 72 % of moisture, whilst the dried material contains about 45 % of grease.

The dense sludge forming in the cylinder can be either subjected to a digestion process, which reduces its volume considerably, admitting of a three to four months storage without removal, or the sludge can be run off in a fresh state every one to three days and digestion carried out in special chambers.

The removal of sludge can be effected by vacuum, sludge pump, or by the head of water in the tank, without interrupting its working.

The digested sludge dries into a spadeable state in sludge drying beds in from three to ten days.

When dry it is used by farmers for warming cold soils, and for rendering heavy arable soils more friable.

The fresh sludge is either dug into the soil or mixed with other substances which make it pressable, the pressed cake being used as manure.

The efficiency of the plant is said to be high, whilst little space is required. A reduction of from 70 % upwards in the suspended solids can be obtained, according to the strength and character of the sewage.

Results appear to have been obtained at Quedlinburg, Brussels and Nordhausen, showing a reduction in suspended solids of 94 % to 89 %.

It is claimed that a Kremer apparatus with tank capacity of from 25 to 30 cubic metres can clarify 800 to 3200 cubic metres of sewage per 24 hours.

As regards cost, under conditions obtaining in Germany, they are given as follows :

Tank with cross section of 4 square metres—about £300⎫ without sludge
Tank with cross section of 5 square metres—about £450⎬   digestion
Tank with cross section of 6 square metres—about £600⎭   chambers.

Adjacent sludge digestion chambers cost from £2 to £4 per cubic metre of capacity.

The above figures of cost do not include sewage inlets to tank, or keeping down water during construction, and a normal subsoil is assumed, with soil easily excavated.

The maintenance costs, including repayment of interest, redemption of capital and depreciation, range from 3d. to 5d. per head of population.

The actual working charges are under 1½d. to 2½d. per head.

Fig. 21 shows a plan and section of the Kremer clarification tank and the method of construction.

The sewage is brought to the tank by the channel aa, and enters it by the side inlet channels bb, at the foot of which the guide plates cc deflect the sewage upwards in the section of the tank lettered dd, causing the lighter solids, such as fat, to separate out and rise to the surface ee.

The body of the tank ff acts as a settling or clarification chamber, where, by reason of the reduction in velocity, the flocculent and heavy matters sink to the bottom. gg consists of an almost entirely submerged rectangular wall or scumboard, under the lower edge of which the tank liquor rises, flows over the continuous weir or sill (I) into the channel h, and thence into the outlet at m.

[1] Tetrachloride of carbon has been employed for extracting the grease, but benzene would answer equally well.

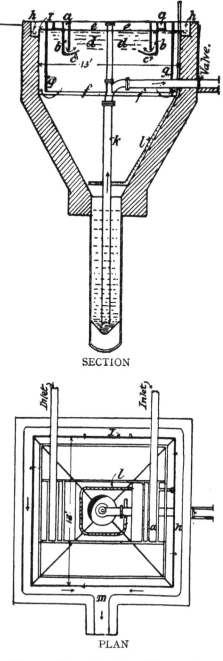

SECTION

PLAN

Fig. 21. Plan and section of Kremer tank

The sludge gradually becomes consolidated in the sludge cylinder, k being a sludge pipe for drawing off the denser sludge by the head of water, without shutting down the tank.

A sparge pipe (l) is provided for loosening the sludge from the walls of the cone, causing it to fall into the cylinder.

It is understood that the process is in successful operation at Nordhausen, Weimar, Gotha, the experimental station in Brussels, and the abattoirs at Lille and Stuttgart.

The Kremer process with separate digestion of the sludge in adjoining chambers is in use at Nordhausen and also at Brussels.

The Company also have another process, which is a combination of the Kremer method with that of Dr Imhoff; in consequence of patent rights, this process cannot be used abroad.

The Kremer-Schilling method is a fat extraction process for removing greasy matter from the sewage, and it is shown in plan and section on Fig. 22.

The grease is retained between the baffle plates.

It is in operation in this country at Withington near Manchester, where, during the year ending March 1911, the grease collected from an average daily flow of 4¾ million gallons, amounted to nearly 1 cwt. per day.

During the year ending March 1913, the total quantity of greasy matter collected was 10·1 tons, which were sold for £33. 9s. 5d.[1]

The Fieldhouse tank. This form of tank was designed with a view to producing a uniform type of tank liquor, containing a minimum of suspended solids, the incoming sewage being forced to mingle with the liquor already in the tank by outward diffusion as it travels towards the overflow sill. The length of overflow sill is of benefit in avoiding the production of currents and eddies.

Fig. 23 shows the general arrangement of the tank, the method of operation being as follows:

The sewage enters at the pipe M, and flows to the inner or roughing chamber A, where the bulk of the heavy solids are deposited, falling to the under side of the inverted cone C, the object of this cone being to prevent stirring up of the deposit, and also to form an annular space E where depositing solids can settle, to be subsequently withdrawn through the valve D.

---

[1] City of Manchester, Rivers Department. Annual Reports for the years ending March 1911 and 1913. Henry Blacklock and Co. Ltd. Manchester.

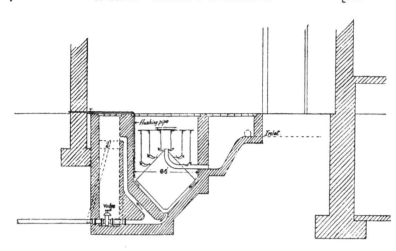

SECTION AB.

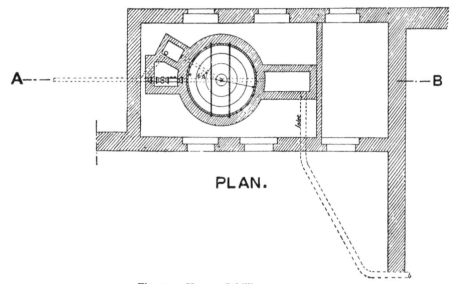

PLAN.

Fig. 22.   Kremer-Schilling apparatus.

The sewage leaves the inner tank A through a number of outlets H to the outer tank B, these outlets being so designed as to cause uniform displacement, and to deflect the finer depositing solids towards the collecting chambers (containing penstocks N) in the deposit chambers, before passing under slide or scumboards J, and over the sill K into the channel L.

The scumboards J dip below the liquid.

From the point of entrance to the point of exit, the liquid is continually spreading outward, covering a larger area, and consequently diminishing its velocity as it approaches the overflow sill or weir K.

The deposit forming in tank A is removed by opening the valve D, when the head of water drives the deposit down the sludge pipe F, the inverted cone C tending to prevent a column of liquid flowing down the pipe, and also deflecting the liquid on to the sloping sides of the sludge well, scouring the deposited solids from them as the sludge is driven out.

The outer tank B is divided into a number of sections according to the size of the tank ; at the bottom of each section a chamber is constructed with a valve N opening to the sludge pipe F. The bottom of each section is formed with inclined faces, to allow the solids to be deposited near the valve N, ready for withdrawal when the valve is opened.

The outer inclined face I is formed at a sufficient inclination to obviate accumulations of solids, thereby preventing likelihood of any decomposing sludge being again thrown into suspension near the sill K.

Removal of scum. The outer tank B is divided into sections by radial scumboards J, and end slides or scumboards T, which form traps and prevent wind from breaking up any scum, and from causing the tank liquor to flow over the sill unequally.

When it is desired to remove scum or floating matter, the slides S_1 and S_2 in the collecting channel are first shut down ; the end slides T in each section are next lifted out or shut down below the surface, when the floating matter is forced over the weir, into the channel, and thence to the sludge tank, or to the land as found convenient. This plan has been found to work satisfactorily at Guildford during the past 18 months. It is only found necessary to shut down the slides T and to head up the tank when the scum is allowed to accumulate in large quantities, which is not advisable.

An example of the Fieldhouse tank has recently been put down at the Guildford sewage works, and it is understood that it is giving good results.

The principal claims advanced for this tank by Mr Fieldhouse are as follows:

Production of tank liquor of a uniform character containing a minimum of suspended solids.

Facilities for sludge and scum removal, which can be carried out without emptying the tank.

Capacity of tank to deal with large fluctuations in flow, and equalisation of variable liquids.

Comparative absence of smell.

It is further claimed that, taking into consideration the larger volumes of sewage which may be dealt with, the capital cost, as compared with other types of tank, is considerably lower; moreover, that a considerable saving in labour for sludging operations is effected.

Further improvements have recently been patented in connection with the Fieldhouse tank, concerning the scum withdrawal from the inner tank, and the utilisation of the spaces between the pockets and inclined faces of the coves for storage of sludge, scum, and floating débris that may periodically be withdrawn, and allowed to decompose without fouling the tank liquor by the gases that are evolved.

Dibdin slate beds. These may be described as being watertight tanks, filled with horizontal layers of slates to a depth of 3 feet, each layer of slates being about 2 inches distant from the layers above and below it, the layers being kept thus by small blocks or distance-pieces of slate.

The capacity of the beds when new is about 85 % to 90 % of the empty tank capacity.

It is understood that the beds are intended to receive crude sewage, and that they should receive one filling a day to secure the best results, further, that the beds should be allowed to drain thoroughly after each filling.

It will be observed,—assuming one filling per day to be the best way of working the slate beds for a domestic sewage of average strength,—that a total bed capacity equivalent to a 24 hours flow would be needed.

Slate beds are in use at High Wycombe, Halstead, Haileybury College, and elsewhere.

Settling towers. These have been used to a considerable extent in Germany and America, but do not appear to have found much favour in England. They consist of cylindrical tanks, often raised above the surface level of the ground, the solids in the sewage settling to the bottom of the tank and being drawn off whenever necessary by suitable appliances.

Chemical precipitants, such as lime and alumino-ferric, are sometimes employed to hasten the settlement of the solids.

Their efficiency in general is said to be less than that of settling tanks ; on the other hand, the removal of the sludge —which contains a large percentage of water—is more easily carried out than with settling tanks.

The cost of settling towers is higher than that of tanks, but they take up little space, and can be economically constructed where the level of the ground water is high.

In most settling towers the bottom of the tank is formed in the shape of a cone, the sludge drain being placed at the apex. The sewage enters the tank by a pipe which is carried down the centre of the tank, ending in a funnel-shaped outlet at a point a little above where the cone commences : the sewage in rising up through the tower meets with a zone of falling suspended matter. The outlets to the tower are generally several in number, spaced round the circumference of the tower at the top, and the outlet pipe itself is submerged about 12 inches to avoid carrying off scum. In some towers a separate funnel-shaped outlet pipe is provided at a slightly higher level than the ordinary outlet, to carry off grease. Unless settling towers are kept very clean, and frequently sludged, septic action is very apt to arise, especially in hot weather, resulting in the rising of large masses of scum to the surface of the tower.

Bacterial clarification of sewage. Messrs Fowler and Mumford[1] have recently suggested the possibility of utilising the reactions of a facultative organism occurring in iron (ochre) water from coal pits, for bringing about clarification of sewage. The process proposed comes in after the grosser suspended solids have been removed from the sewage, either by ordinary settling tanks, Imhoff tanks or Dibdin slate beds, the object being to keep the liquid portion of the sewage as fresh as possible. The resulting tank liquor would then pass into a second tank, where the particular organism would be introduced together with a small dose of ferric salt, and air blown through the liquid until clarification commences. Time for settlement is then to be allowed to admit of precipitation of the coagulated matter, after which the clarified liquid could be filtered or discharged direct as the case may be.

The authors anticipate that the clarified liquor resulting from the above process could be oxidised at a very rapid rate. The experiments carried out so far appear to indicate that approximately one grain of iron salt per gallon would be the maximum dose needed, whilst a total of 12 hours tankage— six hours aeration followed by six hours settlement—would suffice, whilst there does not appear to be any difficulty in maintaining the organism once it has been established in the tank. As Messrs Fowler and Mumford remark, the conditioning factor is the cost of an air blast, and they suggest that much of the required power could be obtained (1) from gas collected from the fermentation of the main bulk of the sewage solids, either in Imhoff tanks or some similar process, or (2) from the fall available from the aerating tank. In conclusion, the authors of the paper say, " The advance claimed in the present communication is the use of a specific organism found in nature, together with iron salts, to effect the clarification of the effluent —that is, the coagulation of the colloidal matter as distinct from the purification of the effluent taken as a whole.

To use a simple illustration, the addition of a little rennet

---

[1] *The Bacterial Clarification of Sewage*, by Gilbert J. Fowler and E. Moore Mumford. (Paper read at Exeter Congress of the Royal Sanitary Institute, 1913.)

does not appreciably alter the composition of milk as a whole, but separates it into a solid and liquid portion. The endeavour of the authors has been to obtain a similar result in the case of a sewage tank effluent ; to collect the precipitated colloids, and purify the liquid portions by high speed filters, or it may be in large tanks stocked with suitable aquatic plants."

Aeration of sewage and tank liquors before filtration. Several attempts have been made to aerate filters artificially by means of blowing air into them, but so far the results obtained have not been commensurate with the cost involved.

A somewhat different plan was tried in some experiments carried out in 1912 by the Massachusetts State Board of Health at Lawrence, U.S.A. and published by Messrs H. W. Clark and G. O. Adams in the *Engineering Record*. In this case air was mixed with the sewage *before* treatment on the filters, and it is stated that when similar sand filters were called upon to treat the same sewage, from six to eight times more of aerated sewage could be efficiently purified than of ordinary sewage. With ordinary percolating filters, aerated sewage could be treated at three times the rate of unaerated sewage. Aeration was carried out in a tank containing slabs of slate about 1 inch apart.

Details of cost are unfortunately not given.

BIBLIOGRAPHY.

Allen, Kenneth. *Sewage Sludge.* McGraw-Hill Book Company, London and New York. 1912.

Baker, M. N. *British Sewage Works.* The Engineering News Publishing Company, New York. 1904.

Bar, W. M. and Buchanan, R. E. *Production of excessive hydrogen sulphide in sewage disposal plants, and consequent disintegration of the concrete.* Iowa State College of Agriculture. Bull. No. 4, Vol. x. Jan. 1912.

Bell, H. D. *Second, third, fourth and fifth Annual Reports on the Stratford-on-Avon Sewage Works.* Stratford-on-Avon.

Calmette. *Recherches sur l'épuration biologique et clinique des eaux d'égout.* Vol. iv.

City of Leeds. *Reports on Sewage Disposal* (1898, 1900, and 1905) by Col. T. W. Harding and W. H. Harrison. Jowett and Sowry, Leeds.

Crimp, W. Santo. *Sewage Disposal Works.* C. Griffin and Co., Ltd., London. 1894.

Dunbar and Calvert. *Principles of Sewage Treatment.* Griffin and Co., Ltd., London. 1908.

Fuller, George W. *Sewage Disposal.* McGraw-Hill Book Co., New York and London. 1912.

Hazen. *Experiments on chemical Precipitation of Sewage.* State Board of Health, Massachusetts. 1890.
Journal of the Association of Engineering Societies, Vol. xxxvii. 1906.
Kershaw, G. Bertram. *Modern Methods of Sewage Disposal,* Chapter x. Griffin and Co., Ltd., London. 1911.
Massachusetts. *State Board of Health.* Forty-third Annual Report.
Royal Commission on Sewage Disposal. Fifth Report, 1908. Appendix iv to Fifth Report. Seventh Report, Vol. iii. part 2. Fifth Report, Appendices i and ii.
Saville. *Boston Society of Civil Engineers.* 1910.
Schmeitzner, Dr Ing. Rudolf. *Clarification of Sewage.* Constable and Co., London. 1910.
Surveyor, The. July 18th, 1913.
Venable, W. M. *Sewage.* John Wiley and Co., New York. 1908.

CHAPTER V

SLUDGE DISPOSAL

The sludge problem. In many instances at the present day, the chief difficulty is not so much how to produce a satisfactory effluent, but how to get rid of the sludge produced by preliminary processes.

Ordinary domestic sewage contains large quantities of greasy matter, and this renders difficult the disintegration or powdering of sludge for easy manipulation for agricultural purposes. Further, the grease contained in the sludge is a drawback when used as a manure, making the soil after a time impervious to air and water. Again, ordinary sewage sludge produced by various processes may contain anything roughly speaking from 80 % to 95 % of moisture, and it is difficult to handle when in the wet sloppy condition.

Sludge presses, which were introduced in England nearly 40 years ago, furnished a process capable of reducing the moisture to such an extent as to produce cakes of sludge which could be easily handled, but unfortunately the process is a somewhat costly one. The old method of running sludge in the liquid state into lagoons, is open to the objection that the drying process in such circumstances is very slow, being largely dependent upon the weather ; every shower providing additional moisture for the sludge to suck up, whilst nuisance is often created during the drying period.

It should be carefully borne in mind that formerly, when land treatment was practically the only sewage purification process, settling tanks were sometimes absent, and when used, the suspended matter left in the tank liquor as it went on to the land was usually greatly in excess of what would now be permitted to pass on to artificial filters or contact beds. Consequently, the practice of providing a tank liquor as free as possible from suspended matter, in order to ensure its proper purification by artificial methods, has resulted in the production of large volumes of sludge.

The composition of sewage sludge varies greatly both hourly, daily and yearly, and may perhaps best be described as consisting mainly of the suspended matter removed from the sewage, chiefly mineral and cellulose matters. Further, the character of the sludge varies greatly according as certain factors are present or absent. It is difficult to deal with in the raw state owing to the amount of moisture present and the putrescible substances which soon cause a nuisance.

Factors influencing sludge production. It may be well at this point to discuss several of the factors influencing the production of sludge. Foremost of these is the nature of the sewerage system. If this is on the combined system, all road water will mingle with the sewage, and a large quantity of small gravel and heavy detritus will be washed from the roads into the gullies. If these latter are not cleaned out regularly, the grit and gravel will in course of time wash out of the gullies into the sewers. The nature of the street or road surfaces also affects sludge production, *i.e.* gravel and macadam roads produce much sludge, especially if the roads have a steep gradient ; wood-paving, asphalt, and tar macadam on the contrary, do not of themselves produce much sludge-making material, but any dust and débris blown on to them are washed into the gullies in times of rainfall. Again, the amount of traffic on the roads, wheeled or otherwise, affects the quantity of sludge, together with the amount of rainfall.

Where the partially separate system of sewers is in use, the heavy gritty matter found in sludge from a combined system of sewers is, or should be, a minimum ; as a general rule, however, it will be found that a good many road gullies are connected to the foul water sewers. Grit chambers will remove a certain amount of the heaviest mineral matters, but some of it is bound to find its way to the settling tanks. It must, however, be remembered that with the partially separate system of sewers, owing to the smaller average daily volume of sewage, the volume of sludge produced *per million gallons of sewage* may approximate to that obtained with the combined system of sewers.

Proportion of mineral to organic matter in sludge. This is a very important question, since the mineral matter contained in sludge, such as grit, fine sand, earth and coal dust must be disposed of somehow, and cannot be appreciably reduced.

Numerous observations have shown that, although individual sewages vary considerably, and precise figures universally applicable cannot be given, roughly speaking about 40 to 60 % of the solids contained in sewage sludges consist of mineral (inorganic) matter, which may be regarded as irreducible, the balance of 60 to 40 % being organic.

Whatever the process of sludge disposal therefore, there will always be this 40 to 60 % of mineral matter to dispose of ; possibly it will be arrested in the pump well or by grit chambers or in the tank process ; or again, it may have to be barrowed from the surface of contact beds, or removed by washing the material, or it may pass through the beds, and be held back in the effluent settling tanks or straining filters, or in the case of land treatment it may require periodical removal from the carriers, but in all cases the mineral matter will be there, and it has to be reckoned with.

It is frequently urged that with the separate or partially separate system of sewers, there will be little or no mineral matter in the sludge, but this is by no means the case.

Although the mineral matter contained in the sewage will, as a rule, be less *during wet weather* with the separate or partially separate system than with the combined, yet the presence of

certain trade wastes may increase the volume of sludge very largely. Again, dust and fine sand, coal dust, etc., are blown down yard gullies and on to back roofs of houses, all tending in the aggregate to increase the volume of sludge, nearly all of this added matter being mineral. Faeces again, contain a certain amount of mineral matter and other highly resistant substance. It is, however, from the daily domestic work that the largest quantity of grit in the aggregate enters sewers.

People going in and out of houses carry in dirt and grit on their feet; this is swept up by the servants, and very frequently the dustpan is emptied down the w.c. as being the nearest and most convenient means of disposal; further, sand is largely used for scouring kitchen utensils, but the largest amount of grit is derived from the washing of vegetables ; it will be found that the grit derived from this particular source often amounts to 1 oz. per house per day. A population of 10,000 inhabitants would indicate some 2000 houses, say 2000 ounces of gritty matter reaching the sewers daily, or about 125 lbs. daily ! or 20 tons per annum, equivalent to 200 tons of 90 % wet sludge containing mineral matter only, or say 500 tons of ordinary sewage sludge if organic matter be included, from this one source alone. It is therefore clear that whatever the sewerage system, and whatever the method of treatment, this 40 to 60 % of mineral matter will have to be dealt with and disposed of in its entirety by one means or another, and it cannot be appreciably reduced. The weight of sewage sludge varies somewhat, an average weight for a cubic yard being about 1790 lbs. or four-fifths of a ton. The late Mr Santo Crimp's[1] formula showing loss of weight of sewage sludge at varying degrees of moisture will be found useful : it is as follows :

$$W_2 = \left(\frac{100 - P}{100 - Q} \right) W_1.$$

$W_1 =$ original weight of wet sludge.
$W_2 =$ weight of sludge cake produced.
$Q\ \ =$ Percentage of moisture after pressing, and
$P\ \ =$ percentage of moisture in the wet sludge.

[1] *Sewage Disposal Works.* Griffin and Co., Ltd., London.

Disposal of detritus from grit chambers. There is not much difficulty as a rule in disposing of detritus, as it is always relatively small in volume compared with the sludge. If it contains little organic matter it can be spread out in layers and weathered for some weeks, when it can be utilised for road binding purposes, gritting tarred surfaces and the like. In some cases it may be convenient to empty it on to a draining bed which can also be used for screenings ; both screenings and detritus being removed together in an iron tumbril cart and disposed of at frequent intervals.

Volumes of sludge produced by various tank processes. In the Leeds Report[1], Col. Harding and Mr Harrison, comparing various methods of tank treatment, give the following table, the first column giving the sludge deposited in the tanks, and the second column the sludge left in the tank effluent :

Grains per gallon	Sludge	Effluent
Chemical precipitation	49	3
Stagnant natural settlement	36	6
Flowing ,, ,,	32	10
Septic settlement	16	13

The Sewage Disposal Commission in their Fifth Report give the theoretical quantities of 90 % moisture sludge likely to be produced per million gallons of sewage by settlement, chemical precipitation and septic tanks as :

1. Quiescent chemical precipitation   ..   17 tons
2. Continuous flow chemical precipitation 16   ,,
3. Quiescent settlement 12   ,,
4. Continuous flow settlement 11   ,,
5. Open septic tanks   ..   ..   .. 6·5 ,,

These figures give the sludge likely to be produced per million gallons of *dry weather* sewage flow, but if storm sewage were included, the amount of sludge produced per million gallons of the average daily flow (all weathers included) might easily be doubled. It should be further noted that it is assumed in the foregoing figures that the suspended matter remaining

[1] City of Leeds, *Report on Experiments in Sewage Disposal*, by Col. T. W. Harding and Mr W. H. Harrison, Leeds, 1905.

in the tank liquid is low enough to admit of favourable treatment upon percolating filters.

Very much depends upon the design and use of grit chambers if used, as to how much sludge will be produced, but speaking quite broadly about 15 to 20 tons of sludge may be produced per million gallons of sewage (storm sewage included) per annum with sedimentation, from 30 to 40 tons with chemical precipitation, and from 10 to 15 tons with septic tank treatment. It is, however, quite impossible to give more than very approximate figures, since local conditions vary so much, quite apart from the meteorological conditions of one particular year as against another, and the above figures must only be taken as being roughly approximate.

Gas evolved from septic tanks. Gas from septic tanks has been used for lighting purposes on the sewage works at Exeter; and, at Chorley, gas for illuminating purposes was obtained from the pressed sludge cake.

It should be borne in mind that the gas evolved from septic tanks and cesspools is highly inflammable, especially when diluted with ordinary atmospheric air; as, for example, when the manhole covers of closed septic tanks have been removed for some hours, and it is highly dangerous to bring a naked light near. Explosions from this cause have occurred with septic tank gas at Exeter, Sheringham, Ilford, Cromer, and other places.

Treatment of crude sewage upon land. This method of sludge disposal is rather apt to be lost sight of. There are, however, several farms where this has been in operation for many years, the crude sewage flowing on to the land without tank treatment of any sort. Nottingham sewage farm is a case in point.

There are, unfortunately, few farms either possessing suitable soils and subsoils, or sufficiently isolated to render this procedure practicable, but where it can be properly carried out there can be little doubt that this is an ideal form of sludge disposal.

Lagooning of sludge. This system of dealing with wet sludge consists in banking in areas of land with earthen embankments from 18 inches to 4 feet high or over, or in excavating areas below ground level, the sludge from time to time being run into the lagoons thus formed, and allowed to dry by evaporation and drainage until it becomes spadeable, when it is either removed by farmers or tipped. It will be noticed that lagooning of sludge is only, so to speak, an intermediate stage, and is not synonymous with actual sludge disposal.

Details of sludge lagoon construction. An improvement on the ordinary form of lagoon is sometimes employed, consisting in a layer of clinker, gravel, ashes, or other suitable materials some 6 to 18 inches deep according to circumstances, spread over the bed of each lagoon, thus enabling the moisture to drain away more rapidly than would otherwise be the case. Sometimes, where the lie of the ground allows, underdrains are laid under the lagoons, but when this is done, the liquid from the drains should always be re-treated upon the land, as the liquid draining from the sludge is exceedingly strong and polluting. Fig. 24 shows a good method of lagoon construction; the lagoon floor has a slight fall, so that any liquid prevented by the sludge from draining off through the clinker and sand bed, will flow off longitudinally and pass through the clinker banks.

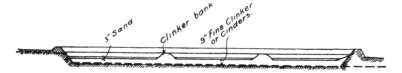

Fig. 24. Longitudinal section of sludge lagoon.

With very greasy sludges bottom drainage is of little use and the supernatant water must be removed from the top. A length of $1\frac{1}{2}$ or 2 inch hose pipe can sometimes be utilised to syphon this off from small lagoons.

In some instances sludge lagoons or drying beds have been formed with an entire flooring of perforated tiles; it will generally be found, however, that a layer of clinker or ashes 12 inches deep with a 6 inch layer of soil makes the best bed for the sludge, both from the point of view of quick drying, and also of easy removal from the bed when dry. The layer of soil prevents the clinker, gravel, or ashes from becoming clogged with the sludge, whilst at the same time, when the sludge comes to be removed, shovels do not catch against the clinker, and the bed of the lagoon can be left perfectly clean.

Sludge lagoons should vary in size and in the number of units, according to the volume of sludge to be dealt with.

It is an advantage, where farmers fetch the bulk of the sludge, to have a cart entrance to each lagoon, provided with two permanent grooved concrete posts holding sliding wooden shutters of sufficient length to allow a cart to pass between, and of adequate height to retain the sludge in the lagoon : the expense and trouble of breaking a way through the embankment and making it up again whenever a lagoon is emptied are thus avoided.   Another plan is to construct all the walls of the beds with planking running in grooved posts.   This method is in use at South Norwood : the wet sludge either gravitates or is pumped into the lagoons to a depth of from 6 inches to 2 feet[1], when it is left to dry, a process which may take from a few weeks in hot weather to several months in wet ; and during the drying process there is considerable risk of a nuisance from smell, especially in hot weather, whilst flies are attracted.

In some cases, where the lagoons are large relatively to the volume of sludge, the practice is followed of running several doses of sludge into them at intervals until the sludge is two or more feet deep.   The better plan would appear to be to have the lagoon units sufficiently numerous to allow of one filling of sludge only, to be removed as soon as it is dry enough to spade.   If several batches of sludge are run in at intervals the bulk of the moisture—after the first batch—has to find its way through the sludge already lying in the lagoon.

The lagoon system is only suitable for disposal works which are placed well away from dwelling-houses, since it is difficult to avoid considerable smell at certain times of the year.

Remedies for smell from sludge lagoons.   Fine ashes, peat dust, etc., can be used in hot weather, and sprinkled over

[1] Other things being equal, the deeper the lagoon, the less the area exposed, and the slower the sludge dries ; the shallower the lagoon, the quicker the sludge dries, but the greater the exposed area, and consequent risk of smell.

the surface of the sludge ; this keeps down the smell to a large extent. Another method is to employ milk of lime to be added to the sludge as it flows to the lagoon. A further method is to dust bleaching powder over the surface of the sludge as it lies in the lagoon ; the bleaching powder is best and most economically applied to the sludge as a dry powder. This method has been used at the Cambridge Sewage Farm. It sometimes happens, however, that the farm manager, having become so used to the smell of the farm, or having lost his sense of smell, objects to the use of bleaching lime because it is slightly irritating to the throat. If added to the sludge in transit, as a solution, its action is used up very quickly, and it is of little use by the time the sludge has reached the lagoon, whereas dusting the surface of the quiescent sludge tends to oxidise the surface layer and thus prevents smell.

Several deodorants have been tried abroad, amongst others one called " faciloil," which forms a film on water or wet sludge, preventing the escape of any smell[1]. The eggs and larvae of insects are said to be killed by it, whilst at the same time it prevents insects gaining access to the sludge. The faciloil is used with a special sprayer. It was used at Frankfort, where it was found that a dose of from ·11 to ·18 gallon per square yard sufficed, the cost of the disinfectant being about 9s. per 100 lbs.

Use of sludge lagoons abroad. Abroad, sludge lagoons or beds are in use at many places. At Leipzig, a portion of the sludge is treated in specially drained earthen lagoons.

The sludge becomes spadeable in summer in about two months, in winter from four to five months.

In selecting the site for sludge beds, due regard should be paid to the direction of the prevalent wind, and the situation should be a sunny and a windy one, well removed from public roads or footpaths.

Much will depend upon the nature of and moisture in the sludge—apart from weather conditions—as to the length of time required for drying.

The average length of time requisite for drying Emscher tank sludge is said to be five days, and only one to two days in favourable weather.

Septic tank sludge at Halberstadt removed from the tanks at intervals of about eight weeks, required 14 days for drying in favourable weather. It should be observed that both in the case of the Emscher Association and Halberstadt.

[1] Allen, *Sewage Sludge*, p. 60.

the sludge is delivered into the beds in thin layers, whereas at other plants where the sludge is run into the beds to a depth of from 2·3 to 3·3 feet, the drying process usually takes some six to nine months.

Imhoff considers that for septic tank sludge 275 square yards of sludge beds are requisite per cubic yard of sludge received daily, whilst for sedimentation sludge 458 square yards are required for a similar amount.

Composting. A method which can sometimes be suitably carried out in conjunction with sludge beds, is to mix some waste material—such as house refuse, street sweepings, etc.—with the sludge with the object of rendering it easier to handle. This was done for some time at Oswestry with satisfactory results, the mixture being disposed of to farmers. In this particular instance, a large cinder tip existed on the site of the works and this material was worked into the sludge.

In a similar manner, stable and farmyard straw litter and manure can be incorporated with liquid sludge in moderate-sized drying beds. A layer of manure is placed on the bottom of the beds, wet sludge is run in to a depth of some 3 to 4 inches over the manure, and the bed is then filled up with alternate layers of manure and sludge. This method was employed by Col. Jones, V.C. more than 20 years ago at the Aldershot Camp Farm.

It should be observed that a particular method of sludge treatment—say lagoons or drying beds, which would be quite permissible in the case of an isolated sewage farm serving a small town—might be quite inadmissible near a large town, not only on account of the high value of the land, but on account of the nuisance from smell and risk of costly litigation arising therefrom.

Regarding the term " nuisance," as applied to smell, this word has recently been defined by the law as something materially interfering with the ordinary comfort physically of human existence. As to what degree may be " material," however, the law is discreetly silent.

Use of sludge for filling in waste land. Sludge can be employed for filling up waste land, old brickyards, etc., either in the liquid state, mixed with other substances, such as house refuse, or simply in the form of pressed cake.

The latter method was adopted at York some years ago by

Mr Creer, then the City Engineer. A large heap of pressed sludge cake had accumulated in the open, causing considerable nuisance to the neighbourhood, until the plan was devised of tipping it some 5 to 6 feet thick on an uneven field adjoining the works, a 24 inch layer of soil being placed over the sludge, the soil in turn being turfed. The nuisance from smell was entirely done away with by this means.

Where pressed sludge cake can be dealt with by filling in waste land, it would seem to be sufficient to press down to say 60 % moisture, allowing for the sludge cake to dry to some extent in the atmosphere.

A somewhat similar practice to that followed at York has been carried out at Providence and Worcester, U.S.A. At Providence, up to July 1908, pressed cake was used for filling up low-lying land, whilst at Worcester, Fuller[1] states that the sludge cake is disposed of with little or no nuisance by conveying it by trolley car to vacant land, about a mile distant from the disposal works : a small proportion of the cake is carted away by farmers.

Disposal of sludge mixed with other refuse has been suggested in the case of Toronto.

At Hanover, the semi-dried sludge from the centrifugal machines is used for filling up low-lying ground.

The employment of wet sewage sludge, it may be observed, for filling in depressions in waste land could not be recommended where any houses adjoin the dump site.

At Messrs Steiner's dye works near Accrington the sludge produced is used for filling up a small valley close to the settling tanks, the sludge being conveyed by a cable-way.

With sludges from certain manufacturing processes, e.g. that of paper-making, the sludge is not nearly so offensive as ordinary sewage sludge.

Flooding land with sludge. This operation consists in covering land with liquid sludge to a depth of some 2 inches to 4 inches.

To obtain the best results by this plan, it is essential that the weather should be fine, and further, that the land should have been freshly ploughed.

The method is open to the same objection as lagooning—more so, in fact, as the exposed surface area of sludge is far greater.

[1] *Sewage Disposal.*

This method of disposal was carried out some years ago for a portion of the sludge at the Beaumont Leys Farm, Leicester Corporation; Bolton and Birmingham have also disposed of their sludge in this manner. It should be noted, however, that at Leicester the sludge areas were a long distance away from dwelling-houses other than those belonging to the farm. The sludge was raised by a chain pump driven by a portable steam engine, the sludge flowing along the ordinary carriers to the sludge areas, which were usually steam cultivated before the application of the sludge.

At Cambridge, the manager has tried the experiment of flooding sections of porous gravelly soil with sludge, allowing it to dry, and then cutting it up into cubes by spade labour, when it is left to dry and finally disposed of to farmers.

It should be noted that it is useless to bury sludge deeply, i.e. 3 to 6 feet deep in the ground, under the impression that it will ultimately disappear, and the ground become available for re-sludging. Sludge buried under such conditions will continue to decompose very slowly and will give off gas for years after it has been buried, and it very often forms an impervious layer in the subsoil. The more lightly the sludge is buried, the quicker will be its decomposition and ultimate disintegration.

It is perhaps advisable to point out that sludge should not be disposed of on land which is likely to be irrigated, before the sludge has become innocuous and thoroughly incorporated with the soil; many bad effluents can be traced to this cause.

Shallow burial of sludge. This is quite one of the best methods of sludge disposal where there is plenty of land available: the process consists in cutting trenches in the soil some 12 to 15 inches deep and 18 inches to 2 feet 6 inches wide; the sludge is then run into the trenches, and after the bulk of the moisture has disappeared, the soil is covered in over the sludge. The trenches should be got ready some days before the sludge is run in, in order to allow the soil to become as dry as possible. Fig. 25 shows a plan and section of the sludge disposal area at Hatfield.

It is of great importance with this system to cover the sludge lightly, and to resist the temptation to make the trenches

either too wide or too deep.   If there is much smell from the
sludge when it is first run into the trenches and there are
dwelling houses in the neighbourhood, bleaching powder can
be dusted over the trenches.   Soot, it may be noted, is useful
for a similar purpose, and in the case of sludge from breweries
has been found to be superior to lime.

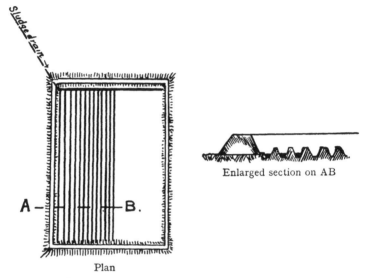

Fig. 25.   Sludge area at Hatfield sewage farm.

The chief objection to this method of disposal is that during
wet weather, it is difficult to get the trenches filled in rapidly,
and smell may arise from the uncovered sludge.

After the trenches have become fairly dry, say after a
month or six weeks in summer, the area can be ploughed and
cropped, when it can again be used for receiving sludge ; it
is, however, better to allow a period of 12 months, before more
sludge is again applied.

Sludge pressing.   This process, broadly speaking, removes
from the wet sludge about 30 % to 35 % of the moisture, leaving the sludge in the form of cakes, and easy of manipulation :

in other words, it will convert 100 tons of wet sludge into about 20 tons of cake and 80 tons of water.

Fig. 26 illustrates diagrammatically a plan and sectional elevation of a sludge pressing plant designed by the well-known firm of Messrs S. H. Johnson and Co., of Stratford, London, in which the mixers and air compressors are driven by self-contained electric motors ; the plant can, however, be worked equally well by self-contained steam engines or by belt from a central power motor.

The sewage arrives at the works by the channel A, and passes through the screen B, the spaces between the screen bars being $\frac{1}{2}$ to $\frac{5}{8}$ inch wide, to arrest substances liable to cause obstruction or damage to the pressing plant ; after passing the screen, the sewage flows along the baffle channel F, receiving *en route* from the channel E a continuous dose of milk of lime of constant strength from the lime mixer C, the flow being adjusted to the character and volume of the sewage.

A second chemical mixer G can be used for preparing a solution of some other precipitant which it may be desirable to use in conjunction with the lime treatment : this second precipitant is added after the milk of lime has become thoroughly incorporated with the sewage.

After leaving the baffle channel, the chemically treated sewage enters the inlet channel H to the precipitation tanks I, I, where the suspended matter in the sewage settles on the floor of the tanks, settlement being assisted by the flocculation caused by the precipitants. When the tanks are sludged the tank liquor is drawn off, usually by floating draw-off arms, the sludge swept to the deep end of the tank, and the sludge valve J opened, the sludge gravitating to the sludge well L through the sludge drain K. As the sludge flows into the well L, milk of lime is added from the mixer M : the object of this being to create a denser sludge, and to facilitate pressing.

The sludge is withdrawn from the sludge well to the sludge settling tank N by the automatic rams O and O_1 which fill by vacuum and work alternately, one filling whilst the other

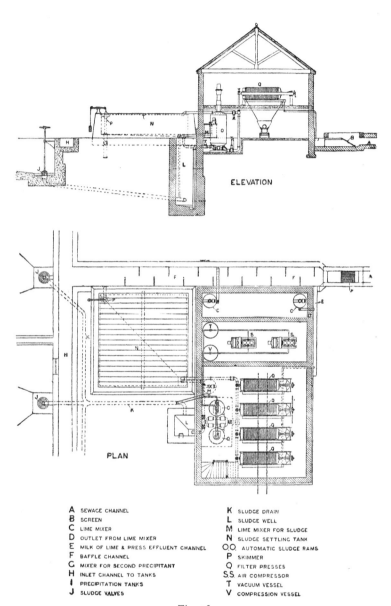

ELEVATION

PLAN

A	SEWAGE CHANNEL	K	SLUDGE DRAIN
B	SCREEN	L	SLUDGE WELL
C	LIME MIXER	M	LIME MIXER FOR SLUDGE
D	OUTLET FROM LIME MIXER	N	SLUDGE SETTLING TANK
E	MILK OF LIME & PRESS EFFLUENT CHANNEL	O,O,	AUTOMATIC SLUDGE RAMS
F	BAFFLE CHANNEL	P	SKIMMER
G	MIXER FOR SECOND PRECIPITANT	Q	FILTER PRESSES
H	INLET CHANNEL TO TANKS	S.S.	AIR COMPRESSOR
I	PRECIPITATION TANKS	T	VACUUM VESSEL
J	SLUDGE VALVES	V	COMPRESSION VESSEL

Fig. 26.

is discharging, a continuous discharge of sludge being secured by the periodical automatic reversal of this action.

The sludge is left in the sludge tank for about 12 hours, to allow the limed sludge to consolidate, when the top water is drawn off by the skimmer P, the liquid being returned to the sewage channel.

The thick settled sludge is then drawn off by vacuum into the rams O and O_1, and forced into the presses Q by compressed air provided by the air compressors S, S_1, these also providing the vacuum for filling the rams with sludge.

The solids present in the sludge are caught by the filter cloths, the press liquor flowing into the trough at the side of each press and thence through the channel E, re-enters the baffle channel F together with the milk of lime from the mixer C.

Pressing is completed when the press liquor ceases to flow from the press chamber outlets ; the press chambers are then opened and the sludge cakes drop into a tip waggon placed under the press.

The filter cloths are then re-adjusted, the chambers closed, and another batch of sludge is pressed, the operations being repeated until the sludge tank N is emptied.

Fig. 27 shows a large filter press made by Messrs S. H. Johnson and Co. This press contains 94 chambers with plates $51\frac{1}{2}$ inches square, fitted with hydraulic opening closing and tightening gear, the opening cylinder being arranged vertically beneath the closing cylinder. The plates of these presses are recessed, a rim projecting all round the periphery on both sides, leaving the body of the plate, which forms the drainage area, in a recess ; the rims are machined, and form the surfaces on which the joints are made between the plates ; the joints are faced by a special method which ensures the joint surfaces being true and parallel to within $\frac{1}{500}$ of an inch.

When the plates are placed side by side in the framework of the press, hollow chambers are formed between the adjacent plates, the chambers being enclosed on all sides by the raised rims of the plates. Each plate has a hole through the centre by which the sludge flows into each of the chambers when admitted through the central hole in the head of the press.

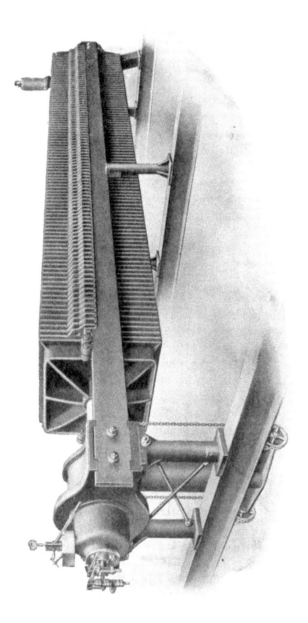

Fig. 27. Filter Press.

A filter cloth is hung over each plate so as to hang down on each side and completely cover the whole of the plate. Each cloth has two holes, corresponding when in position with the hole in the centre of the plate, round which it is secured with a clip.

It will thus be seen that when the plates are all in position in the framework of the press, and the whole tightly screwed up, a number of chambers are formed between the plates, each chamber being completely lined with the filter cloth.

On the sludge being forced into the press all the solid matter in suspension is retained by the filter cloths, upon which it is deposited in a layer, gradually increasing in thickness until the chambers are all completely filled, whilst the liquid portion or filtrate escapes through the cloths to the outlets fitted to each plate.

With well-limed and settled sludge, good firm cakes can be formed of a thickness of $1\frac{1}{2}$ inches, but it is unusual to exceed this dimension, and, if the sludge is of a slimy nature and difficult to press, then press chambers to form cakes only 1 inch thick or less are more suitable.

In the majority of cases the pressure employed in sludge pressing is between 70 and 100 lbs. per square inch, but the press just described can be used with working pressures up to 120 lbs. per square inch.

The sludge can be forced into the sludge presses either by pumps or by pneumatic forcing rams. For small installations, the use of pumps is generally found quite satisfactory, but for large sludge presses the pneumatic system of charging is far preferable to pumps, the pressure being less liable to fluctuate, and the whole operation of charging more easily controlled.

The apparatus consists essentially of one or more closed vessels (variously known as forcing receivers, forcing rams, or montejus) into which the sludge is first run, and then displaced under pressure by compressed air. The simplest form of this system consists of a single forcing ram and air compressor, the sludge being run into the ram by gravitation, displaced by compressed air into the sludge presses, and the air allowed to escape from the ram whilst another charge of sludge is run in.

By using a pair of such rams worked on the twin system, one charging whilst the other is filling, a constant supply of sludge to the presses is maintained.

Where a pair of rams is employed, a great saving of power can be effected by re-compressing the compressed air contained in each ram—after the sludge has been discharged—into the other ram instead of allowing it to exhaust to waste. In this way the same amount of air is circulated in a closed system and used over and over again, being compressed into each ram alternately; the air compressor in such a case being specially designed to operate the rams in this way.

Messrs Johnson's latest improvement of this system is to make the reversal of air pressure in these rams quite automatic so that instead of the air pressure being switched over from one ram to the other when required by a man in attendance, the switching over is done automatically by the flow of the sludge into and from the rams.

For operating these automatic forcing rams, air compressors are supplied, fitted with automatic devices by which the compressor is so controlled that it handles only just the quantity of air necessary to operate the rams at the rate required by the sludge presses.

When a battery of presses is first started the filtration is very rapid but it gradually slows down as the chambers become nearly filled, and it is evident that when the presses are taking the sludge at a slower rate, the volume of air required is much smaller than when the presses are taking the sludge at the maximum rate. The controlling devices automatically adjust the supply of air to suit the rate of flow of sludge.

The air compressors may be driven either by belt, steam or electricity, but in either case a pneumatic installation in which these automatic rams are included requires very little supervision.

In order to make the sludge easily pressable it is a general practice, as has already been pointed out, to add to the sludge a proportion of lime in the form of milk of lime, usually about

1 % of dry lime on the weight of the sludge. Sludge thus properly limed and settled should be pressed into good firm cakes in about 1 hour to 1½ hours.

If the sludge is not properly limed the time required for pressing will be considerably extended.

Where it is required to recover grease from the sludge, lime treatment is omitted, the sewage being cracked with acid to separate out the sludge, from which the grease is extracted by an injection of steam into the sludge presses whilst the pressing operation is proceeding. By this method the time required for pressing is considerably extended and may occupy 12 hours or even longer.

Trade effluents containing grease, such as wool washings, are treated in a similar manner. Sludge presses are also used for dealing with the sludge obtained from other waste effluents, such as from paper mills, tanneries, etc., the process being practically the same as for sewage sludge, but the method of precipitation of the sludge and chemicals may be varied in order to give the best results in any particular case.

Regarding the power required for sludge pressing plant, this is approximately 8 to 15 B.H.P. per ton of pressed cake produced per hour, the smaller figure obtaining for large installations, whilst for small plants the power consumed is proportionately greater. It should be observed too that the power required depends to a very great extent upon the " pressability " of the sludge, together with the percentage of water contained in the wet sludge prior to pressing.

The subjoined table gives particulars of the cast iron " Pyramid " sludge presses made by Messrs Johnson, together with useful data concerning the output of this type of press.

The weight of the pressed cake varies according to the degree of moisture it contains ; 12 cwt. per cube yard being an average weight.

The quantity of lime added to the sludge before pressing varies according to the nature of the sludge ; 1 % of the weight of the sludge is perhaps an average amount, calculated as dry lime.

With septic tank sludge and some sedimentation sludges

TABLE XVII. *Giving particulars of cast iron " Pyramid " sludge presses.*

Size of Plates	Number of Chambers	Filtering Area Sq. ft.	Thickness of Cake	Capacity of Chambers Cu. ft.	Weight of pressed cake per charge Cwts.
	12	88		3·4	2·3
	18	132		5·1	3·5
24 ins. square	24	176	1 in.	6·8	4·7
	30	220		8·5	5·9
	36	264		10·2	7·1
	18	168		8·1	5·6
27 ins. square	24	224	1¼ ins.	10·8	7·5
	30	280		13·5	9·4
	36	336		16·2	11·3
	24	260		14·0	9·8
30 ins. square	30	325	1½ ins.	17·5	12·2
	36	390		21·0	14·7
	48	520		28·0	19·6
	24	420		24·0	16·8
	30	525		30·0	21·0
36 ins. square	36	630	1½ ins.	36·0	25·2
	48	840		48·0	33·6
	60	1050		60·0	42·0
	30	615		37·0	25·9
40½ ins. square	36	738	1½ ins	44·4	31·0
	48	984		59·2	41·4
	60	1230		74·0	51·8
	36	1200		72·0	50·4
50¾ ins. square	48	1600	1½ ins.	96·0	67·2
	60	2000		120·0	84·0
	72	2400		144·0	100·8

very much more lime may have to be added. When the sludge has been obtained with a heavy dose of lime, less lime will need to be added for pressing purposes. The lime added for pressing purposes should be intimately mixed with the sludge to obtain the best results.

The cost of pressing depends mainly upon (1) cost of lime in the locality, (2) amount of precipitant added to sewage, (3) nature of sludge, (4) quantity of grease present in the sludge, (5) amount of lime added to sludge for pressing purposes, (6) the degree of moisture left in the pressed cake, and (7) the size of the installation. An average cost per ton of pressed cake produced may be taken at from 2s. 6d. to 3s. 6d. including all charges. In certain cases where there is plenty of waste

land available, it may be economical to press to say 60 %
moisture, allowing the cake to become air dried. In Table XVIII
taken from the *Fifth Report* of the Sewage Disposal Commission, will be found particulars of the cost of sludge pressing
at various places.

Grease is the chief constituent in sewage sludge which
renders it difficult to press, and this difficulty is accentuated
in hot weather.

In cases where the sludge is found to be difficult to press,
it is often advantageous to pass milk of lime through the filters
and press cloths before any sludge is admitted.

Septic tank sludge is exceedingly difficult to press owing
to the extreme fineness of the particles in the sludge, lime
to the extent of more than 15 % of the pressed cake being
added to facilitate pressing. Difficulty in pressing septic
sludge has been experienced at York, Rochdale, Oldham,
Nelson and Burnley.

At Withington[1], pressing of sludge with fine coal has been
tried, the finest coal being screened out. With 5 tons of coal
to 40 tons of wet sludge, a good cake was obtained in two hours,
containing half its weight of coal. Later experiments showed
that with a proportional addition of lime, the amount of coal
used could be much reduced: 28 tons of wet sludge, together
with 1 ton of fine coal, and $1\frac{1}{2}$ cwt. of lime, produced 5 tons
of pressed sludge, pressing taking $1\frac{1}{2}$ hours.

A large amount of dust is produced during the burning
of the cake.

The writer is not aware whether the pressing of Emscher tank sludge has
been tried on a practical scale: possibly the entangled gas bubbles would allow
of easier pressing in this case.

It should be observed that the percentage of moisture
in pressed cake is not uniform throughout the cake; it is
usually greatest near the inlets to the press cells, *i.e.* where
the last sludge enters; this inconsistency as regards moisture
should be borne in mind when it is proposed to dry the sludge
for artificial manures.

[1] City of Manchester, Rivers Department, *Annual Report for year ending
March* 1911. Henry Blacklock and Co., Ltd., Manchester.

Sludge pressing in America. Sludge pressing is carried out at Worcester and Providence, U.S.A., and Fuller[1] gives details of the process at the latter city.

Here the average daily volume of sludge pumped is 68,679 gallons, an average of 7·93 % of this being dry solids.

The sludge is pumped by two Shone ejectors to storage reservoirs, flowing thence to four rams, each 8 ft. diameter by 12 ft. long. From the rams it is forced into the presses at a pressure of from 60 to 50 lbs. per square inch. There are 18 presses, each containing 43 to 54 plates, producing cakes 36 inches square, and from ¾ to 1¼ inches thick.

Two air compressors of 150 and 50 H.P. respectively worked by electric motors work the ejectors and rams. The presses are in use on an average for about 5·74 hours per day, turning out a daily average of 82·22 tons of sludge cake, equivalent to 22·69 tons of dry solids. The daily cost for light and power is about 24s. 9d. The cost of sludge pressing at Providence for the years 1909 and 1910 is given by Allen[2] as being respectively about 12s. and 11s. per ton of dry solids.

Composition of pressed cake. The following analyses by Dr McGowan[3] show the composition of pressed cake from Chorley and Dorking.

The sludge at Chorley is produced by the addition of 9 grains per gallon of alumino-ferric, whilst that from Dorking is the result of adding 5 grains of lime per gallon : both sewages are domestic in character.

TABLE XIX. *Giving composition of pressed sludge cake.*

	Chorley pressed cake after drying at 110° C.	Dorking pressed cake after drying at 110° C.
Grit, etc. (*i.e.* matter insoluble in HCL after ignition) ..	25·30	6·84
Oxides of iron and alumina ..	9·37	3·46
Lime	10·32	23·16
Phosphoric acid	0·98	0·66
Equivalent to tribasic phosphate of lime..	2·14	1·44
Nitrogen (total)	1·28	0·89
Nitrogen evolved on boiling the sludge for two hours with dilute (·5 %) potash solution	0·13	0·03

Dr McGowan observes that the calculated value of the above two sludges in the form of pressed cake containing 50 % moisture, as judged by their manurial constituents alone, is about 6s. to 7s. per ton, but that, as experience shows, the market value is less.

[1] *Sewage Disposal,* Fuller.   [2] *Sewage Sludge,* pp. 230 and 243.
[3] Sewage Disposal Commission, *Fifth Report.*

Disposal of pressed cake.   Pressed cake, owing to its portability, can often be disposed of for a small sum to farmers where the sewage works lie in an agricultural district.

In the vicinity of large towns there used to be considerable difficulty in obtaining a market for it, since horse manure could be obtained very cheaply.   Possibly with the increase of motor traction, a better market will obtain for pressed sewage sludge.

Many farmers prefer to have the sludge cake broken up before carting it ; this was found to be the case at Burnley, the cake being broken up immediately after pressing, a good market resulting.

At Chorley, the pressed cake is sold to farmers who cart it away for about 10*d.* to 1*s.* per ton.

Mr Allen[1] states that Providence, U.S.A. has recently, as a temporary measure, disposed of its pressed sludge by dumping in Narragansett Bay from a scow 135 feet long × 38 feet wide × 11 feet deep, divided into six compartments and having a capacity of 850 cubic yards when filled level, and 1050 cubic yards when heaped. The scow is towed about 10 miles down the bay, and the contents dumped into a depth of about 65 feet of water.

Disposal of sludge by diffusion in water.   This mode of disposal is carried on by several of the largest cities in the United Kingdom, and is one of the cheapest methods of getting rid of an undesirable product, given proximity to the sea.

In the case of London, some $2\frac{1}{2}$ million tons of wet sludge are disposed of annually at Barrow Deep, about 20 miles south of Southend, in sludge steamers discharging their cargoes over a length of from 5 to 10 miles.

Glasgow discharges some 300,000 tons of sludge per annum between Arran and the mainland.

At Manchester, Salford, Dublin, and Southampton, the same practice is followed.

In America, Boston and Providence are mentioned by Fuller[2] as using this method of disposal, whilst in 1911 it was recommended by the Milwaukee Sewerage Commission, that the sludge should be dumped in Lake Michigan, about 15 miles from the shore.

At Boston U.S.A. the sludge from the deposit sewer is drawn into a sludge tank 50 feet × 10 feet × 15 feet holding 150 cubic yards, whence it is

[1] *Sewage Sludge.*   [2] *Sewage Disposal.*

removed by a scow, which is towed about 20 miles out in Massachusetts bay, and its contents dumped in deep water.

At Columbus, Ohio, sludge is discharged into the Scioto river when flowing with sufficient volume, being stored during insufficient river flow.

At Waterbury, Conn., it was found that when sludge from the experimental tanks was mixed with 1650 volumes of water in the Naugatuck River, no nuisance resulted, and the mixture was found to be non-putrescible.

Incineration of sewage sludge. The large percentage of moisture present in wet sludge renders incineration impracticable, unless some other substance is mixed with it to reduce the water present. Pressed sludge cake has, however, been burnt successfully in several instances, and it is advisable where it is desired eventually to burn the sludge cake, to press thoroughly, and by this means to reduce the moisture to a figure well below 60 %.

The late Mr Charles Jones for some years burnt pressed cake at the Southern Ealing Works, the cake containing about 60 % of moisture. The pressed cake at these works falls from the filter presses into trucks which are conveyed by a hydraulic lift to the destructor. Before being burnt, the pressed cake was mixed with dry house refuse in the proportion of $1\frac{1}{2}$ to 2 parts of dry refuse to 1 of pressed cake.

The steam raised by the burning of the cake was used for lime mixing, sludge pressing, and the production of artificial stone slabs, also for pumping a portion of the sewage. From 2000 to 3000 tons of pressed cake were disposed of yearly by this method during the years 1905, 1906, and 1907.

At Withington[1] pressed sludge cake containing half its weight of coal, with an addition of 2 parts of dry ash-bin refuse, could be burnt rapidly in the destructor, but large quantities of dust were produced. Cake containing 1 part of coal to 2 of sludge did not burn very well when mixed with refuse. The process proved more expensive than when lime was used, even when the coal could be procured for the carting.

As would be anticipated, some sludges containing much organic matter and grease are more easily burnt than those containing large quantities of mineral matter; on the other

[1] City of Manchester Rivers Department, *Annual Report for year ending March* 1911. Henry Blacklock and Co., Ltd., Manchester.

hand, the presence of the grease may cause trouble during the process of expelling the moisture prior to burning.   Unless the moisture can be reduced below 60 % much of the heat created during combustion will be absorbed in drawing off the excess of moisture as steam.

At Bury, pressed sludge cake has been mixed with street sweepings in the proportion of 1 to 2 and burnt in a Horsfall destructor.

Having regard to the trouble caused by grease in sewage sludge when attempts are made to burn it, it would seem desirable that the sewage should in the first instance be subjected to treatment for the removal of grease.

Incineration of sewage sludge abroad.   Incineration of sludge has received much attention abroad, and Allen[1] in his excellent book gives valuable data regarding this method of disposal.   At Frankfort-on-the-Main, briquettes made up from de-watered sludge and air-dried to 10 % moisture, gave an effective heat value of 9910 B.T.U. on an average, with 47 % of combustible material.   Experiments at Elberfeld indicated that sludge with 60 % moisture could be burnt without using coal, by the medium of a forced draught.

Septic tank sludge, as would be expected, yielded lower results as regards heat ; the calorific value of septic sludge at Stuttgart (40 % moisture) being 6456 B.T.U., whereas, with settled sludge containing 47 % moisture, it was 8035 B.T.U.

Sludge of 60 % moisture obtained at Potsdam from the Lignite process gave 5950 B.T.U., and settling tank sludge from Hanover dried at 212° F. gave 15,870 B.T.U. with 28 % ash, and 17,120 B.T.U. with 18·5 % ash.   It is interesting to note that in colliery districts a certain increase in calorific value is found, being caused by the particles of coal present in the sewage.

Experiments carried out on the burning of septic sludge from Emscher tanks containing 46·4 % of moisture showed that it burnt when mixed with from 5 % to 20 % of coal, when 50 % with no commercial value was left as ash.

Allen[2] mentions that at the Philadelphia experimental station, wet sludge was mixed with an equal weight of rice-size anthracite coal, the mixture being 1·57 times the volume of the sludge, and the percentage of moisture being reduced from 91 % to 48½ %.   After being run into a sludge lagoon to a depth of 12 inches and drying for 24 hours, the mixture was further reduced to about 27½ %, and after the lapse of 9 days to 22½ %, the temperature being about 37° F.

The results of the mixing were as follows :

Constituents	per cent.	lbs. per cube yard
Moisture	45·5	1069
Coal	50·0	1175
Dry residue of sludge ..	4·5	106
	100·0	2350

[1] *Sewage Sludge*, Allen, pp. 97–100.   [2] *Sewage Sludge, ibid.* p. 250.

Each cube yard of wet sludge, after drying, with 1760 lbs. of coal, produced one ton of the dried mixture for fuel. The b.t.u.s contained in the materials used were as follows.

In the coal as received—12,065.

In the sludge as burned—1216 to 1265.

The results of burning air-dried sludge with coal are given below:

Weight of sludge broken to 2 inch size, per cube yard in lbs.	710 to 1015
Percentage of water in sludge	15·3 to 40·2
Percentage of dry residue, volatile	24·5 to 30
lbs. of dry residue in sludge used	168 to 233
lbs. volatile matter	48 to 70
lbs. coal burned with sludge	192 to 285
lbs. wet sludge burned per minute	2·66 to 4·15
lbs. volatile matter burned per minute	·555 to ·705
lbs. dry residue burned per minute	2·18 to 2·47
lbs. of coal burned per lb. of wet sludge	·68 to ·895
,, ,, ,, ,, dry residue	·817 to ·945
,, ,. ,, ,, volatile matter	·223 to ·25

The experiment showed that it was possible to burn sludge in this way under boilers.

In some districts in England peat is easily obtainable, and it would seem practicable in the neighbourhood of such localities, to employ dried peat dust to mix with sludge prior to the burning process. Again, sawdust could be employed for lining the sludge drying beds, the layer of sawdust being removed with the sludge, pressed into cake and burnt.

Manufacture of fertilisers from sewage sludge. This subject has for many years received the attention of agriculturists and chemists.

Probably the best-known process is that which has been carried on for many years at Kingston-on-Thames Sewage Works by the Native Guano Company, and called the A.B.C. process. For a number of years the Kingston sewage treatment only went as far as tank purification, the tank liquor being discharged into the Thames; the tank liquor produced was, however, an exceptionally good one. It is now further treated on contact beds.

A full description of the A.B.C. process will be found in the *Fifth Report* of the Sewage Disposal Commission.

The process carried on by the Anglo-Continental Fertilisers Syndicate Ltd. (Dixon's Patent), consists in allowing tank sludge to ferment at a temperature of about 90° F. for a period of about 24 hours, with a small proportion of yeast; the effect of the fermentation is to cause a separation of the sludge from roughly half its volume of water. The sludge rises to the top of the fermenting tank, and the water is drawn off from the bottom.

The general effect is to convert a sludge of 90 % water into one containing 80 %, and it is also claimed that the manurial constituents of the sludge are rendered much more readily available, as the result of the fermentation.

The Company complete the process by drying and disintegrating the sludge, the dried product being used as a base for artificial manures.

The process is to be seen on a working scale at the Dublin Sewage Works.

Very many attempts have been made abroad to produce fertilisers from sewage sludge, in some cases with success. As a rule, the fresher the sewage the better the fertiliser obtained from it, in other cases further chemical manures have to be added.

Farmers do not care to take a sludge which is greasy and therefore cannot be sown, and many sludges contain seeds of various weeds. They are not long in finding out that sludge has to be disposed of by the authority, and in many cases they have to be paid before they will remove the sludge. Again, they will only as a rule fetch it during certain seasons of the year.

Septic sludge is not of much value manurially to farmers, owing to its worked-out condition. Small sewage disposal works in rural districts have not usually any difficulty in disposing of their sludge to neighbouring farmers, but in the vicinity of large cities this is not the case.

There have been very many statistics advanced regarding the colossal waste of manure from sewage disposal works yearly. This may be so, and the figures put forward may be correct, but the cost of getting the sludge into a suitable form for sale and transit and use must be borne in mind.

Good results have been obtained from using sewage sludge at Essen-N.W., Bochum, and Recklinghausen, where it is sold to farmers, and the supply is said to be unequal to the demand.

Recently—1924, valuable work has been done by T. C. Hatton, at Milwaukee, with a view to producing a sludge of greater fertilising value.

Summary of cost of sludge disposal in England. The following statement and table are taken from the Fifth Report of the Sewage Disposal Commission.

Comparative cost of different methods of disposal of sludge.

" The cost of disposing of sludge depends not merely upon the method adopted, but also, and to a large extent, upon the local circumstances of each place. This must be carefully borne in mind in considering the following table."

TABLE **XX.** *Giving comparative cost of the various methods of sludge disposal as instanced by the examples given.*

Method of Sludge Disposal	Number of Examples	Maximum and minimum cost of the process, in pence, per ton of sludge containing 90 per cent of water, including interest and sinking fund and all other charges	Average cost of process in pence, per ton of sludge containing 90 % of water, including interest and sinking fund and all other charges
Covering land with sludge	3	Minimum 1·32d. Maximum 2·8d.	Say 2d.
Sea disposal	6	Minimum 4·1d. Maximum 6·9d,	Say 5d.
Trenching in Soil	3	Minimum 4d. Maximum 7d.	Say 5d.
Pressing. Group I	10	Minimum 4·8d Maximum 7·3d.[1]	Say 6d.
Pressing. Group II	11	Minimum 7·7d. Maximum 12·6d.[1]	Say 11·5d.
Pressing and Burning	1 Experimental	13·3d. (excluding interest and sinking fund)	Say 18d.[2]

Recovery of by-products from sewage sludge. The size of the town from which the sewage is derived, quite apart from the character of the sewage itself, must to a very great extent decide as to whether a special plant is warranted to deal specially with by-products.

For example, it would be unwise, save in very exceptional

---

[1] "Owing to the great variations in the actual figures for interest and sinking fund, mainly because of the different dates at which the sewage works were constructed, we have been obliged, in dealing with 'pressing,' to take an approximate average figure for this item, *viz.*, 9d. per ton of pressed cake, containing 55 per cent. of water, or 2d. per ton of sludge containing 90 per cent. of water."

[2] " This figure is an estimate."

circumstances, to erect a special plant for grease recovery, for
a town of 2000 inhabitants, whereas the provision of the same
plant might be amply justified for a town of say 20,000 inhabitants.

It should be remembered that if sludge contains 10 % of
grease when dried, in its raw state as delivered from the tanks
it may contain 90 to 95 % of moisture, so that the percentage
of grease in the wet sludge will only be about 1 %.

Again, the cost of working any particular recovery process
must depend very largely upon the market value of the by-
product recovered. The price of grease is now (1913) high
(about £8 to £10 per ton), whilst some years ago it was very
much lower. Grease recovery works will, as a rule, take pressed
cake which contains a workable percentage of grease and the
wastes from wool-scouring works. The greases obtained from
the various sludge cakes are blended according to the type
of oil it is desired to produce. At several sewage works, the
greasy scum lying on the surface of the sewage has been saved
for the sake of the large percentage of grease which it contains.
At the Cambridge Sewage Farm, the manager for some years
collected the greasy scum lying on the surface of the sewage
in the settling tank, passing steam through it in old paraffin
tubs, the resulting grease being used as a lubricant for carts.

At Rochdale, grease from the sewage is collected, barrelled
and sold.

All sewages contain more or less grease, principally derived
in the case of domestic sewages, from soapsuds and waste water
resulting from cooking operations.

In the case of sewages containing certain trade wastes
such as wool and piece scouring, the percentage of grease
present is often high—in some cases, notably that of Bradford—
sufficiently high to warrant the provision of expensive special
plant for the sole purpose of extracting the grease.

Grease extraction at Bradford. By the courtesy of Mr
Joseph Garfield, M.Inst.C.E., the Sewage Works Engineer
—Engineer of the new scheme—the writer has been enabled
to give particulars of the new Bradford sludge disposal works
at Esholt. Pending further alterations, a temporary 8 inch

sludge main some five miles long has been laid from the old Frizinghall tanks to the new plant at Esholt. The sludge, which contains about 84 % of water, is fed into this main together with compressed air (initial pressure varying from 30 to 40 lbs. per square inch), the fall from inlet to outlet of the sludge main being some 70 feet.

The press house measures 237 feet × 92 feet, containing no less than 128 sludge presses : the grease house measures 237 feet × 50 feet : it contains 16 grease vats, each having a purifying capacity of 7 tons of grease, with a grease storage tank having a capacity of 1000 tons, together with grease separators, boiling vats and rams.

On arriving at the receiving tanks the sludge is forced by means of compressed air to the boiling vats, where it is heated by steam, and passed into three steel vessels beneath. From these vessels it is forced by compressed air to the filter presses.

The press chambers are 3 feet square, with 47 chambers to each press. The press liquor passes into tanks where the grease which it contains is separated and sent to the purifying vats, the water being pumped back again to the sewage. From the grease vats the grease is either barrelled, pumped into tank waggons on the railway, or sent to the storage vats as the case may be.

At the present time 128 presses produce 16 to 20 tons of grease per 24 hours, having a value of from £8 to £10 per ton, whilst the press cake is sold as a fertiliser at 3s. per ton f.o.v. being loaded direct to the waggons from the presses above.

The press cake only contains from 25 % to 28 % of moisture and no lime ; there is a large market for it as a fertiliser in England and on the continent. Some has been shipped to America.

Experiments initiated by Dr Grossmann have been in progress for some time at Oldham, the grease being removed from the sludge by distillation by steam. This process is described later (p. 154).

Extraction of grease by benzine has also been successfully tried.

Massachusetts experiments. Valuable experiments on the disposal of sewage sludge by destructive distillation have been made by the Massachusetts State Board of Health[1].

The relative volume and composition of the gases from various kinds of sludges were as follows.

TABLE XXI. *Showing relative volume and composition of gases produced by destructive distillation of sewage sludge.*

	Cubic feet of gas per ton of sample	CO₂ (Carbon dioxide)	Illum-inants	O (oxygen)	CO (Carbonic oxide)	H (Hydrogen)	CH₄ (Methane)	N (Nitrogen)
					Per Cent			
Lawrence sludge[1] ..	4900	4·4	2·2	0·3	30·7	34·9	18·6	9·1
Andover sludge[1] ..	6400	7·4	15·1	0·6	14·3	22·9	34·3	5·4
Clinton sludge[1] ..	9100	8·3	6·7	0·0	20·4	33·2	24·5	7·0
Brockton sludge[1] ..	6000	16·5	21·4	0·2	10·3	22·6	29·1	0·2
Worcester sludge[2] ..	8100	14·2	4·9	0·3	29·8	32·6	16·2	2·2
Septic tank sludge ..	4900	7·5	1·0	0·1	24·3	44·0	13·0	10·2
Trickling filter sludge	6000	20·2	17·4	0·3	6·6	32·7	22·8	0·0
Sludge from evaporation of sulphite pulp liquor	11000	21·6	2·1	0·0	20·0	42·0	12·0	0·3
Peat	8400	39·0	4·7	0·2	11·0	28·0	17·1	0·0
Sawdust	12700	18·4	4·8	0·3	28·2	26·9	19·1	2·3
Woodpulp	12000	23·5	1·4	0·0	16·4	44·5	13·3	0·9
Soapgrease	5400	6·8	44·5	0·0	6·2	15·8	26·7	0·0
Soft coal[3]	10200	1·6	2·0	0·1	5·2	62·3	25·7	3·2
Lawrence illuminating gas[4] —		3·4	9·1	0·0	21·5	42·5	19·7	3·8

[1] Settled sewage sludge.   [2] Chemically precipitated sludge.
[3] Average of four kinds of steam and gas coal.
[4] From gas company pipes at experiment station.

It may be added that Esparto sludge, without the " dust," gives a good yield of gas when dried.

Experiments at Manchester[2]. Messrs Crossley Bros. carried out some experiments for the Manchester Rivers Department on the gas produced from Withington sludge cake containing one part of coal to two parts of sludge, together with some dry ash-bin refuse.

They succeeded in gasifying the material up to a moisture content of 50 % to 55 %. The yields showed 80,000 cubic feet of gas per dried ton gasified, having a calorific value of 112 B.T.U. net at N.T.P., and the equivalent of 61 lbs. of ammonium sulphate, when dealing with material of 1·46 % nitrogen content.

[1] 40th *Annual Report*, pp. 497 and 498.
    City of Manchester, Rivers Department. *Annual Report for year ending March* 1911. Henry Blacklock and Co., Ltd., Manchester.

The only difficulty experienced appears to have been th thorough cleaning of the fire, when using a material containin 40 % of ash, for which a specially designed plant would b necessary.

Centrifugalising of sludge. Various types of centrifuga machines have been in use for the drying of sludge at many places abroad. They possess the marked advantage of bringing down the moisture in sludges of certain composition in far less time than is taken by filter pressing, and the working cost does not appear to be excessive when compared with pressing. On the other hand, with some sludges containing much grease, the moisture does not appear to be extracted from sludge to the same extent as with the filter press, difficulty arising by reason of the grease forming a watertight layer on the sludge surface in the centrifugal machine : this was found to be the case with experiments carried out at Cologne, Mannheim and Spandau.

The " colacit " process appears to have been employed successfully with centrifugalising of sludge at Frankfort on the Main, where it was found as the result of experiment that 10 cubic metres of sludge, treated with colacit powder, could be centrifugalised down to 65 % of moisture : the process is stated to have been considerably cheaper than pressing.

The earlier centrifugal machines were constructed somewhat upon the lines of the well-known centrifugal cream separators used in dairies, the heavier matters in the sludge flying to the periphery of the revolving vessel, and the liquid being drawn off by a pipe whilst the machine was running ; cleaning by hand had to be resorted to after each centrifugalisation.

The Schaefer-ter-Meer system appears to have improved considerably upon the earlier types of centrifugal, and with this form of machine the sludge can be filled into it and removed automatically whilst the apparatus is actually running. Installations on a large scale are running at Hanover, Harburg and Frankfort, and a short description of the Harburg plant is given later.

Briefly described, the drum of the centrifugal machine is provided with a central tube through which the wet sludge is admitted, and a number of radial sludge chambers, each one of these being fitted with fine sieves, perforated with openings ·4 inch long and about ·020 inch wide, and having both external and internal valves ; the chambers have a capacity of from 1 to 10 cubic feet. A sludge supplying reservoir is above the machine, and the sludge flows into the chambers whilst they are rotating, the inner valve being open, and the outer slide shut : the heavy solids in the sludge are thrown to the outer part of the chambers, whilst the water, being of lower specific gravity, is separated from the sludge, passing through the sieves and flowing away by an annular channel into the shell of the machine and thence to an outlet. Further sludge then enters the chambers to replace the water lost, the chambers eventually becoming full of the centrifugalised sludge.

When this stage is reached, the inner valve is closed and the supply of sludge is cut off, the centrifugalised sludge in the chambers being separated from the wet sludge in the delivery pipe; the outer valve is then opened and the de-watered sludge ejected by centrifugal force, striking the walls of the shell, and falling in small fragments into wheelbarrows or waggons placed beneath the machine.

As soon as the outer valve has been closed and the inner one opened, the whole process is repeated, there are therefore two separate and distinct cycles or periods which are constantly repeated : (1) the period during which the wet sludge enters the machine and is de-watered, and (2) the period during which the sludge is ejected from the machine.

Whilst the sludge is being ejected, it slides past the sieves, which are placed almost radially, freeing them from the greater part of the solids which may chance to be adhering to them, and which if not removed, might choke the openings and thus impede the free passage of water.

The valves of the machine are actuated by means of oil under pressure, a regulating disc revolving on the stationary shell of the apparatus controlling the admission of oil under pressure into the cylinders actuating the valves.

The drum of the machine is driven by a belt at a rate of about 700 to 800 revolutions per minute, and rotates in a very strongly built shell, enclosed on all sides. The parts of the shell on which the sludge impinges on being ejected are constructed of wrought iron. The vertical journal of the drum shaft rotates in a step bearing on a cushion of compressed oil.

About 70 to 140 cubic feet of wet sludge can be treated hourly by one machine, the de-watered sludge from these volumes weighing 660 to 1000 lbs.

From one cubic foot of wet sludge containing 90 % of water, 8 to 12 lbs. of de-watered sludge are produced, whilst from 40 % to 60 % of all the solids in the sludge is removed. The centrifugal liquor is led back to the settling tanks.

The centrifugalised sludge can be easily manipulated and conveyed where desired : it contains from 50 % to 70 % of water, its volume therefore as compared with that of wet sludge containing 90 % to 95 % water is reduced to about 20 % to 14 % of its original bulk—say $\frac{1}{5}$ to $\frac{1}{7}$. The power required to drive one of these centrifugal machines is from 5 to 10 H.P.

It is found necessary to pass the sewage through a bar screen ($\frac{1}{3}$ to $\frac{3}{8}$ inch spaces) before it enters the settling tanks, so as to remove coarse matter likely to cause trouble during centrifugalising. The sludge should be treated before it putrifies, otherwise the time necessary for centrifugalising must be somewhat extended.

Harburg installation. The following particulars relate to the Harburg installation.

There are four settling tanks, the sludge from these being drawn by suction into a sludge tank, and forced thence by compressed air into a tank[1] above the

---

[1] This tank should hold one day's supply of wet sludge, and serve two machines.

centrifugal machines, of which there are two, with space reserved for two further machines. The liquid separated from the sludge is led back to the main outfall sewer.

This plant has been in operation since the end of 1907, and the entire plant is driven by a direct current motor of 45 H.P. One settling tank is shut off daily, the water drawn off, and the sludge removed and dried; the sludge treated is thus 4 days old ; the amount treated daily is from 530 to 700 cubic feet, the moisture varying from 95 % to 88 %. This quantity of sludge is dried by one machine in from 7 to 8 hours, the total power required for driving the plant being 100 K.W. From ·2 K.W. to ·14 K.W. is therefore used per cubic foot of wet sludge.

Electric energy is obtained from the municipal electric station, the cost per K.W. being about 6d., the cost of power used in drying 100 cubic feet of wet sludge being therefore 8½d. to 12d.

One man attends to the sludge drying plant.

Dr Grossmann's Process[1]. This process devised by Dr J. Grossmann, consists in the removal of grease from the sludge, and the conversion of the sludge into a dry powder for use as a fertiliser. By itself, the powder is deficient in potash and sulphates, and these are added to the fertiliser in proportions adapted to the crop for which the fertiliser is intended. The Grossmann process is in operation at Oldham, the population being about 147,000, and the mode of working the plant is briefly as follows.

The ordinary wet sludge is taken from the settling tanks and deposited in special settling tanks to get rid of as much moisture as possible. After leaving these tanks the percentage of solids is raised from about 10 % to 20 %. The sludge is next dried, being raised by an automatic conveyor to the top of the building, and thence passes by shoots to horizontal heated drying cylinders, six in number, the temperature within the driers being never more than about 212° C. Inside these cylinders, rotating screw conveyors move the sludge along, causing it to fall as a powder into hoppers. Each drying machine is capable of producing about 1½ tons of dried sludge per 24 hours, equivalent to about 15 tons of the original sludge.

The grease is next extracted, and to accomplish this, the dried sludge passes through a cylinder, into which superheated steam enters, together with a slender stream of sulphuric acid :

[1] Abstract from *The Surveyor*, June 13th, 1913.

by means of a revolving shaft and paddles perforated with holes, the steam permeates the sludge, and takes up the grease and fats, being then led to condensors where the grease separates out, and floats upon the surface of the condensed water.

It is understood that the grease obtained by this process contains about 80 % of saponifiable matter : it is sold, and the dried powder as previously stated is disposed of as fertiliser.

The dried sludge as it leaves the final machine is said to contain about 3 to 5 % of phosphates of lime, nitrogen equivalent to 2 % of ammonia, and about 1½ % of potash.

Complete figures of capital cost of plant, working cost, and depreciation over an adequate period would be of interest regarding this process, but so far as the writer is aware, none have been published ; it is, however, understood that the cost of Dr Grossmann's process is considerably in excess of that of a filter press installation ; it must, however, be remembered that in the latter case the pressed cake has to be disposed of.

Manurial value of sewage sludge. This subject was gone into rather fully by the Sewage Disposal Commission, and the results obtained will be found in the Fifth Report and in Appendix IV to that report.

The experiments were carried out at several collegiate centres under the supervision of the Board of Agriculture and Fisheries.

Dr Voelcker's conclusions, drawn from the results of the two years' experiments, were :

(1) " That the different sewage sludges, when used in quantity to supply 40 lbs. of nitrogen per acre, will benefit a wheat crop to which they are applied, increasing both corn and straw to the extent of 10 to 12 per cent. above the un-manured product.

(2) " That the increase of produce in the first crop (based on the results of the experiments of 1907 and 1908) will not be as much, by 5 or 6 per cent., as that obtained with ' artificial equivalents ' supplying the same constituents in equal amount.

(3) " That, after taking a wheat crop, sewage sludge or its equivalents in artificial manures leave practically nothing over for a second corn crop.

(4) "That, of different sewage sludges tried, those which show the most benefit for a wheat crop to which they are applied, and which leave most remaining over for a second corn crop, are those which are moist in character, and which contain much lime.

(5) "That nitrogenous organic matter is not the determining factor in the value of sewage sludge, but that it is in an inert condition which requires the use of lime to bring it into action.

(6) "That 10s. a ton, on the farm, is an outside figure for the value of such sewage sludges as have been examined, even when a crop subsequent to that to which the sludge has been directly applied is also taken into account."

Taking the experiments as a whole, it may be said that they tend to confirm the generally accepted impression that sewage sludges are beneficial as farm manures. Further, owing to the low price at which sludge can be obtained, it can be applied in large quantities per acre, the cost of carriage being the chief desideratum. At the Cambridge Sewage Farm, the air-dried sludge is easily sold to the neighbouring farmers at 3s. per load. They send their own carts for it, and the supply is not equal to the demand. It has also been used by market gardeners, and, when sparingly used, it was found to be highly beneficial to various garden products.

BIBLIOGRAPHY.

Allen, Kenneth. *Sewage Sludge.* McGraw-Hill Book Company, New York and London.

Bell, H. D. *Stratford-on-Avon Sewage Works.* Annual Reports on Stratford-on-Avon.

Crimp, W. Santo. *Sewage Disposal Works.* Charles Griffin and Co., Ltd., London. 1894.

Dunbar, Professor. *Principles of Sewage Treatment*, translated by H. T. Calvert. Griffin and Co., Ltd., London.

Eddy and Fales. *Journal of the Association of Engineering Societies*, vol. XXXVII. 1906.

Fuller, Geo. W. *Sewage Disposal.* McGraw-Hill Book Company, New York and London. 1912.

Kershaw, G. Bertram. *Modern Methods of Sewage Disposal*, chap. XI. Charles Griffin and Co., Ltd., London. 1911.

Leeds, City of. *Reports on Sewage Experiments*, 1898, 1900 *and* 1905. Jowett and Sowry. Leeds.

Manchester, City of. Rivers Department. *Annual Report for* 1911. H. Blacklock and Co., Ltd., Manchester.

Massachusetts State Board of Health. *Reports.*

New York Department of Health. 1907.

Royal Commission on Sewage Disposal. *Fifth Report.* Appendices 3, 4, and 7 to *Fifth Report.*

Schmeitzner, Dr Ing Rudolph. *Clarification of Sewage*, translated by A. Elliott Kimberley. Constable and Co., Ltd., London. 1910.

The Surveyor, June 13th, 1913. London.

Venable, W. M. *Sewage Treatment.* John Wiley, New York. 1908.

Water and Sewage Purification in Ohio. State Board of Health, Ohio. State Printer, Columbus, Ohio. 1908.

Wilson, H. M. and H. T. Calvert. *Trade Waste Waters.* Charles Griffin and Co., Ltd., London. 1913.

CHAPTER VI

LAND TREATMENT

Land treatment of sewage. This method of purification where the soil and subsoil are of a suitable character, and the volume of sewage treated per acre is not excessive, may be looked upon as the best means of producing a high-class effluent, containing a minimum of suspended solids, and a low figure for the 5 days dissolved oxygen absorption test.

Both broad irrigation, as it is termed, and filtration have been practised for very many years abroad and in the United Kingdom, the Craigentinny meadows near Edinburgh and the Ashburton water meadows being frequently quoted by various authorities as two of the earliest examples of land treatment of sewage in this country.

Surface irrigation and filtration. The terms " broad irrigation" and "intermittent downward filtration," probably arose from the fact that in the first case the sewage was spread over a considerable breadth or area of land, whilst in the latter case large volumes of sewage were concentrated at intervals over smaller areas of land, which of necessity had to be of a permeable character. Further, in the former case under-drainage was the exception, whereas with filtration it was in the majority of cases a necessity. Moreover, there is greater scope for crops with sewage irrigation than with filtration, owing to the smaller dose of sewage per acre in the former case. Again, land used for irrigation should have a slight fall, whereas land used for filtration must be practically level, and as a rule embanked to retain the sewage during filtration. It would seem, however, that the term " land treatment of sewage " might suitably be employed to embrace both systems, differentiating between the two where needful by the words " irrigation" and " filtration."

Broad irrigation so-called, and filtration have many features common to both processes, and in many cases it is by no means easy to decide where the one begins and the other leaves off ; the former cannot be carried on without a certain amount of filtration (usually lateral) occurring; similarly, filtration cannot be carried out without broad irrigation taking place to a certain extent.

Croydon (Beddington) and South Norwood irrigation farms are still in operation after some fifty years of use, but of late years the Croydon sewage has received tank treatment and artificial filtration through percolating filters before passing over the land, whilst at Norwood the tank liquor is dealt with by single contact before irrigation over the land.

The Nottingham Sewage Farm has been in use as a filtration farm for upwards of 30 years with good results as regards sludge disposal and the purification of the sewage. Cambridge, Grantham, Kidderminster, Stourbridge and Aldershot Camp Farms are also good examples of land treatment of sewage.

As regards the purification of sewage by land treatment, this is a process of indirect oxidation by bacteria. The suspended matter in both surface irrigation and filtration is strained out, at or near the surface of the soil, the impurities in solution being converted finally to carbonic acid, nitric acid and water through the agency of bacteria present in the soil.

Soils differ very greatly as regards their purifying powers, and it has been shown that this power depends very largely upon their physical condition, rather than upon their chemical composition.

Irrigation of, and filtration through, land. Theoretically, with land irrigation, the depth of liquid over the area treated should be uniform ; in practice, as every farm manager is aware, it is anything but uniform, and even supposing it to be uniform, the texture of the soil and subsoil is as a rule very far from being so, consequently the rate of treatment is not constant per unit of the area irrigated.

With filtration, however, these variations are greatly lessened. As a rule, filtration areas are laid out level or nearly so, with embankments to retain the sewage, which is flooded on to a particular area until, maybe, an average depth of from 3 inches to 6 inches of sewage or tank liquor is standing on the land. In fact, sewage filtration is analogous to water filtration, with this exception, namely that sewage carries a very large amount of matter in suspension as compared with raw drinking waters.

Like the water filter of sand, filtration areas used for sewage treatment gradually acquire a film of suspended matter strained out of the sewage, which regulates the rate of filtration in exactly the same manner as the film of the water filter. Further, in course of time when the film impedes filtration too much, both water filters and sewage filters need the removal of the film. In the former case, the film is usually scraped off, and after several periodical scrapings, the thickness of sand lost by scraping is made up with fresh sand. With a sewage filtration area the same end is usually accomplished by ploughing, since the effluent is not used for drinking purposes, and it is not disadvantageous to allow the suspended matter to become mixed with the upper portion of the filtering soil, where the organic matter is speedily oxidised and becomes beneficial to further working.

Although it is perfectly true that suitable land can, given good management, yield excellent results when treating crude sewage, yet, as has already been mentioned, there is risk of smell with this method, and it is essential that the land used in this way should be some considerable distance away from dwelling houses.

Preliminary treatment. Preliminary tank treatment of the sewage by one or other of the methods mentioned in Chapter IV is desirable in most cases, the particular method depending upon the type of sewage dealt with : for example, continuous flow settlement will very often do all that is required in the case of a purely domestic sewage of average strength, whereas, with a sewage containing brewery or tannery wastes, precipitation with lime will probably give the best results, since the use of lime tends to keep down the smell, whilst acting beneficially on the land.

Preliminary treatment of the sewage considerably lightens the work of the land, whilst tending to keep down any smell, but it is by no means necessary or even advisable to reduce the suspended solids in the tank liquor to the same figure as would be advisable for filtration through fine percolating filters.

Extent of removal of suspended matter. The extent to which it will be necessary to remove suspended solids, will depend very largely upon the nature of the land to be used. If this consists of a light barren sandy soil, then a maximum amount of suspended matter (apart from paper, faeces, etc.) may be allowed to pass on to it, and the land will benefit both from an agricultural point of view and also from the purification standpoint. If, on the other hand, the land is of a clayey nature, the solids passing on to the land should be limited to a fairly low figure, the actual amount depending upon the average depth of surface soil overlying the clay.

Purification effected by soil. The Rivers Pollution Commissioners in their First Report issued in 1870, made several experiments on the degree of purification effected by passing sewage through different soils.

The apparatus consisted of several glass cylinders $10\frac{1}{4}$ ins. diameter and 6 feet long, open at each end, and standing on a shallow earthenware tray ; a length of glass tubing, open at both ends, was passed down the centre of each cylinder to within about 3 inches of the lower extremity, the object being to provide aeration.

A 3 inch layer of small pebbles was placed at the bottom of the cylinder, and over this was placed a 5 foot layer of the soil to be experimented upon, whilst in some cases a 1 inch layer of fine sand was placed on the top of the soil, to prevent the coarse suspended matter in the sewage from passing into the soil, leaving a space at the top of the cylinder for the sewage which was applied in equal quantities morning and evening. The effluent was collected in the earthenware tray, flowing thence into a vessel.

When Beddington (Croydon) soil was used, the purification was effective when the sewage was filtered at the rate of 7·6 gallons per cube yard of soil per day.

Barking soil, however, was found to act in an entirely different manner, this soil possessing the property of absorbing a large amount of fertilising ingredients from the sewage.

The Commissioners observed: "It is scarcely possible to overrate the agricultural value of this property in a soil which is destined for irrigation. This quality, however, greatly detracts from its efficiency as a continuous purifier of sewage filtered through it. The application of 3·8 gallons per diem to each cubic yard, for about 12 weeks, showed a continuous increase of organic impurity in the effluent water, which at the end of that time was rapidly approaching in quality to unchanged and unpurified sewage."

The best results were obtained from Dursley (Gloucestershire) soil.

One cubic yard of this soil was found to cleanse satisfactorily 9·9 gallons of sewage per 24 hours, or nearly 100,000 gallons per acre per 24 hours, on the assumption that the underdrains were laid 6 feet deep.

One cubic yard of sand or of Hambrook soil it was found, would not continue satisfactorily to purify more than 4·4 gallons of London sewage per 24 hours.

The Commissioners go on to say, "At the conclusion of the long series of experiments, there were no symptoms of clogging up or diminution of activity, and the effluent water was always bright, inodorous, and nearly colourless. The cleansing power of a soil seems to be more closely connected with physical conditions as regards porosity and fineness of division than with its chemical composition.

Thus the Beddington and Barking soils, whilst similar in chemical composition, are most widely dissimilar in their action upon sewage. Again, sand and Hambrook soil act very similarly upon sewage, whilst they differ considerably in chemical composition ; and lastly, the Hambrook and Dursley soils do not differ very widely in their chemical composition—nevertheless, the latter has more than twice the purifying power of the former."

It should be observed in connection with the above experiments that the results obtained by the Commissioners from soil carefully filled into glass cylinders and of fairly uniform composition throughout, and carefully dosed with measured quantities of sewage, would naturally be expected to yield better results than those obtained under actual working conditions.

It must be remembered that if, say 10,000 gallons of sewage are applied to an acre of land per 24 hours, probably no two square yards out of the 4840 would receive exactly the same amount, and when some little depth below the surface soil is reached, the discrepancies would tend to be even greater.

As showing the difficulty of preparing an artificial soil for purposes of experiment in imitation of a natural soil, some experiments by Messrs Gilbert and Lawes[1] may be quoted.

They endeavoured to fill, by calculation, a number of tubes, 5 feet deep and 2 feet in diameter, with the soil of the immediately adjoining field in its exact natural condition.

After putting in 3 feet of soil, pouring a great deal of water through, and applying a weight of more than a ton for many months, the soil had not sunk down to the 3 feet by about 6 inches. " It was almost impossible by artificial means to get a soil like the natural one."

Physical characteristics of soils and subsoils. The size of the particles composing a particular soil and subsoil vary greatly, and it is upon the relative size of these particles to one another, in the main, that the purifying power of the soil will depend. If the particles of a light sandy soil were

---

[1] *Evaporation and percolation,* paper by Charles Greaves. *Excerpt. Mins. of Proc. Inst. C.E.,* xlv. Session 1875–76. Part III, pp. 54, 55.

all of about equal size, the interstices between the particles would amount to approximately 40 % of the total content per unit volume of the soil; this, however, is never the case in practice, although in the case of a fine sand, the particles approximate in size fairly closely.

Again, assuming the particles of soil to be of uniform size, the interstices would be the same, irrespective of whether the particles are small or the reverse.

In nature it is found that the particles of soil vary very greatly as regards size, small particles filling up the spaces between the larger particles, so that with natural soils, the percentage of voids will be found to fall considerably below 40 %.

Accordingly as the soil is fine or coarse, so will the passage of air and water through it be retarded or accelerated, and a rough estimate of the water capacity of a soil can be obtained by filling a vessel containing a known volume of soil with a measured quantity of water.

A fine soil, owing to the very large number of small particles of which it is composed, contains an enormous surface area, and this surface area when wet exerts a considerable power known as surface attraction, whilst capillary action is also increased—or the power of the soil to cause motion of the water contained in it—through the fine hair-like channels existing between the particles of soil.

It has been found to be the case that the effective size of granules of sand in a water filter is very closely related to the rate of filtration through it, and so it is with the filtration through soil.

In order to give some idea of the surface area of some soils it may be observed that a single cubic foot of sand composed of grains $\frac{1}{100}$ inch in diameter (treating the grains, for purposes of calculation as spheres), would possess a total surface area of some 5000 square feet, equivalent to about 3 acres of surface area per cube yard, or about 14,520 acres per acre of sand 3 feet deep !

When sewage is applied to a light porous soil, the top layer of soil acts as a fine sieve and strains off all but the finest suspended matters, and each one of the small particles of soil —if the filtration is uniform—becomes surrounded by a film of liquid, surface attraction and capillary action take place, and the sewage matter in solution will be retained by the absorptive power of the soil and oxidised, to be finally removed by plant life, or to pass away in the underdrain effluent as nitrates.

If, however, the soil is an exceedingly fine one, there will be considerable obstruction to filtration, further, such soils are usually deficient of aeration.

A soil should possess a certain amount of " retentive " power, but not sufficient to require a depth of several inches head of sewage to displace the liquid already held in the soil.

It has been found that temperature influences the rate of filtration through soil, the rate increasing with a rise in temperature, and falling with a decrease owing to the increase in viscosity of the liquid being filtered.

Ripening of soils. It should be borne in mind that soil, like the material used in filter and contact beds, takes time to ripen before it gives the best results, and it appears to be a slower process in the case of land, possibly consisting in the re-adjustment of the soil particles to meet altered conditions, and also in the formation of humus. After a soil has been sewaged for some time, the period largely depending upon the temperature, the particles of soil at the surface become coated with a gelatinous substance apparently akin to that which eventually covers the material of filters and contact beds, after they have become matured.

It is said that saline solutions have the effect of carrying down the finest particles of soil, and since sewage contains saline matter to a considerable extent, this process may occur when land is put under sewage.

Samples taken from some new barren sandy soil which was being sewaged at the Aldershot Camp Farm, showed that it would take some considerable time before the resulting effluent reached the degree of purification effected by the older land.

This maturing process which land undergoes has also been noticed at the Wolverhampton farm and elsewhere.

Depth of surface soil. It is the surface soil with land treatment which bears the brunt of the work in effecting purification of sewage. Aeration of the soil is greatest near the surface, whilst bacterial activity diminishes as greater depths are reached.

With clay soils, the depth of surface soil is of special importance, and a rough rule for estimating the volume of settled sewage which such soils will purify per acre per 24 hours, is to divide 30,000 by the depth of the surface soil in inches expressed as the fraction of 36 inches : thus, a surface soil of say 6 inches, will deal with $\dfrac{6}{36} \times \dfrac{30,000}{1} = 5,000$ gallons.

Various soils and subsoils. Speaking broadly, nearly all soils and subsoils consist of clay and sand with a certain amount of humus and some lime.

The soils ordinarily met with and likely to be used for sewage treatment may be classified as follows.

1. Sand, containing about 5 % or less of clay.
2. Light loam containing about 15 % of clay.
3. Loam　　　　　,,　　　,,　　　50 %　　,,
4. Heavy loam　　,,　　　,,　　　75 %　　,,
5. Stiff clay　　　,,　　　,,　　　90 %　　,,
6. Marl—clayey soil with about 15 % of carbonate of lime.
7. Calcareous soil—soil containing more than 20 % of carbonate of lime.
8. Chalk.

The best soils for the purification of sewage liquor are found on the Bunter sandstone formation, and consist of light porous soil overlying a subsoil of gravelly sand ; such soils are well aerated, and eminently suited for sewage purification.

Alluvial tracts in river valleys are also sometimes good for sewage treatment.

Sand. Of the above soils, fine barren sand with a subsoil of the same character is about the worst that could be used for sewage treatment, and the Bagshot sands of the Aldershot district may be cited as an excellent example ; such soils are usually very deficient in lime, and until they have been under cultivation for some time, equally so in humus. Owing to the subsoil being also for the most part composed of very fine closely compacted sand, aeration is very defective.

If such land is employed for the treatment of sewage, it should be underdrained, and the sewage applied in moderate doses, until the formation of a few inches of top soil has commenced. Further, frequent ploughings in of sludge on areas of land not actually used, but destined to be used for irrigation purposes, will hasten the production of humus, and benefit the land both from an agricultural and sewage purification point of view. Sandy soils are almost invariably greedy of manure, and can assimilate large quantities ; lime or chalk should also be frequently applied to sandy land in heavy doses.

Chalk was applied to the sand land added to the camp farm, Aldershot, with good results. One particular difficulty experienced there was the existence of a layer of iron oxide " pan," which was a great obstruction to filtration, until the underdraining operations broke it up.

Light loam. A deep layer of light loam superimposed upon a well-aerated sandy gravel subsoil, such as exists over a large portion of the Nottingham Sewage Farm, forms excellent land for sewage purification purposes.

Loam and heavy loam. The former soil, although not so good as light loam, yields a good degree of purification when treated with sewage, providing the surface soil is of sufficient depth and the subsoil is of a suitable character.

Heavy loam has been used successfully for sewage purification at the Rugby and other sewage farms. As a rule, however, the subsoil of a heavy loam soil is too dense to admit of much filtration taking place, and the bulk of the purification is effected by lateral filtration through the soil. Heavy loam soils can be lightened by admixture with ashes, sludge, etc., whilst dressings of lime are of benefit. " Plough pan[1] " is apt to occur on these soils, necessitating after a time either deep cultivation or subsoiling.

[1] Plough pan is a hard stratum formed in the soil by the constant sliding action of the ploughshare at one depth ; in course of time it forms a layer almost impervious to water and the roots of plants.

Clay soils. The volume of sewage which can be properly purified upon clay soils depends upon the layer of top soil, which is rarely deeper than say 6 inches, consequently a large area of land is necessary if surface irrigation is adopted. Unless the land can be obtained very cheaply and is " side-lying " with plenty of fall to re-treat the drain effluents, it will usually be more satisfactory to employ one or other of the artificial processes of sewage treatment.

It is possible to lighten clay land by burning it with small coal or slack, and ploughing it into the land, but this is an exceedingly costly process.

The clay can also be burnt and the burnt ballast used for contact material, but unless very carefully burnt and the soft portions rejected, it is apt to prove unreliable after a few years working, and to revert to clay.

Peat. Peat is almost useless for sewage purification owing to its great retention of moisture. Water from peat frequently has an acid reaction, and is very slightly antiseptic.

Although useless for sewage purification purposes owing to its retention of moisture and lack of aeration, and unsuited for carrying permanent works by reason of its instability, it has been usefully employed on sewage works in many ways : —in the form of peat dust for sprinkling over sludge, and also for forming a covering for lightly roofed septic tanks, whilst a 6 inch layer of peat and peat dust is of use in straining and distributing sewage liquors over a limited area of land ; for example, the distribution of waste liquids from creameries over land used for filtration. Dr Fowler has also shown it to be of use in distributing raw sewage upon filters (cf. p. 270).

Chalk soils. Chalky soils, if of sufficient depth, can be used for sewage treatment. There are several sewage farms on chalk, of which the Winchester and Luton farms may be cited.

Pure chalk, save in exceptional circumstances, should not be used for sewage treatment, unless there are very good reasons for supposing that no drinking water supply is likely to be contaminated thereby.

The chalk formation is especially prone to contain cracks and channels, through and along which the sewage may travel for some considerable distance without any real purification being affected.

Artificial preparation and lightening of soils. This procedure was much in vogue before the advent of artificial processes of sewage treatment, where heavy clay soils were concerned. In most cases, however, at the present day, it would be more economical to adopt one or other of the many artificial processes available, unless the land can be obtained at a very low price.

As a rule, house refuse and cinders are the materials used for lightening the soil, the cinders being spread over the surface of the land and ploughed in, this having the effect of lightening the soil, in the same way as gravel tends to improve the aeration of an otherwise somewhat heavy soil.

This method has been used on the London clay soils at the Wimbledon and South Norwood Sewage Farms in the past, with beneficial results. At Wimbledon, the surface of the land was ploughed to a depth of about 9 inches, and whilst in this condition, it was covered with a thick layer of screened town's ashes. The usual agricultural operations were then carried out, a porous layer of top soil resulting, about 12 inches in depth, lateral filtration occurring when the land was sewaged.

Weathered grit-chamber sludge is also eminently suitable for the lightening of heavy soils.

The sludging of certain lands at the Beaumont Leys (Leicester Corporation) Sewage Farm has resulted in greatly improving the surface soil, which was formerly a dense heavy clay.

Evaporation, transpiration, and absorption. These are natural processes which have a considerable influence on sewage purification on land, particularly when crops are grown. The amount of water given up by some soils under certain conditions by these three processes being by no means a negligible factor.

By evaporation is meant, broadly speaking, the vaporisation of water from the surface of the soil ; and by transpiration, the exhalation by plant life of water which it has taken up.

The loss of water in dry weather from soils by evaporation proceeds at a rate chiefly dependent on the quantity of water

present, and one would therefore naturally expect more evaporation from sewaged land than from ordinary farm land. Further,
fine soils lose water much less rapidly than those of coarser
texture, since the water retaining powers of a soil are intimately connected with the total surface area possessed by
the particles of soil. Temperature plays an important part
in evaporation, a rise in temperature lowering the viscosity
of the water, and thus permitting a freer flow through the soil
particles.

Mr W. Clifford[1], A.M.Inst.C.E., in a paper entitled " Land
Filtration Effluents," gives some interesting figures relating to
the variations in quality and rate of flow of land effluents from
the Wolverhampton Sewage Farm.

The area of land used for one of a series of experiments
consisted of 7700 square yards, under drain at an average
depth of 3 feet 6 inches; the soil consisting of clayey
loam, whilst the subsoil was stony sandy clay. This area was
under second year rye grass when the experiment was made in
May 1911, and by courtesy of Mr Clifford and the Royal
Sanitary Institute the summarised results are given below in
tabular and diagrammatic form.

TABLE XXII. *Showing evaporation at the Wolverhampton
Sewage Farm.*

Period	Day	Volume of liquid irrigated, gallons	Volume of effluent drained away, gallons	Volume of effluent as a percentage of the liquid irrigated
Irrigation ..	Fri., Sat., Sun.	6329o	2797o	44·2 } 55·3
Resting ..	Mon., Tues.		7135	11·1
Irrigation ..	Wed., Thurs.	46246	22228	50·2 } 66·9
Resting ..	Fri., Sat., Sun.		7380	16·7
Irrigation ..	Mon., Tues.	4527o	16355	36·1 } 49·9
Resting ..	Wed., Thurs.		6060	13·4

The total volume of effluent during the 14 days was equal
to 56·2 % of the irrigated liquid.

At Hatfield, Hertfordshire, in moderately warm weather,
only about one gallon of effluent leaves the farm out of six
gallons of tank liquor distributed over it, and in hot weather

---

[1] *Journ. Roy. San. Inst.*, vol. XXXIV. No. 10. London, Nov. 1913.

there is no effluent leaving the farm. At Luton, and Henley,
and many other sewage farms, the effluent is all absorbed.

At Rugby, for a short period in early summer, about 75 %
of the sewage left the farm as effluent, the rate of treatment
per acre being about 40,000 gallons per acre per 24 hours.
The. soil is loamy.

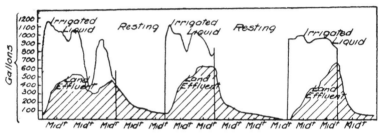

Fig. 28.   Diagram showing Evaporation at Wolverhampton Sewage Farm.

This diminution in volume of effluent should be carefully
borne in mind when dealing with the various merits and de-
merits of sewage farms.   With artificial processes on the other
hand, the volume of effluent leaving the works is practically
the same as the sewage arriving on the works.

The following diagram shows the loss by evaporation,
absorption and transpiration at the Coventry Sewage Farm over
a period of 30 days.

Careful gaugings by means of three automatic gauges were
made by the author of all the volumes of effluent leaving the
farm, the daily volume of sewage pumped to the farm being
accurately known.   The rate of treatment per acre per 24 hours
was between 40,000 and 50,000 gallons, and the soil is for the
most part light with sand and gravel.   The total loss from the
causes mentioned above, amounted as will be seen to about
30 %.   It should be noted, however, that heavy rainfall
occurred during the period of experiment, and that 30 % is
probably a good deal below the actual percentage of loss on
the sewage flow, apart from rainfall.

It must, of course, be borne in mind that the figures given
for the flow of effluent from sewage farms, refer to the ordinary

or normal working of the farms, and that frequently only a fifth or a sixth of the total irrigable area of a farm is under sewage at one time. If the whole area were under irrigation at one time, there would in many cases be no flow of effluent at all.

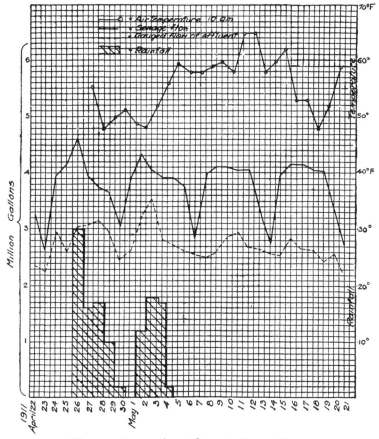

Fig. 29. Evaporation at Coventry Sewage Farm.

Relative areas necessary for surface irrigation and filtration. The relative areas necessary for surface irrigation and filtration will vary somewhat according to the character of the soil and subsoil over the whole irrigable area. Assuming this to be of a fairly uniform character, the ratio of area necessary for surface irrigation to that requisite for filtration will be from about 2–4 to 1, according to the quantity and nature of the crops grown.

It often happens in practice that the soil and subsoil are extremely variable, even in the limited area of one field, and it is often necessary to lay out one portion of the farm for surface irrigation, and another part, possessing a more porous soil and subsoil, as filtration areas, whilst certain areas which may possibly be somewhat unsuitable for purification purposes, can be used for sludge disposal.

Surface irrigation permits a wider range of crops to be grown than filtration, and the effluent leaving the farm in dry weather will always be considerably less than the volume of sewage arriving for treatment ; more labour in distribution will, however, be needful if the best results are to be achieved.

A gentle surface slope is best for surface irrigation, a gradient of about 1 in 300 being perhaps the best, although average slopes of 1 in 100 have been used successfully: if the gradient is much steeper than 1 in 100 trouble is apt to occur in times of storm.

When filtration is used, the cost of the laying out of the land, other things being equal, will in most cases be far in excess of that usually required for surface irrigation, although in some cases, notably at the Cambridge Sewage Farm, the natural lie of the land lends itself admirably to filtration purposes with comparatively little levelling or laying out beyond underdraining.

Rate of treatment of sewage upon land. The area of land required in a particular case is naturally governed by the rate at which it can purify sewage, and this in turn depends mainly upon the strength of the sewage, the nature of the soil, and the preliminary treatment which it receives ; the question of the ultimate destiny of the effluent, and the degree to which it is necessary to push the purification, also have to be considered.

It is generally admitted that good land with suitable soil and subsoil, can purify at a given time about 30,000 gallons of well-settled domestic sewage per acre per 24 hours by filtration. This does not mean that a plot of land can continue to treat sewage for months at the rate of 30,000 gallons, but allows for proper intervals of rest.

In the case of a surface irrigation farm, the usual practice is to sewage separate sections of the farm alternately, thus allowing a period of rest for the land. The quantity of land under sewage at any one time will vary according to the kind of soil present, but, as a rule, not more than one-fourth to one-sixth of the total irrigable area should be under sewage at any one time in dry weather, whilst with a filtration farm about one-third is usually sewaged at one time.

The several volumes of sewage or tank liquor being dealt with per acre by several sewage farms, may be compared by taking the daily dry weather flow per 24 hours, and dividing this by the total irrigable area, the result will be the number of gallons treated per acre per 24 hours, *assuming the whole irrigable area to be under sewage at one time.* As has just been pointed out, this does not occur in practice, but this does not invalidate the comparison ; it must be recollected that in storm times, very much larger volumes will be dealt with per acre, even allowing for the fact that more land is brought into use, and if the normal dry weather volume treated per acre per 24 hours is 12,000 gallons, the total average daily volume per acre, including wet weather flows of sewage, will probably approach if not exceed an additional 50 %, *i.e.* 18,000 gallons in all.

It has always been assumed, apparently with a considerable amount of reason, that the volume of sewage is of more importance than the strength of sewage where land treatment is in question.

Unless the land is very porous it will not take even with filtration more than a certain volume of sewage per acre, and with surface irrigation, the volume treated per 24 hours cannot be increased to nearly the same extent as with filtration, if satisfactory results are looked for. The old method of taking the population draining to the works as a basis of the area of land required is seldom used now, and has rightly been abandoned, since the number of gallons of sewage per head of the population and the strength of the sewage are the main points, and these, taken in conjunction with the quality of the soil and subsoil, should be the determining factors.

If then, the limiting dose of settled sewage is about 30,000 gallons per acre per 24 hours for the best land, it follows that this figure will have to be considerably diminished if land of inferior grade is to be used, and when a dense clay soil is in question the dose of sewage which can be purified per acre is so small that, as has been pointed out, it would usually be more economical to look out for some other method of treatment.

The limiting dose of sewage for clay lands with only a few inches of surface soil, is probably not much in excess of 3000 gallons per acre, and in dry weather this means that there will not only be very considerable difficulty experienced in spreading a volume of 3000 gallons of sewage over an acre of land (about one-eighth of an inch in depth over an acre in 24 hours), but that if this can be accomplished, there will be little or no run-off of effluent except in rainy weather. What is done as a matter of fact in such cases, is to put the 3000 gallons on about one quarter of an acre, thereby quadrupling the *actual* rate of treatment " per acre per 24 hours."

The volume of sewage or tank liquor which land of intermediate grade between good and clay lands will treat satisfactorily, must be largely a matter of personal judgment, founded on an intimate experience in the treatment of sewages of various characters and strength, and coupled with very careful examination of the prospective soil and subsoil to be utilised.

One point requires emphasising, *viz.*, that the total irrigable area of a farm should be very considerably in excess of the area required for purification purposes at any one time ; otherwise the land recently sewaged will not have a sufficiently long resting period before it receives another dose of sewage. This is of especial importance where crops are grown, as the general tendency—especially if the farm is sublet—is to cramp the irrigated land to avoid risk of damage to crops, and it may be pointed out here that the larger, within limits, the "resting" surplus irrigable area is, the better is the chance of the crops proving remunerative.

In vol. IV, part I, issued by the Sewage Disposal Commission, the writers of the General Report deal with the question of the volume of sewage per acre land can purify as follows:

*　　*　　*　　*　　*　　*　　*　　*

"To summarise all our results within the limits of a few sentences is impossible, but we may say in conclusion, and speaking in general terms, that we doubt whether even the most suitable kind of soil worked as a filtration farm should be called upon to treat more than 30,000 to 60,000 gallons per acre per 24 hours at a given time (750 to 1000 persons per acre) ; or more than 10,000 to 20,000 gallons per acre per 24 hours, calculated on the total irrigable area (250 to 500 persons per acre). Further, that soil not well suited for purification purposes, worked as a surface irrigation or as a combined surface irrigation and filtration farm, should not be called upon to treat more than 5000 to 10,000 gallons per acre per 24 hours at a given time (125 to 250 persons per acre) ; or more than 1000 to 2000 gallons per acre per 24 hours, calculated on the total irrigable area (25 to 50 persons per acre). It is doubtful if the *very worst* kinds of soil are capable of dealing satisfactorily even with this relatively small volume of sewage. The population per acre is calculated on 40 gallons of sewage per head per day. It is here assumed that the sewage is of medium strength, and is mechanically settled before going on to the land."

Treatment of sewage upon land in Germany and America. As regards the volumes of sewage usually treated by land in other countries, it may be observed that the Metropolitan Sewage Commission of New York in one of their reports give estimates based on treating the sewage of that city by irrigation upon sandy soil at Long Island, at an average rate of 12,000 gallons per acre per 24 hours, which, viewed in the light of English practice, seems a low figure, having regard to the weakness of most American sewages : it should be pointed out, however, that the sewages employed for the Massachusetts experiments were by no means as weak as has generally been assumed in this country.

Fuller[1] notes that in America, irrigation of land has little standing " as an independent method of purifying sewage in the humid regions of the Eastern and middle sections.   Its use is an accidental feature at a few intermittent sand filtration plants.

" In the arid regions there are almost no instances of broad irrigation or sewage farming that are carried out in a sanitary way, giving a permanently satisfactory means of sewage disposal."

Sand filtration on the other hand, appears to have had a considerable vogue in the States, especially in the N.E. section, where suitable sandy soil frequently occurs ; and satisfactory results have been obtained where proper management has been forthcoming.

Fuller states that an average provision may be taken as an acre of filter surface for each 600 to 700 persons, depending upon the nature of the filtering material.

He also states that " with good management, the quality of the effluent is the best that can be obtained for a given cost under many conditions."

These views coincide with data obtained from English practice.

Laying out of land for sewage treatment. This demands a good deal of care and labour if the land is to be made the most of.

Where the land is to be used for irrigation, after selecting the site for the effluent outfalls, one of the first points is to decide upon the site for the tanks, if they are used.   These will be on the highest portion of the irrigable area, but not necessarily at the highest level of the farm.   In some cases land which cannot be utilised for irrigation purposes, has to be taken as part and parcel of a sewage farm, and, in other cases, a neutral zone surrounding the farm is insisted upon by neighbouring landowners.

If the land is used for surface irrigation, it is essential that all hollows should be filled up to obviate the risk of sewage stagnating in the low places ; a very large hollow can sometimes be drained and the effluent re-treated lower down the farm.   In some valleys where the contour of the land is steep, the best results will be obtained by laying out the land in terraces ; this, however, entails a somewhat heavy expenditure in excavation and cartage.   In certain cases the best results will be obtained by combining surface irrigation with filtration, utilising the gently sloping land for surface irrigation, and the steeper slopes, after terracing (see Fig. 30), for filtration

[1] *Sewage Disposal.*

purposes. Or again, the upper portion may lend itself to being underdrained, the drain outlets being brought out lower down the farm, and the drain effluent being re-treated by surface irrigation over land where there is not sufficient fall to admit of underdrains. Much will depend upon the nature of the soil and subsoil. At Hatfield in Hertfordshire, the writer adopted the plan of underdraining the upper portion of the irrigation area, which had a fairly rapid fall for about half its depth ; the drain effluent was then brought into a surface carrier and irrigated over the lower plot. This plan has been carried out at several farms. At Rugby, before percolating filters were installed, the underdrain effluent used to mix with the tank liquor midway down the farm, the mixture being irrigated over the remaining area of land near the foot of the farm.

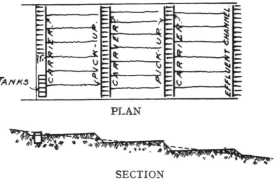

PLAN

SECTION

Fig. 30.   Terracing of land.

When the site for the tanks has been decided upon, it is advisable to fix upon the site for sludge disposal ; and if practicable this should be so placed as to be as far as possible removed from public roads, footpaths, and streams ; further, if it can be contrived, the sludge should gravitate from the tanks to the sludge area.

If the area of land reserved for sludge disposal is surrounded with a slight embankment, this is often advantageous, and it can be planted with Austrian Pines and Scotch Firs or other non-deciduous trees or shrubs. No underdrains should be laid under land used for sludge disposal, unless the effluent from them can afterwards receive treatment, and it is of importance that the sludge area should be set quite apart for the time being from that used for irrigation or filtration purposes.

Position of carriers, size of plots, etc. A point requiring a good deal of consideration is the position of the main and subsidiary carriers, for distributing the sewage or tank liquor over the prepared land, and unless this is carefully done, it may not be possible to irrigate the land satisfactorily, the land nearest the tanks receiving too much liquid, whilst remoter plots do not get their fair share.

As to how many carriers will be required, much will depend upon the method of treatment adopted, the contour of the land, and also whether this is divided by hedges or ditches into separate fields or plots, or whether it is all open land.

In the case of a large sewage farm, especially when used for surface irrigation, the plots are usually large in size, to minimise labour in sewaging, and also to admit of steam ploughing and cultivation when needed. If the land is to be used for filtration purposes, the size of the plots, embankments, etc. should be decided upon, and the lines of the main carriers fixed, before the farm is laid out. With filtration farms, the plots are usually much smaller than with surface irrigation farms. If surface irrigation is desired, the size of the plots is not of such importance, as the watermen attending to the distribution will see to the sewaging of the whole of a plot of land, or only part of it as the case may be, by restricting the sewage flow with hand sluices, sods, etc.

It should be borne in mind that carriers and distribution grips obstruct ploughing operations, and they should therefore be planned keeping this fact in view.

Roads should be laid out for the purpose of access to the various fields, and as a rule a 12 foot road will be found ample. A road should be laid to the sludge area for the purpose of allowing farmers to remove sludge if necessary.

When cattle are likely to be kept upon the farm, and farm buildings will be required, the latter can usually be arranged for on surplus land which is not dosed with sewage, and convenient of access to a main road.

If practicable, it is desirable that the manager of the farm should be present when the laying out, underdraining, etc., are in progress, since he will then obtain an insight into the nature of the various soils and subsoils of the land he will presently be called upon to sewage. It is seldom the case that the soil and subsoil are uniform over the whole area of even a moderate-sized farm, and with a farm of, say, 1000 acres it is of comparatively rare occurrence ; in consequence of this fact, it will be found that some of the land can only take perhaps half or two-thirds the dose of sewage per acre per 24 hours that the best land on the farm can deal with satisfactorily. Consequently, a good manager will direct his sewaging operations accordingly, and if he has seen several cross sections of the soil and subsoil, he is in a position to make immediate use of this knowledge.

Underdraining of irrigated land. The underdraining of land destined to be used for sewage treatment stands on quite a different footing from the underdraining of ordinary farm lands. In the latter case, the farmer's main object is to remove to the nearest watercourse as quickly as possible (1) any rain or flood water which would otherwise stand on the land too long, or (2) to lower the level of the subsoil water in lands which tend to become waterlogged.

In other words, the farmer tries to induce a maximum amount of filtration to the underdrains, since he is not concerned with the quality of the underdrain water, and speedy disposal of it is his chief requirement. With underdrains for land which is sewaged on the other hand, the case is altogether different ; the main object of the underdrains here is to bring the sewage or tank liquor, as the case may be, intimately into contact with as large a surface area of soil and subsoil particles as possible, and thus obtain a far higher degree of purification than could possibly be obtained by passing it over the *surface* of the soil. Further, it is essential that air shall have free access to the soil and subsoil between the intervals of irrigation, and it cannot do this if the subsoil is waterlogged, and unless drains are provided in the case of certain closely compacted soils, waterlogging at the surface often occurs and the land is very slow in " drying-off," whilst in the absence of under-drainage, the application of sewage to land in large volumes is apt to cause the ground water level to rise.

Again, an attempt to rush the sewage through to the under-drains would defeat its own object, since it is desired to obtain the longest contact economically practicable of the sewage liquor with the soil particles. When the land intended to be used for sewage treatment is of a porous gravelly nature, it is possible in rare cases, when the subsoil water lies at an exceptionally low level, to dispense with underdrains, but even in such cases, where it is practicable to bring the underdrain effluent to the surface, and re-treat it upon a further area of drained land, better results will be obtained. In some instances, unless underdrains are provided the effluent is apt to make its appearance where it is not wanted, for instance in public roads, and an intercepting drain is necessary. Sometimes, when a pumping main is being laid along a public road to tanks and an irrigation area bordering on the road, the nature of the sub-soil on the irrigation area is such as to cause the effluent water to follow the pipe trench, as being the line of least resistance, causing trouble when the road over the trench comes to be rolled and re-surfaced.

It is generally safer to be able to see the kind of effluent which is passing away from a sewage farm, than to rely upon absorption and dilution to effect an uncertain amount of purification. If the sewage or sewage liquor is dealt with on coarse gravelly soil where it percolates through so quickly that little purification is effected by the time the drains are reached, that land is seldom suitable for sewage treatment, and the use of it even without underdrains will not improve matters. Another point in which the draining of sewaged land differs from drainage of farm lands, is the much greater depth at which the drains should be laid in the former instance. With land used purely for agricultural purposes, drains are often laid just clear of the plough, and in few instances will the drains be found deeper than 2 feet 6 inches. To lay the drains deeper would only mean considerably increased cost, with little if any resulting advantage to the farmer.

Where land is used for sewage treatment, however, the converse holds good : the depth of drains will be determined by the porosity or otherwise of the soil and subsoil, but if the drains can be laid at an average depth of from 4 to 6 feet, so much the better, since increased duration of contact with the soil is thereby assured. The atmospheric air will dry the surface of the land, whilst the drains should carry off the liquid in the intermediate zone between the surface soil and the drains, and they will also tend to lower the level of the capillary zone lying beneath the drains and above the subsoil water level, thus assisting aeration. As soon as the liquid has passed through the necessary depth of soil, the drains should carry it away as quickly as possible.

It will often be found in practice that some of the drains at their highest—or possibly their lowest—ends, may, owing to the configuration of the land, be rather near the surface of the soil ; in such cases it is usually practicable to put an extra 12 inches or so of cover over each drain, extending for about 3 feet on either side of the drain. When the drains are shallow at the end of the plot furthest from where the sewage comes on, the sewage will already have attained some degree of purification by flowing over the surface of the land before the shallow drains are reached. In some cases it is advisable, where the underdrain effluent is brought to the surface and re-treated upon a drained area, to interpose a band of un-drained land between the two drained areas.

In ferruginous soils a layer of " pan," consisting of gravel, sand, etc., closely cemented together with oxide of iron, very frequently occurs at various depths below the surface soil, and until this is broken up good results are seldom obtained with sewage treatment, since the subsoil never becomes thoroughly aerated. The operation of underdraining breaks up this hard pan, and improves the land tenfold for purposes of sewage purification.

Great care should be taken over the filling in of the various lines of drains, and after the land has been sewaged for some days, the sewage should be taken off, and the lines of drains carefully gone over, any mole runs or subsidences being filled in, as these cannot as a rule be found out until the filling becomes saturated.

For tributary drains 3 to 4 inches in diameter agricultural tiles are as good as any for most soils and subsoils, since the joints occur at frequent intervals, but in very porous soils containing fine sand, it may be found necessary to place a thin layer of peat or turf immediately above the drain joints, to prevent the sand entering the drains, and in course of time choking them.

Drains will be found to answer best when laid transversely to the general slope of the land and the flow of the sewage. The practice of filling in drain trenches with porous material such as clinker or gravel in order to induce filtration cannot be regarded as sound, even if the drain effluent is re-treated. In most cases this means that the land immediately over the drains is treating sewage or tank liquor at far too high a rate to ensure good results, and the drains ultimately become choked with sewage fungus.

Drains can be laid in parallel or " herring-boned." In the former case, should anything go wrong with one of the drains, the sewage can be shut off from each line of drains consecutively, until the drain yielding the bad effluent is discovered.

The fall given to the subsidiary drains should be as much as can be afforded, there is then little likelihood of their becoming choked with sand or fine silt.

The main or master drains should be stoneware socketed pipes, and manholes should be provided at intervals for cleaning purposes, and also for judging of the quality of the effluent. Where manholes are not provided, air vents should be constructed at the head of each master drain, and if these are formed by pipes, the socket end of the last pipe should be carried well above the surrounding ground, and protected with an iron grating.

The distance apart at which tributary drains should be laid will be governed by the nature of the soil and subsoil, quantity of liquid applied, etc. It may be noted though, that it is far better to place the drains too far apart in the first instance, rather than too close together ; intermediate lines of drains can easily be added subsequently if found necessary.

Underdrainage of clay soils. Clay soils, owing to their tendency to crack in hot weather when the sewage is temporarily off the fields, should only be underdrained when the effluent from the drains can be picked up and re-treated, and there is seldom sufficient fall available for this.

At the Beaumont Leys Sewage Farm where the Leicester sewage is treated, and where there is plenty of fall available, this method of underdrainage has been carried out. The land was prepared for sewage by deepening the old ditches and cleaning them out to form main effluent channels to the streams : the underdrains of each field have separate outfalls brought out to the surface of the next lowest field, and so arranged that should a bad effluent reach the drains through cracks in the clay, it can be re-treated a second or a third time as the case may be. This is left to the discretion of the watermen ; but, as a general rule, an effluent is not passed off the farm until it has been treated at least twice.

The underdrains are ordinary agricultural butt tiles, laid from 24 feet to 99 feet apart, and averaging 4 feet in depth. Where additional underdrains are needed they are now put in at a depth of 3 feet. The diameter of the underdrains varies : 4 inch to 6 inch main drains are employed. Formerly, the drains when made, were filled in with top soil only, they are now filled in with the same soil as that excavated. The general system of underdrainage consists of 4 inch butt land tiles, connected to a 6 inch main drain laid along the lowest side of the field. At the lowest corner of the field this 6 inch main drain is provided with a valve chamber and free outfall on to the next field below, so that the drain effluent can, if necessary, be re-treated on the surface, or diverted into the ditches if adequately purified. If the plots under irrigation are large and long, only two may be used ; if, on the other hand, they are small plots, then three or even four plots are used. Surface effluents are carried across the ditches where necessary by means of wooden troughs.

Carriers. The distribution of sewage or tank liquor over land requires careful manipulation, especially in the case of surface irrigation, where much of the distribution of the sewage must of necessity devolve upon the watermen, and they require close supervision by the manager, otherwise sewage is apt to go astray at night.

The type of distribution channel or " carrier " employed varies according to circumstances ; in the case of a small flow of sewage, stoneware pipes laid on a bed of concrete, with suitable outlets to the land and provided with hand sluices, are probably as good as any.

Carriers formed by ditches cut in the earth itself or embanked, are objectionable, and tend to become deeper after each cleaning out: further, vermin often cause leakages. There is, however, no objection to using small channels cut in the soil for use as subsidiary carriers or grips, as the position of these can be frequently changed. Larger carriers are usually constructed of brickwork or concrete, and can be either semi-circular or half-hexagon in cross section.

The cross-sectional area of the main carriers will be governed by the maximum quantity of sewage and storm water likely to be brought down in times of heavy rainfall, and it may be observed that this will sometimes occur when the flow of the sewage itself is at its maximum. Large carriers require little fall, and can be laid almost level, the fall being just sufficient to allow them to run dry when needed. Where a sudden drop in a carrier is required, this can be effected by means of ramps, a sluice gate being placed just above the ramp. Owing to the rise and fall of sewage in carriers, a deposit or crust forms in time against the brickwork, and in hot weather this should be scraped off from time to time, and the sides of the carrier wel brushed to below the water line ; all sludge and débris from the carriers should be thrown out some distance from the carrier edges or carted away. A good deal of settlement of suspended solids occurs in carriers, since these act in much the same way as elongated settling tanks, and whenever gas bubbles begin to rise from the sediment, the sewage flow should be cut off, the carrier emptied, and the sediment or sludge brushed out.

Whether the main carriers are constructed of brickwork or concrete, the sides and invert must be smooth, and not left with any excrescences liable to catch up any floating matter in the sewage.

A good type of main carrier is shown in Fig. 31.

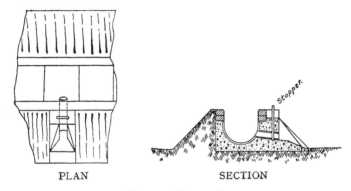

PLAN   SECTION

Fig. 31.   Main carrier.

Occasionally, where a slight dip in the surface of the land takes place, a length of closed pipe carrier can be used in the form of an inverted syphon, but the necessity for this can often be obviated by continuing the carrier in embankment for a little distance.

Where large carriers cross under roads, short inverted syphons may be necessary, or the road can be raised to allow headway for the carrier to pass under it.

In some cases piped carriers are used with outlets on to the land, and sometimes sluice valves with outlets are placed on the pumping main itself : when this method is employed, it is often convenient to connect the sluice valve outlet to a distributing chamber, having one or more outlets connected up to subsidiary carriers, the outlet to each carrier being regulated with a hand sluice.

Closed carriers are difficult to clean out, and when the sewage is being held up in them to sewage high-lying ground, stagnation and settlement are apt to occur in the lower length of the carrier.

Carriers formed of perforated pipes laid 12 inches to 18 inches below the surface of the soil have been used in certain instances, usually when a strongly-smelling liquid is to be distributed.

If this method is adopted, it is very necessary that the tank liquor to be distributed should contain a minimum quantity of suspended solids, otherwise such carriers will rapidly become choked.

A useful adjunct to large carriers is an electric or other alarm, adjusted to warn the watermen when the carrier is flowing full or thereabouts.

Outlets to carriers.   The outlets from the main carriers to the subsidiary carriers, or to the land, as the case may be, can be suitably provided with hand sluices, disc valves, or in the case of very large carriers by penstocks. Frequently, with carriers of fairly large dimensions, the outlets, if opening directly on to the land, will cause holes to be scooped out in the soil, where the sewage will stagnate and smell in hot weather.

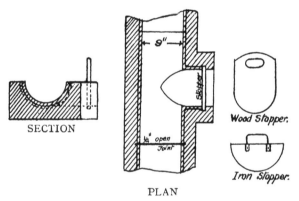

Fig. 32.   Carrier outlet.

This can be obviated by suitably placed slabs of stone or concrete upon which the sewage falls and flows off on to the land. With half-pipe carriers bedded on concrete, a quarter-inch open joint may be kept between two pipes at intervals, to admit of a thin sheet iron stopper being inserted when necessary (see Fig. 32).

Subsidiary carriers. These can be formed of half pipes bedded on concrete, junction blocks with sluice ways similar to those shown in Fig. 33 being used where a smaller branch carrier is required, but wherever it is possible to have carriers of a temporary character they should be plough-formed and trimmed to shape by spade labour, since these do not interfere with agricultural work in the same way as would carriers constructed of stoneware or concrete. With filtration pure and simple, few subsidiary carriers are required as a general rule, except in the case of large farms, but with surface irrigation the more complete the arrangements for distributing the sewage are, the better—with good management—will be the distribution, and consequently the purification attained.

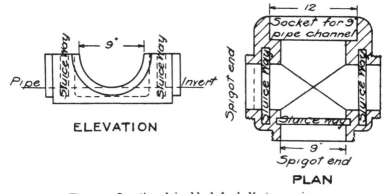

ELEVATION　　PLAN

Fig. 33. Junction sluice block for half-pipe carriers.

When the land to be sewaged is uneven in contour, small distribution grips can be cut in the soil, giving them a very slight fall ; this form of distribution answers particularly well where grass on a moderately heavy soil is concerned.

When the sewage is treated over two or three plots in succession by surface irrigation, " pick-up " carriers or grips will be needed at the foot of each plot, and they may be formed by earthen trenches.

As regards the periods for which carriers will run without cleaning, much depends upon the temperature of the air, nature of the sewage and carrier, etc. As a general rule in practice, carriers are not cleaned out nearly as often as they should be, and on some farms it is rarely or never done, the impression being that so long as sewage is covering the sludge lying on the invert of the carriers, that this will keep down the smell. The gas bubbles rising, however, not only often cause smell, but they carry up much sludge into suspension, and this passes on to the land, with the result that in course of time a coating of black sludge accumulates on the surface of the land adjoining the carrier outlets.

Effluent outfalls. The selection of a proper site for the effluent outfall or outfalls demands a good deal of consideration, since the great desideratum is to bring about the fullest dilution with river water as quickly as possible, and the rate of mixing will depend upon velocities, nature of river bed, absence or presence of eddies, depth of water, etc. In the majority of cases, a river or stream is accessible, but in some instances only a ditch or even a dry channel may be available; in this last case, however, the soil and subsoil are generally of so porous

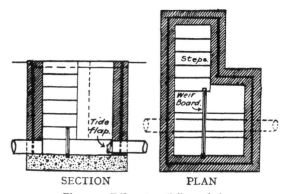

SECTION   PLAN

Fig. 34.   Effluent outfall manhole.

a character that the effluent is lost by absorption before it has travelled far: or again in some instances, particularly in districts overlying the chalk, it may be that the channel is dry for a number of years, when for a short period bourne water causes a flow in the channel.

In the case of large sewage farms, several effluent outfalls may be indicated, and there can be little doubt that in most

cases several outfalls of moderate size are preferable to one
large outfall, since they have the effect of thoroughly mixing
the effluent with the diluting water.

If in any way practicable, manholes should be provided on
each effluent outfall before the effluent is discharged into the
river or stream, so that samples can be taken of the effluent
before admixture with the diluting water; further, it is of great
advantage to be able to insert a weir board in the manhole
when necessary for gauging purposes. When there is sufficient
fall for this, a manhole of the type shown in Fig. 34 will be
found convenient for small outfalls.

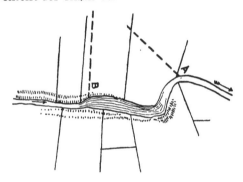

Fig. 35. Good and bad positions for effluent outfalls.

With wide and deep rivers, and where there is a large volume
of effluent, it will usually be found best to carry the outlet
pipe to midstream, or at all events to where the current is
strongest, and further benefit will result if the outfall pipe is
provided with multiple outlets, ensuring fairly complete mixture with the river water in a short distance, and in addition
equable distribution of suspended solids contained in the
liquor discharged. The multiple outlet method is of special
advantage where sewage or tank liquor is to be discharged into
a river without any further treatment. Backwaters and bays
in rivers should be rigidly avoided, even at the expense of a
longer outfall pipe or channel, since in both cases suspended
matter is sure to settle and accumulate in such places. Further,
in sluggish places a dense growth of water plants is liable to
accumulate, and this may not always and at all seasons of the

year be desirable ; water weeds are apt to arrest and entangle floating debris, whilst they afford moorings for grey growths. In Fig. 35 suitable and unsuitable positions for effluent outfalls are shown at points *A* and *B* respectively.

As a general rule it will be found best to have a submerged effluent pipe, especially if sewage or tank liquor is to be discharged.

When the river is subject to tidal action or rapid fluctuations in stage, tide flaps should be provided at the extremity of the outfall pipes, and provision made for adequate storage of the effluent.

Cost of laying out land. The cost of laying out land for filtration or surface irrigation will vary in almost every case, and no average figures can be given. The land used for surface irrigation may need very little levelling, in which case it may cost as little or even less than £2 per acre, or it may involve a great deal of excavation and filling in, and the cost may be considerably in excess of £10 per acre, quite apart from underdrains and carriers.

If the land is utilised for filtration, the cost of laying out will almost certainly largely exceed the cost for surface irrigation, since many more underdrains and permanent subsidiary carriers will be necessary, and in most cases a good deal of embanking as well.

As a rule, after a farm has been working for some little time after completion, various little points crop up, necessitating slight alterations and improvements, but these are usually so small that they are paid for out of revenue, no application being made by the authority to the Local Government Board to sanction a loan.

Planting of trees and shrubs on sewage farms. When a sewage farm is situated near a highway it is often desirable to plant hedges of trees for the purpose of shutting off any odours that may arise during spells of hot weather, or during sludging operations.

If this is done, and it is an excellent practice, the trees should be evergreens and not deciduous, possibly the best varieties to grow on the flat being Austrian Pines and Scotch

Fir, whilst on embankments Laurels answer well. The young trees should have been twice, or better still, thrice transplanted, when they are about 1½ to 2 feet high, costing about 350s. per 1000 ; and if it is proposed to plant a belt of them, they may be filled in and screened by Scotch Firs, (costing about 50s. per 1000), until they have become fair sized trees, when the Scotch Firs may be cut out. Scotch Firs being very much less expensive than Austrian pines, economy is effected in this manner. If the site is an exposed one the pines should be planted about ten feet apart, and each of them should be carefully staked.

Trees, in the case of artificial sewage works, tend to keep swarms of flies and midges within certain limits.

At the Cambridge Sewage Farm there are over a hundred cricket-bat willow trees growing. They are planted round various sections of the farm.

Sewage works can perhaps hardly be regarded as flower gardens, but in many cases excellent results have been achieved at a very small outlay, by judicious planting with flowers. Buxton, Exeter, Lincoln and Maidstone are cases in point. Double gorse and varieties of broom will be found to be useful shrubs to grow where the soil is sandy and poor.

Labour required for distribution of sewage. This will depend very much upon the method of treatment adopted, and the way in which the land is laid out in the first instance ; with surface irrigation, the number of men employed in distributing sewage (or watermen as they are termed technically) is more than is required for a filtration farm, not only on account of the greater variety of crops grown, but because the cutting of grips for distribution and setting of stops goes on, or should go on, almost incessantly, bringing fresh land into use, and resting land that has been used. In any case with a farm laid out for surface irrigation more men will be required than would be requisite for an ordinary agricultural farm of similar acreage.

The following tabular statement shows approximately the number of watermen employed at various farms, and the acreage of the farms.

TABLE XXIII.   *Showing number of watermen employed on various farms.*

Place		Irrigable Area (acres)	Number of watermen employed
Beddington	..	420	8
Leicester ..	..	1350	21
Rugby ..	..	35	1
Nottingham	..	651	6
Cambridge	..	80	1
Hatfield ..	..	24	1 (manager) and 1 occasional labourer

With the exception of Cambridge and Hatfield, the above figures relate to the year 1902.

Area under irrigation at one time. The flow of sewage arriving at the farm will be the chief factor in determining the area under irrigation ; *i.e.* during storm times, with a surface irrigation farm, it is impossible to avoid using a larger area; with filtration farms, where the various plots are embanked, the depth of liquid on the plots is often increased without extending the area sewaged, although better results would be obtained by increasing the area treating the sewage, instead of increasing the rate of filtration on the dry weather area.

Many other factors influence the extent of area under irrigation at any one time, *e.g.* agricultural operations, particular season of year, crops, etc.

In winter, during severe frosts, it is necessary on most farms to increase the irrigable area considerably, but this can usually be done without much difficulty, since crops do not interfere.

Stubble land, when it can be reached by sewage, is useful during hard frosts, the short stalks supporting a table of ice, under which the liquid continues to flow on the land. With filtration areas, when severe weather is anticipated, it is often advisable to plough the land in advance, the furrows and ridges acting in a precisely similar manner to the stubble. It is chiefly in summer time when rye-grass is the principal crop grown, that any want of land for irrigation is felt most, since it often requires as much as ten days to dry off, and allow the crop to be cut, dried and gathered. The main difficulty facing a farm manager, is the dealing with large volumes of storm water on land in times of heavy and continued rainfall, and instead of treating, as is sometimes done, six volumes of sewage and rainwater, it would be far better for the river into which the effluent goes, to treat only three times the dry weather flow as suggested by the Sewage Disposal Commission, and to pass the balance through " stand-by " tanks, direct to the river.

The subjoined table gives an idea of the average areas irrigated at one time at nine English sewage farms.

TABLE XXIV. *Showing average area sewaged at various farms.*

Place	Average area irrigated at one time (acres)	Total irrigable area (acres)	Percentage of the total irrigable area actually irrigated at one time
Leicester	337	1350	about 25 %
Nottingham ..	300	651	,, 46 %
Beddington.. ..	70	420	,, 16 %
S. Norwood.. ..	50	152	,, 33 %
Aldershot Camp ..	40	120	,, 33 %
Cambridge	25	80	,, 31 %
Altringham.. ..	17	35	,, 48 %
Rugby	7	35	,, 20 %
Hatfield	8	24	,, 33 %

Resting and working of land. This is a matter which requires most careful consideration, since the purification effected is very largely influenced by it ; put into other words it means rate of treatment per acre, or volume of sewage treated per acre. If, for instance, 20,000 gallons of sewage are run on to a plot on alternate days for 12 hours daily, the land is really treating at the rate of about 40,000 gallons per acre per 24 hours whilst the sewage is actually on the land. Again, the intermittency of treatment may take several forms : that is to say, the sewage may be applied in heavy doses with long periods of rest, or in frequent light doses with comparatively short intervals of rest, and between these two extremes will lie the most suitable rate of intermittency, which can only be determined by the manager in each particular case by a system of trial and error. Much will depend upon the character of the sewage, amount of storm water dealt with, kind of preliminary treatment, method of treatment on the land, *i.e.* whether surface irrigation or filtration, the contour of the area under irrigation and many other factors, chief of which is the fact that different areas of the irrigable area may require very different treatment, according to the nature of the soil and subsoil.

Generally speaking, land is kept under sewage for far too long periods without rest, and this is generally due to the fact that the area of land available is too small, or that the sewage is not moved about often enough, because this entails a good deal of labour. Again, the methods employed in cold weather may need to be considerably modified to meet the requirements of hot weather.

When the land is used for filtration only, the best results will, as a rule, be obtained when the sewage or tank liquor is applied in rather heavy flushes for from say, 6 hours to 12 hours, allowing a rest of from 18 to 12 hours. After a particular plot has been in use in this manner for perhaps a week or a fortnight it will become necessary to give the land a thorough rest of perhaps a week or longer, before it again receives sewage, and in the interval of rest it will probably be convenient either to plough or harrow the surface soil, weather permitting.

From what has been said, it will be seen that there are really two kinds of rest which land should receive, (1) the frequent intervals of short periods of rest between successive sewagings, and (2) the prolonged periods of rest (or drying-off) at longer intervals of time.

With some kinds of retentive soil, it is advisable to apply the sewage in a heavy flush for the first day, gradually reducing the dose subsequently, and with some clayey soils in very hot weather (especially when the land is underdrained) it may be advisable to apply a light dose of sewage in the daytime when the sun is hot, cutting off the supply in the late evening, for as long as the drought lasts ; this will reduce to a large extent the liability of such soils to crack in continued hot weather, sometimes resulting in the escape of an imperfectly purified effluent from the farm.

It is usually quite obvious when land requires a rest, the

surface becoming coated in places with a greyish black sediment, or growths of algæ, with ponding showing in places, and signs of grey growths at certain points : such visible signs taken in conjunction with the appearance of the effluent and effluent channel, are danger signals to the manager that the land is being unduly burdened, and that a thorough rest is imperative.

Sewage-sick land. This is a term used with reference to land which has been overdosed with sewage for some time, and has become what is called "sour."

Some kinds of land, such as that of the greater portion of the Nottingham sewage farm, recover with a very short interval of rest, and in most cases where land becomes sewage-sick, a thorough rest usually effects a cure.

Frequently, however, the recovery can be hastened and the land benefited in addition, by the application of dressings of lime, at the rate of about $1\frac{1}{2}$ to 2 tons of lime per acre. The lime sweetens the soil, and also assists the process of nitrification.

If the sour land can be thrown out of use for some months, and a crop taken in the meantime, so much the better.

In connection with some investigations at the Cambridge sewage farm, Purvis, McHattie and Fisher were led to consider some of the sections which were reported to be sick or getting sick[1]. Analyses of the effluents from these plots showed that they were good effluents, and that some cause was at work which interfered with the filtration of the sewage. It was proved that the surface of such sections was covered by a deposit of the suspended solids, which had not been very completely removed in the settling tanks, and which formed an excellent ground for the growth of various kinds of algae, thereby causing further resistance to filtration. The cause was a physical one primarily. By increasing the tank capacity, so that a greater proportion of the suspended solids was separated, is one obvious remedy ; and this is further strengthened by scarifying and ploughing followed by short periods of rest. This can be done when the season is favourable. The year's rest and cropping is unnecessary, and the economic saving is

[1] *Jour. Roy. San. Inst.* (1911), vol. XXXII. p. 439.

considerable. The sewage should be turned on to each section in regular rotation, and not remain on for more than eight hours at a time, and when the rate of filtration becomes slower, due to the above causes, the land is scarified and ploughed and allowed to stand for a short time for aeration.

Ridge and furrow method of irrigation. Fig. 36 gives a section showing the ridge and furrow method. In this case the beds or " ridges " usually run from four to eight feet or so wide, the intervening feed channel being some four or five feet wide; the sewage or tank liquor, as the case may be, flows down each of the channels to a depth of about nine inches or one foot, and is drawn up into the beds or ridges by capillary action. With a fine soil, the liquid rises up in the beds to a point considerably above the level of the liquid in the channel.

Fig. 36.   Ridge and furrow irrigation.

The position of the beds should be changed from year to year, but care should be taken when this takes place that the underdrains, if there are any, do not come immediately under the feed channel

This method is a very good one for growing vegetables intended for human consumption, as the liquid in the trenches or channels is never in contact with the leaves of the growing plants.

Sewage farm crops. In the case of a sewage farm laid out exclusively for filtration, the range of crops which can be grown will naturally be limited, and if the area is small in proportion to the flow of sewage, it can scarcely be cropped at all. Surface irrigation alone, or in combination with filtration, permits of a variety of crops being grown on the irrigable area.

Rye-grass, mangolds, cabbage, kohl-rabi, peppermint and comfrey will stand very large doses of sewage upon most soils, whilst lucerne flourishes on sandy soils, and where the area under sewage is ample, market garden produce such as brussels sprouts, celery, carrots, beet, and cauliflowers can be grown with advantage.

Permanent pasture will stand a certain amount of sewage, if the bulk of the suspended solids are first removed, but continuous sewaging tends to exterminate the finer grasses, coarser kinds replacing them to the detriment of the pasture.

Rye-grass.   Italian rye-grass and mangolds are perhaps more frequently grown upon sewage farms than any others.

Rye-grass is usually sown on sewage farms about August or September, to admit of the young plants hardening off before frosts set in, the sowing being at the rate of about six bushels per acre, and irrigation with light doses of sewage or tank liquor can be commenced after the young plants have become thoroughly rooted.

As many as six or seven cuttings of rye-grass may be obtained from the same plot in one year from a freshly laid down area.   After the plot has been in use for some two to three years the grass goes off, and the land should then be broken up, ploughed, and re-sown.   Frost is apt to play havoc with young rye-grass if it happens to be under sewage at the time. Before the grass is cut the sewage is generally taken off it for from seven to 14 days to allow the ground and crop to harden One great advantage of rye-grass as a sewage farm crop rests in the fact that it can be sewaged almost continuously throughout the year once it has become established.

Large quantities of rye-grass are grown yearly on the Beddington sewage farm, and the method of laying out the land there consisted in cutting grips some 50 feet apart along the line of greatest fall of the land, which was slightly hollowed between the grips, causing the on-coming sewage to spread itself evenly over the surface of the ground.   The grips end about 50 yards or so from the foot of the plot, and from this point to the pick-up trench at the foot of the plot the land is level.

Mangolds.   Both the globe and tankard mangolds thrive excellently upon sewage farms, where the soil is moderately light. They appear to do best when sown upon ridges or "bouts," and when grown in this manner, the uniform application of the sewage is easier than when the crop is grown on the flat; further, the plants are not at any time in actual contact with the sewage, and the ridges, after they have been sown, can be irrigated shortly after the sowing has been made, whereas, if sown on the flat, this has to be postponed until the young plants are well up. Weeds then begin to make their appearance, and these are usually cleaned off at the same operation as the thinning process, the ridges being afterwards earthed up again with a ridging plough. One great advantage that a sewage farm possesses over an ordinary farm is that in the former case the seeds can always be supplied with the moisture requisite for germination, and there is not the same chance of their "missing," as would occur on an ordinary farm should a drought set in after sowing, as was the case in many parts of the country in 1913. Again, the temperature of the sewage probably hastens growth quite as much as the manurial ingredients it contains[1]. The cost of destroying weeds is a heavy item in a sewage farm balance sheet, and they grow with surprising rapidity in hot weather. On the other hand, with a filtration farm, it seems quite likely that a dense growth of chickweed effects a most useful purpose, not only by reason of the transpiration effected through its medium, but by tending to keep down smell in hot weather; moreover, the presence of plant life extracts manurial constituents from the soil.

Peppermint. Of late years peppermint has come to be quite a common plant on land which is sewaged, the plants being disposed of to firms which distil oil of peppermint from the stems and leaves. Peppermint plants cost about 30s. per 1000 the roots being planted in March (in ordinary seasons) in lines some 14 inches apart, the same distance being kept between the rows. The crop is usually sold as it stands, and

[1] It would appear probable that farmyard manure, mixed as it usually is with straw litter, is almost as valuable for its protective action as for its manurial constituents, the straw protecting both seeds and roots of plants from extremes of heat and cold, and, in addition, conserving the moisture in the surface layers of soil.

is harvested when just coming into bloom, generally about August. Weeds should be carefully kept down if a heavy crop is desired. Peppermint is a profitable crop to grow, as much as £16 or even more having been realised per acre.

Lucerne. This crop has been grown with success on the Paris sewage farms, and has also been tried on an experimental scale at Hatfield. French lucerne seed is the best, the plants produced from it standing frost better than seed from Germany or Holland.

The roots of lucerne sometimes penetrate as much as eight to ten feet in depth in light sandy soil, and land should not be underdrained where this crop is grown year by year, since the roots would probably end by blocking the drains ; the same remark applies to osiers, which are exceedingly deep rooted plants. Lucerne requires potash, phosphates and lime, and likes a deep calcareous loam with a deep and open subsoil. The crop will last seven to ten years, but four to five years is a more usual period ; an average crop would be 18 to 24 tons per acre, and a heavy crop, 30 tons ; it should be cut before it comes into full flower. The land on which it is sown should be clean.

Osiers. These cannot be regarded as a suitable crop for sewage farms, although they are often to be seen there. They seem to have a way of attracting all the bindweed in the neighbourhood, and, in course of time, the bed becomes a dense tangled jungle, frequently employed as a receptacle for all surplus sewage, storm water, and sludge, often creating a nuisance in hot weather. Osiers grown under these conditions are generally very brittle, and realise very poor prices when sold. When the sewage receives efficient preliminary treatment, osiers could be grown on sewage farms provided the management is first class, but they only appear to do well in cold damp soils, gravelly and sandy soils being of no use. The best kinds of osier for sewage farms are the " New Kind," Merrin's osier, and the Golden osier.

Fruit trees. These might be grown upon sewage farms more frequently, since they can do with a good deal of manure, and screenings may be employed for this purpose with great benefit.

The Lincoln and Cambridge sewage farms have a number of fruit trees upon them ; at the latter farm the trees are planted in the embankments of the carriers which intersect the filtration areas.

Grain crops. Unless there is a very large surplus area of land, cereals are inadmissible on a sewage farm ; indeed, if grown, the straw is generally so long that the crop usually becomes " laid " after rain and wind, and is frequently rendered useless for anything but straw.

Disposal of sewage farm crops. In the vicinity of large towns there is not much difficulty in finding an outlet for various crops at good prices, and on a good many English sewage farms a certain area is devoted to the growing of market garden produce, such as celery, cabbage, brussels sprouts, carrots, etc. This procedure has been followed for many years at the Lincoln sewage farm. Mangolds and rye-grass may, however, be termed the staple sewage farm crops, and mangolds can nearly always be disposed of profitably, whether the farm is situated in a rural or urban district, and in dry seasons sewage farms have a considerable advantage over the ordinary farm, which suffers from lack of moisture.

When rye-grass is the main crop grown on a sewage farm, there is sometimes a difficulty in disposing of it quickly enough, unless stock are kept upon the farm itself.

Local prejudice sometimes exists against the consumption of sewage farm produce either by human beings or by cattle, but this seems to be gradually dying a natural death.

Passing of land effluents through fish ponds. This practice is in operation at the Berlin sewage farms, where the fish are kept in ponds which are supplied with sewage effluent, the fish being sold for edible purposes.

The passing of effluents through shallow ponds planted with various water plants and stocked with fish, might usefully be carried out on most sewage farms, since with surface irrigation farms there is usually plenty of opportunity for forming a series of shallow ponds, without sacrificing any appreciable fall.

The effluents from artificial processes would probably benefit to a greater extent than land effluents by such treatment, since the quantity of suspended solids and small worms in such effluents is usually rather high, whereas in the case of good land filtration effluents, they are an almost negligible quantity.

With artificial processes, however, it is generally of great importance to reduce the area required for the purification works as far as possible, and straining filters or humus tanks would probably be less trouble than fish ponds

The point is, however, well worth considering in the case of new works.

EFFECT OF POLLUTED WATERS UPON FISH LIFE. It may not be without interest to mention some facts concerning the effect upon fish life of waters polluted by trade wastes, sewage, and effluents, carried out at the Lawrence Experimental Station of the Massachusetts State Board of Health, and set out in a paper by Messrs Clark and Adams[1], entitled "Studies of Fish Life and Water Pollution."

Very briefly, the writers observe that from a scientific point of view there are many questions to be considered in connection with fish life and pollution, the most important being :

(1)   The amount of pollution that a stream may receive without decreasing the dissolved oxygen of the water to such a degree that fish can no longer live in the water;

(2)   The effect of the various constituents of sewage and trade wastes upon fish life, and the effect of these various constituents upon fish even when a plentiful supply of dissolved oxygen remains in the water after receiving these wastes ;

(3)   The amount of oxygen consumed by the fish themselves, and

(4)   The rate of absorption of oxygen by polluted water.

The experiments were for the most part carried out in five-gallon glass aquaria, and the fish used were the commonest of the locality, viz. chub, carp, shiners and suckers, weighing from 1 to 8 ounces each.

It was found (1) that the fish placed in undiluted Lawrence sewage, containing from 50 to 100 % saturation of dissolved oxygen, died a few minutes after immersion.

(2)   That when equal volumes of sewage (freed from suspended matters) and water were employed and kept aerated, fish life could exist almost indefinitely, but with a larger volume of sewage of the strength used, the longest period for which the fish lived was an hour or so.   Even in the equal mixtures of sewage and water, a number of fish soon died, but those that did survive, lived in the mixture for fourteen days, and apparently could have continued to live for an indefinite period.

(3)   Effluents from contact and percolating filters, kept aerated, supported fish life for fourteen days, no ill effects being noted during that period.

[1] Paper presented at the Eighth International Congress of Applied Chemistry, 1913.   Boston, Mass.

Further experiments were made to ascertain the degree of dilution necessary to support fish life under stagnant conditions, *i.e.* no dissolved oxygen being introduced artificially as in the previous experiment.

It was found that (1) only 10 % of sewage could be mixed with 90 % of water to produce conditions under which the fish could survive in good condition for 14 days. (2) That only 25 % of water was required in 75 % of the best percolating filter effluent to secure similar results, whilst with contact effluents, equal volumes of tap water and effluent were necessary.

It is important to note that in these last experiments, the dissolved oxygen present in the mixtures when the fish were first introduced was ·50 part per 100,000. During the progress of the experiment this became reduced in the water plus effluent mixtures to as little as ·11 part per 100,000, and in the sewage plus water mixture to ·14 part per 100,000, with no apparent discomfort to the fish.

It was noted that the greatest consumption of oxygen by the organic matter present in the mixtures occurred in the first few hours, and that if the initial supply of oxygen was sufficient to last through this early period, the oxygen would then be increased by absorption from the air.

Six experiments were carried out with well purified, highly nitrified effluent from sand filters; the fish lived for from three hours to three days after being introduced, but it is pointed out that all the effluents but one were slightly acid, the exception being alkaline and containing much matter in suspension. On the removal of the suspended matter the fish suffered no discomfort.

Further experiments with various chemicals likely to occur in trade wastes, showed iron salts, caustic and carbonate alkali to be exceedingly injurious to fish life.

An interesting statement is made by the authors of the paper on the amount of oxygen consumed by fish.

Several experiments were carried out on this question, and averaging the results, it was found roughly speaking that the entire supply of oxygen in solution in a gallon of water at 60° F. (about 1 part per 100,000 or 7 cc. per litre) would be breathed in one hour by a weight of fish equal to 1 lb. In other words, 1000 lbs. of fish life would in some 15 days exhaust the dissolved oxygen in a layer of water one foot deep and one acre in extent saturated at 60° F., assuming that dissolved oxygen was not added by absorption from the air.

Other experiments were made in connection with the liberation of oxygen by green growths in the presence of light.

In one of these experiments an aquarium was filled with tap water, and seeded with green growth, the dissolved oxygen and CO_2 at the start being respectively ·18 and 1 parts per 100,000 ; at the end of seven days they had become 1·14 and ·0 parts per 100,000.

In another experiment a small fish was put in a bottle of water containing green growths, the bottle then being tightly stoppered. In the absence of liberation of oxgyen by the growths, the oxygen originally present in the water would have been used up by the fish in 38 hours; it lived, however, for eight days.

In a similar experiment carried out in cloudy weather, the fish present consumed the oxygen in four days.

The importance of green growths and water plants to fish life can scarcely be over estimated.

Probably the time when fish are most susceptible to pollution of various kinds, is just after the spawning period, when they are in a debilitated condition.

Land effluent temperatures. Until comparatively recently, but little interest was evinced in the temperatures of effluents throughout the various seasons, but their daily record is only a matter of a few minutes, whilst in view of the important part played by temperature in sewage purification processes, the information thus obtained may prove exceedingly valuable in after years.

Surface irrigation effluents will be found to follow the daily temperature of the air fairly closely, whilst effluents produced by filtration through soil give a much more even curve. It is quite possible from a series of air, sewage, and effluent temperatures, to judge fairly closely the relative proportions of filtration and surface irrigation effluents.

The diagram given on page 204 shows the mean monthly temperatures of air, sewage, and effluent at Nottingham (filtration) and Beddington (surface irrigation) sewage farms from 1900 to 1901 ; it will be observed that the air and effluent temperatures in the case of the Nottingham farm, cross one another twice in the course of the year, *viz* about October and March, whilst from about October to March the temperature of the effluent is warmer than that of the air. In the case of Beddington, the effluent temperature follows that of the atmosphere, and the air and effluent temperatures again approximate as in the Nottingham diagram, about October and March, but they also approach one another in the hot months of the year

The crossing of air and soil temperature curves in October and March is a fact well known to meteorologists, and it would seem that suitable land used for filtration purposes possesses a distinct advantage in very cold weather over land used on surface irrigation principles, for, on the assumption that in the case of surface irrigation, nitrification is at a very low ebb during severe weather, it would seem to persist under the surface layers of soil, as effluents containing nitrates were

taken at the Nottingham sewage farm during very severe
frosts in 1899 (22 degrees of frost were registered on one
occasion).

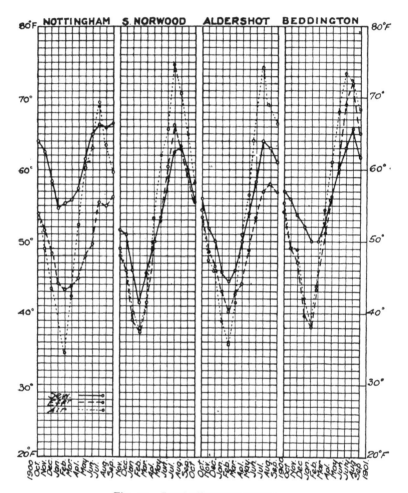

Fig. 37.   Land effluent temperatures.

Temperatures of rivers and streams.   Whilst speaking of
the temperatures of effluents it is perhaps not inappropriate
to touch upon the temperatures of rivers and streams also,

and considering how intimately connected is the growth of plant life and self-purification of rivers, it seems curious that this matter has hitherto received so little attention.

During the cool months of the year, it is an undoubted fact that a river or stream can receive more pollution without becoming a nuisance to the senses, than would be possible in hot weather ; in other words, a river receiving a constant degree of pollution throughout the year, may have an unpleasant smell and appearance in the hot weather which would be totally absent in the winter.

Clean well aerated river water has a content of roughly about 7 cc. of oxygen per litre (equal to one part per 100,000) at a temperature of about 60° F., but it varies considerably according to the temperature of the water as will be seen from the following table:

TABLE XXV. *Showing oxygen held in solution by water at various temperatures.*

Temperature in degrees Fahrenheit	cc. of oxygen held in solution by 1 litre of water (Winkler)	Temperatures in degrees Fahrenheit	cc. of oxygen held in solution by 1 litre of water (Winkler)
32·0	10·2	51·8	7·7
33·8	9·9	53·6	7·5
35·6	9·6	55·4	7·3
37·4	9·4	57·2	7·2
39·2	9·1	59·0	7·0
41·0	8·9	60·8	6·9
42·8	8·7	62·6	6·8
44·6	8·5	64·4	6·6
46·4	8·3	66·2	6·6
48·2	8·1	68·0	6·4
50·0	7·9		

Thus there is a difference in oxygen content for 36° F. (32° F. to 68° F.) of 3·8 cc. or nearly 4 cc. So that it would appear that in cold weather, rivers can theoretically receive more pollution without smell arising than in the summer months.

The reason why the Sewage Disposal Commission adopted the figure of 65° F. for the standard test for dissolved oxygen, was because daily records of the temperatures of various rivers and streams in England (in non-manufacturing districts) showed that it was unusual for a river to exceed it.

The temperatures of some of the rivers referred to, together with the air temperatures, are given in the diagram on Fig. 38.

It is fortunate that during the hot months, when objectionable features would otherwise be apt to arise in a polluted river, this is counterbalanced by the rapid growth of aquatic plants and algae ; these have been shown to have the power of abstracting ammonia, chlorides and nitrates from the water. Again, insect life is most active when the temperature is high.

Grey growths, and some of the algae, appear to exist throughout the year, but much more sparsely in cold weather, whilst in favourably sheltered positions, aquatic plants, such as *Callitriche verna* and *Ranunculus aquatilis*, live through the winter with scarcely any alteration in appearance.

In hot weather, the quantity of oxygen given off by dense beds of water plants in sunlight is very large, and analyses of certain river waters have shown as much as 12 cc. to be present per litre as a result of flowing over such beds. In regard to the purification of sewage effluents; which goes on naturally when poured into rivers, it was found by Purvis and Rayner[1] that the river Cam, for example, purified itself chemically fairly well within a moderate distance from the effluent outfall. As regards the numbers obtained for the two ammonias and the oxygen absorbed from potassium permanganate, they found that the chemical purification was fairly good at a quarter to half a mile below the outfall. At the same time it should be stated that *Bacillus coli*, coming from the effluent, was traced to three or four miles below. These chemical results were confirmed later by Purvis and Black[2], who conducted a series of experiments on the amount of oxygen dissolved in the river Cam above and below the effluent outfall. They found that at a quarter of a mile below the outfall the self-purification of the river had gone on so well that the river could at no time be called a "bad" river, as defined by the 8th Report of the Royal Commission on Sewage Disposal (1912), vol. I. p. 5. They showed that the amount of oxygen in the stream was of

[1] *Jour. Roy. San. Inst.* (1913), vol. XXXIV. p. 479.
[2] *Proc. Camb. Phil. Soc.* (1914), vol. XVII. p. 353.

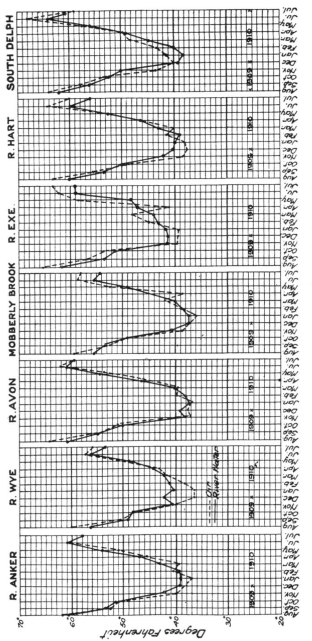

Fig. 38. Mean monthly air and river water temperatures.

prime importance in this purification, and that as the number of hours of sunshine increased, the amount of oxygen in the river given off by the aquatic plants also increased; and also that in the winter the water at the lower temperatures dissolved more oxygen from the air than at the higher summer temperatures, notwithstanding the fact that the number of hours of sunshine was considerably less with the corresponding lessened influence on the power of aquatic plants to give off oxygen. So that there is a definite balance of the various influences.

It is chiefly during the daytime that effluents are likely to deteriorate in the case of artificial processes, the sewage from which they are derived being then strongest, and the increased supply of oxygen derived from water plants must be of great benefit at such times. At night time, when the effluent would probably be at its best, the river water would presumably lose a certain percentage of the oxygen given off by the plants in sunlight, but on the other hand the water, being cooler, would hold more oxygen in solution.

A good deal of stress has been laid on the fact that sooner or later the weeds must decay and then cause nuisance, but as a general rule this does not occur until late autumn, and then floods frequently occur, scouring out the river bed, whilst the normal flow of the river for this period of the year is usually considerably higher than during the summer months.

It is quite possible that before many years are past it will be realised that a thorough examination of the flora and fauna of a river, will yield even more valuable results as to the actual state of that river, than chemical analysis unsupported by riverside observation.

A river of sterile tap water would scarcely be regarded favourably by farmers who possess meadows which are habitually flooded once or twice yearly by rivers containing manurial constituents, and are rendered valuable land by that fact. Further, if such a river were possible, it would be unable to support plant or insect life and therefore fish life.

Annual volume of sewage and rainwater dealt with per acre per annum by sewage farms. Few people realise what the aggregate volume of sewage *and* rainwater dealt with on a sewage farm comes to in the course of a year, and it may be useful to show this in diagram form.

The diagram reproduced in Fig. 39 is a modification of one prepared by the author for Vol. IV of the Sewage Disposal Commission's Fourth Report. The original diagram showed graphically the depth in feet of sewage— *based on the dry weather flow*, plus the depth in feet of the average annual rainfall.

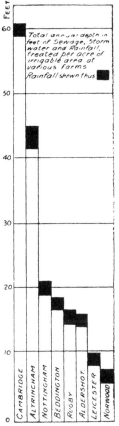

In the diagram given below, the extra volume of storm water over and above the dry weather flow of sewage, is in the case of each farm taken at an increase of 50 per cent. on the dry weather flow of sewage. The volume of sewage and storm water flow treated per acre per annum of the irrigable area is shown by a black line, the average annual rainfall being shown in black.

It will be seen that in the case of the Cambridge farm, the volume of sewage and storm water treated per acre of irrigable area, is about 30 times the rain falling in a year upon the same area. At Altrincham a volume of sewage and storm water about 12 times greater than the rainfall passes through each acre of land in a year, and at South Norwood, where surface irrigation is employed, and the land is heavy, an acre of irrigable area receives in the course of a year about four times as much sewage and storm water as rainfall.

Fig. 39. Annual volume of sewage and rainfall dealt with per acre per annum at certain sewage farms.

Cattle on sewage farms. Cattle should rarely be permitted to roam loose on land used for sewage treatment, on account of the damage they do to land—especially heavy soils—by " pocketing " it with footprints, in which the sewage or tank liquor after application to the land, stagnates and smells when the field is dried off. Cattle also do damage to carriers, grips, and fences. Where surplus land is available on the farm, or where the cattle are stall fed, this objection naturally does not arise, and heavy crops of rye-grass can be disposed of regularly where cattle are kept.

Subletting of sewage farms. As a general rule, sewage farms should not be let, and much trouble frequently arises from letting the farm to a tenant whose sole interest is the production of heavy crops, the purification of the sewage being quite a secondary matter. From the point of view of the farmer, the greatest quantity of sewage generally requires treatment when the crops are least in need of it.

If the farm is a small one, and can be let to a tenant who possesses ample means, and who also takes a real interest in the treatment of the sewage, it is, of course, a different matter altogether, and in such a case the tenant will probably be in a position to put a large amount of horse labour to work ploughing and cultivating, and to get the work completed during the somewhat infrequent opportunities which occur on a sewage farm for these operations, whereas, if the horse labour is hired, it has to wait the convenience of local farmers, and this does not always fit in with dry spells.

In any case, if a farm is sublet, it should not be for a longer period than say 12 months to commence with, by way of trial, with six months notice on either side, and the distribution of the sewage should be in the hands of the local authority's manager ; further, it should be clearly pointed out in the agreement that no claim can be considered in respect of crops damaged by the application of sewage, and the crops should be limited to mangolds, rye-grass and the like ; cereals should not be permitted. The tenant should also be made responsible for any damage to carriers, manholes, etc., caused by his labourers in the course of agricultural operations.

Smell from sewage farms. This question may be dealt with here as affecting not only land treatment of sewage but also artificial processes and sewage works in general.

Whatever smell there may be from sewage works in general,

is sure to be accentuated in hot weather, and especially on calm days when there is much moisture present in the air, and a light gentle breeze to carry the smell to houses near.

Special conditions favourable to the production of smell, are the presence of certain trade wastes in the sewage, such as brewery and tannery wastes, and it is often necessary to add certain chemicals to the sewage during its preliminary treatment.

Where sewage farms are concerned, the smell usually arises from one of three operations, namely, (1) sludge disposal, (2) irrigation of the sewage on the land, or (3) the preliminary tank treatment.

In the first case, if the smell is from the sludge when it is draining in lagoons or trenches, prior to removal or trenching in, a light sprinkling of lime or bleaching powder will generally remedy the matter.

In the second case, dirty carriers, and land which has been too heavily sewaged, are often a cause of smell, and the smell of dirty land in process of drying off under a hot sun is perhaps one of the most frequent causes of smell. The remedy is to be found in keeping the carriers clean, giving longer periods of rest to the land, or, if necessary, extending the irrigable areas, whilst moving the sewage from one plot to another at frequent intervals.

In the third case, if the smell is from the tanks themselves, it can often be reduced by using certain chemicals, such as lime, at the expense, however, of producing a larger volume of sludge, which in turn may cause nuisance elsewhere.

At Hatfield, the treatment of sewage containing brewery waste which had become septic by passing through a tank and a long inverted siphon of too large diameter, formerly caused an intolerable nuisance when distributed on the land. In the new works carried out by the writer, the sewage is pumped to quiescent settling tanks on the farm, so designed as to be capable of being used as precipitation tanks in very hot weather. The distribution of settled sewage instead of septic liquor had the effect of reducing the smell to a minimum

Septic tank liquor is particularly prone to cause nuisance from smell in hot weather, especially if it contains even a small proportion of brewery or tannery waste, and if it is treated by sprinkling on percolating filters.

Much naturally depends upon the size and situation of the works where a particular process is carried on, as to the degree and extent to which smell may carry ; for example, a small sewage works treating 100,000 gallons of sewage per day, may be practically unnoticed a short distance away, but with a large works treating 1,000,000 gallons of an identical sewage, the case would be altogether different.

When, however, a site for sewage works can be secured in an isolated position, it is always well to consider it thoroughly, even though the cost of utilising it be greater than the cost of a site nearer to dwelling houses.

Sewage farms in relation to health. All the reliable data available afford the strongest presumptive evidence that no injury to health occurs to men who work upon sewage farms. It may be said that they work there day after day, and become more or less inured to it. This, however, can scarcely be the case, as during busy times, in addition to casual labourers, the same outside labourers are often engaged year after year, and they do not appear to suffer in any way ; indeed, it will be found on inquiry that men employed upon sewage farms enjoy particularly good health.

Taking the case of the Berlin sewage farms in 1905, when there were about 4200 persons residing on the farms ; a report dealing with the subject of effect of the sewage farms on health says, " We can only repeat here what we said in previous reports—that the sewage treatment has had no injurious effect upon health." Dr Carpenter, as far back as 1887, showed conclusively that " in no single instance out of nearly 100 cases in which sewage has been utilised by broad irrigation, has any fact been proved to establish the allegations of insanitariness which are sometimes raised against them."

In the Fourth Report of the Sewage Disposal Commission (vol. IV. part 1), the same view is expressed :

" As regards the likelihood of sewage farms being dangerous to health, we can do no more than tentatively express the opinion that no convincing proof has yet been furnished of *direct* or widespread injury to health in the case of well-managed farms.

"It may be possible that the foul emanations from a badly managed or over-sewaged farm constitute an indirect source of danger to health by lowering the vitality of weakly and susceptible individuals."

Management of sewage farms. When the sewage farm is completed and the sewage being treated on the land, the efficiency of the process will depend very greatly, in fact almost entirely, upon the management of the farm, and it is no exaggeration to say that a badly laid out farm under a first class manager, will yield consistently better results than a well laid out farm, the working of which is bad. Few things are more disheartening to those who have been responsible for the proper laying out of a farm, than to see their work nullified by incompetent and ignorant usage. The main points for the manager are : (1) to produce as economically as possible an effluent of such quality as will in no wise cause injury to the river or stream into which it flows ; (2) to endeavour as far as practicable to keep down smell from the farm ; and (3) to get the best results he is able from the crops, always bearing in mind the fact that the farm is primarily for treating sewage, and not for growing crops for sale, and that therefore, should any question arise of damaging crops or turning away a bad effluent, the purification of the sewage must come first and the crops must come last.

Further points which should receive consideration from the manager are statistics of various kinds relating to flow of sewage[1], filling and emptying of tanks (quiescent flow), length of time tanks are run before being sludged, volume of sludge produced, storm water dealt with, length of time various plots are kept under sewage ; daily rainfall and temperatures should also be taken in the case of large farms, and many other points, too numerous to mention, will occur to a good manager, such as the recording of dates and times at which certain trade wastes come down.

As regards tests which a farm manager might be expected to be familiar with, the writer uses as a rough field test for effluents a small pocket set consisting of a test tube and pipette

---

[1] This is of especial value when the sewage contains much subsoil water.

together with two small bottles of reagents ; these can easily
be carried in the pocket when visiting a sewage farm, and if
necessary the bulk can be still further reduced by carrying the
two solutions in one bottle. The apparatus is shown in Fig. 40.

Two solutions are required : (1) $\frac{N}{80}$ permanganate (= 0·395
gm. $KMnO_4$ per litre), and (2) dilute sulphuric acid (10 volumes
of H_2SO_4 *added to* 90 volumes of water).

The test is carried out as follows :—25 cc. of effluent are

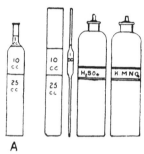

A
Fig. 40.   Effluent testing
apparatus.

poured into the test tube (*i.e.* up to
the first mark), 10 cc. of the dilute
sulphuric acid are then added, bringing the level of the liquid up to the
second graduation.   One cc. of the
permanganate solution is then added.
If the mixture in the tube is not
decolourisèd, or only just decolourised in three minutes, the effluent
may be termed a good one.   If 2 cc.
of permanganate are added and become decolourised in three minutes
the effluent may be termed poor to bad.   The pipette could be
dispensed with by forming the test tube in the manner shown
at A in Fig. 40, but it would be more difficult to fill and to
keep clean.   The writer is indebted to Dr George ˙McGowan
for working out the chemical part of the test[1].

Perhaps the very best test the manager possesses as to
the quality of the effluent he is producing, is to be found in the
condition of the channel, river, or stream, which receives the
effluent.

It will be found in practice that an effluent registers its
character fairly accurately on the bed and side of the channel
streams, and so long as these remain clean, and grey growths
are absent, or at all events do not extend for more than a
short distance below the effluent outfall, the effluent is in all

---

[1] More complete tests are described in *The chemical examination of water,
sewage, foods and other substances*, by J. E. Purvis and T. R. Hodgson, one of
the volumes in the Cambridge Public Health Series.

probability causing no injury. Green algae in moderate quantity are generally a sign that the effluent is a good one ; it is
when they become replaced or covered by grey growths in
abundance that trouble is to be anticipated.

What has been said as regards management of sewage
farms applies equally to artificial processes.

Cost of land treatment of sewage. Given a sufficient area of
good land, well laid out in the first instance and suitable for
sewage purification, coupled with intelligent management, a
sewage farm should nearly pay for the cost of labour and
management during normal seasons, whilst in dry seasons a
small surplus over the cost of the year's working of the farm
will sometimes result.

It must be carefully borne in mind, however, that the main
point by which a sewage farm should be judged is not by the
favourable showing as regards receipts at the end of the year's
working, but by the proper purification of the effluent, absence
of smell, satisfactory disposal of sludge, and general way in
which the farm is worked

It is usual to compare the costs of various processes of
sewage treatment by showing the cost involved for treatment
per million gallons, based on the dry weather flow, sometimes
coupled with the cost of treatment per head of the population
sewered.

This method, it may be observed, would hold good were
the sewages treated and the effluents produced similar in each
case ; otherwise this procedure may sometimes prove misleading. It is hardly possible to give any figures including
interest on capital expenditure which are not liable to mislead,
since so much depends on the cost of the land in the first instance,
and also on the money required to be expended before it can
properly be used for sewage treatment.

The Sewage Disposal Commission in their Fifth Report
say ·

" Assuming that really suitable land can be purchased at
£100 per acre, land treatment of sewage is probably cheaper
than artificial treatment, but where the soil is not suitable,
and on which only a comparatively small volume of sewage can

be treated per acre, the cost of land treatment would probably be greater than most of the artificial processes.

" The differences in cost are, however, small, and it is evident that in deciding between the two methods regard must be had to local conditions. If, for instance, £200 per acre had to be paid for land, the cost of land treatment would materially exceed the estimates given, which have been based on an assumed price of £100 per acre.

" As a general rule, an effluent from good land, properly worked, contains practically no suspended solids, but this cannot be said of artificial filters, even assuming that settlement of the effluent in tanks is adopted. This might be a factor of considerable importance in the case of some streams."

Good examples of (1) the treatment of crude sewage upon land, can be seen at Nottingham, Grantham and Stourbridge ; (2) tank liquor upon land at Woking, Altrincham, Cambridge, Aldershot Camp, Coventry and Hatfield.

BIBLIOGRAPHY.

British Association. *Rep.* 1871, pp. 176–177.
Clifford, William. " Land filtration effluents." *Journ. Roy. San. Inst.*, Vol. xxxiv. No. 10, London, Nov. 1913.
Crimp, W. Santo. *Sewage Disposal Works.* Chas. Griffin and Co., Ltd., London (1894).
Fortier, S. *Farmers' Bulletin*, 404. U.S. Depart. of Agriculture, p. 28.
Dienert, F. *Hydrologie agricole.* J. B. Baillière et fils, à Paris (1907).
Fream. *Elements of Agriculture.* John Murray, London (1892).
Fuller, G. W. *Sewage Disposal.* McGraw-Hill Book Co., New York and London (1912).
Institute of Civil Engineers. *Excerpt. Min. Proc.*, Vol. xlv. Session 1875-6. Part 3.
Jones, V. C., Col. A. and A. Roechling. *Sewage Treatment.* E. and F. N. Spon, London (1902).
Kayser, E. *Microbiologie Agricole.* J. B. Baillière et fils. Saint Germain, à Paris (1911).
Kershaw, G. Bertram. *Modern methods of sewage disposal*, chap. xii. Chas. Griffin and Co., Ltd., London (1911).
Klein, P. *Météorologie Agricole.* J. B. Baillière et fils, à Paris (1912).
Massachusetts State Board of Health. *Studies of fish life and water pollution*, by Messrs Clark and Adams.

Purvis, J. E., McHattie, A. C. N., and Fisher, R. H. J. "Sewage Sickness in land filtration." *Journ. Roy. San. Inst.*, Vol. XXXII. No. 9 (1911), p. 439.

Purvis, J. E. and Rayner, A. E. "The chemical and bacterial condition of rivers above and below the sewage effluent outfall." *Journ. Roy. San. Inst.* (1913), Vol. XXXIV. p. 479.

Purvis, J. E. and Black, E. H. "The oxygen content of the River Cam above and below the sewage effluent outfall." *Proc. Camb. Phil. Soc.* (1914), Vol. XVII. p. 353.

Risler. *Archives des sciences de la Bibliothèque Universelle*, September, 1869.

Risler and Wery. *Irrigations et drainages.* J. B. Baillière et fils, à Paris (1909).

Rivers Pollution Commission, 1st *Report*, 1870.

Royal Commission on Sewage Disposal. *Fifth Report, Fourth Report,* Vol. I : *Eighth Report*; *Seventh Report* Appendix, Vol. II : *Fourth Report*, Vol. IV.

Tillmans, J. *Water purification and sewage disposal*, translated by Hugh S. Taylor. Constable and Co., London (1913).

Whitney. *Bull.* No. 4. U.S. Weather Bureau.

Wilson, H. M. and Calvert, H. T. *Trade Waste Waters.* Chas. Griffin and Co., Ltd., London (1913).

CHAPTER VII

CONTACT BEDS

Preliminary treatment. Unless exceptionally coarse contact material is used, or probable ultimate clogging of the beds recognised, it is necessary to give the sewage some form of preliminary tank treatment, before passing it on to the contact beds.

Crude sewage was formerly treated without any preliminary settlement upon contact beds at Hampton, Maidstone and other places, but the beds soon became clogged with suspended matter and lost capacity rapidly, and it is now recognised that efficient preliminary treatment is essential if the life of the beds is to be of anything more than comparatively short duration. Removal and washing of contact material is a lengthy and somewhat costly business, as will be seen later, and in the vast majority of cases, at all events, it is far cheaper to prevent the suspended solids entering the beds by means of one or another form of tank treatment, than to remove the whole of the contact material with the suspended solids or sludge, to wash and screen out the sludge, and to replace the material in the beds, making good, in addition, the deficit caused by loss and disintegration of material.

The extent to which the suspended solids will require removal will depend very largely upon the size of the contact material employed ; the finer the material, the less suspended solids should the liquids contain.

Regarding this point, the Sewage Disposal Commission say (Fifth Report) :

" No rule can be laid down as to the extent to which the suspended solids should be removed from sewage before it is filtered, but, speaking generally, if it is proposed to use filters of fine material, we think it will be found most economical to adopt some form of tank treatment which will yield a tank liquor fairly free from suspended solids ; whereas, if coarse filtering material is to be used this is not so essential.

" If much suspended matter is put on fine filters they are likely to choke very rapidly unless the rate of filtration is very slow."

A good deal also depends upon facilities or the reverse for getting rid of the sludge as to how far the suspended matter in the tank liquor should be reduced before it is treated upon contact beds. The foregoing remarks also apply to the preliminary treatment of sewage before it is passed on to percolating filters.

Description of contact beds. Contact beds consist of watertight tanks provided with inlets and outlets for sewage or tank liquor, underdrained, and filled with hard durable material, such as clinker, coke, broken stone, etc., the size of the material varying according to several factors, such as nature of sewage, character of preliminary process, etc. The sewage or tank liquor is run into a contact bed (the outlet valve or valves being first closed) until the liquid is almost level with the top of the contact material, when the inlet valve is closed and the

liquid is left in " contact "—hence the name contact[1] bed—for
a certain period, after which the outlet valve—placed at the
foot of the bed—is opened and the liquid run off, the bed then
standing empty for a certain time ; when it is re-filled the same
cycle of operations being repeated.

The agents by which the purification is brought about are
the same as in the treatment of sewage by land and percolating
filters, *i.e.* mechanical, chemical, physical and biological.

When the sewage or tank liquor is only passed through one
bed it is termed single contact ; save in exceptional circumstances, however, single contact is not sufficient to produce
a satisfactory effluent, and the first contact bed effluent is
usually passed through a second, and, more rarely, a third bed,
the method of working the second and third contacts being
similar in all respects to that of the first.   Double contact, as
the name implies, means the passing of the liquid to be purified
through two beds, and triple contact the passing of the liquid
through three beds in series.   Since the outlet valve is at the
lowest point of each bed, and an average depth of contact
material is four feet, it follows that a good deal of fall is needed
for double contact and still more for triple contact.   It is usual
to have the material in the second or secondary contact beds
of somewhat finer material than that of the first or primary
beds, whilst the material in the tertiary beds is of still finer
medium, the decrease in size of material pre-supposing a pro-
gressive decrease in the suspended solids present in the effluent
after each contact.   Further, a much greater combined surface
area of particles is secured by the use of fine material, and
the greater the surface area, the greater will be the proportion
of colloidal matter removed.

Since the flow of sewage to the works is continuous in a
gravitation scheme, it follows that there must be a sufficient
number of both primary and secondary beds, to admit of
other beds being filled, whilst the bed first filled has time for
running off and resting, before being ready for a second filling.

---

[1] The word " contact material " is used when referring to contact beds
in preference to the word " filtering material," the latter phrase being applied
to the material of percolating filters.

A conventional plan and section of double contact beds is shown in Fig. 41.

Contact beds may be said to have been the forerunners of percolating filters, and their working, save in a few instances, notably at Manchester, does not appear to have received the same attention as percolating filters, failures in many instances being due to faulty methods of working, inferior material, etc.

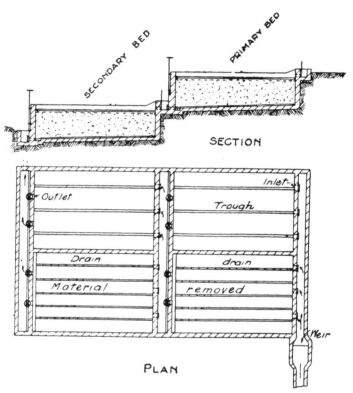

Fig. 41. Conventional plan and section of double contact beds.

It is true that many contact bed installations have been altered to percolating filters, but this is sometimes due to the fact that the contact beds were not fairly treated in the first instance, too much being expected of them.

Action of contact beds. Concerning the action of contact beds, reference may be made here to the Fifth Report of the Sewage Disposal Commission, where it is stated :

" Our knowledge of the action of a contact bed is very incomplete, and little is known as to the manner in which the organic substances of sewage are broken down during the first stages of fermentation[1] into carbon dioxide, ammonia, etc. The purifying agents seem to be not only bacteria, but also worms, larvae, insects, etc., and we can offer no opinion as to the respective amount of work done by each set of agents. It has been observed that at some places large numbers of worms are present, while at others there are comparatively few. Little is known of the kind of bacteria essential for purification, or as to their mode of action, and we are not able to state whether they act chiefly during the period of contact or during the period of rest, or aeration, after the filter is emptied. There are, however, grounds for thinking that the resting period is the more important phase of the cycle.

" The generally accepted theory as regards nitrogenous matter seems to be that the ammonia is extracted from the liquid during the period of contact, and oxidised during the period of rest, and that the resulting nitrate and nitrite are diffused through the liquid of a subsequent filling. All the ammoniacal nitrogen, however, does not appear in the effluent in the oxidised state, for there is always loss of nitrogen, as nitrogen gas, during the process.

" The withdrawal of suspended and colloidal matter from the sewage during its passage through the bed appears not to be a simple mechanical effect of the material, for a mature contact bed, not clogged, will withdraw more suspended matter from the sewage than another bed similar in all other respects, but not matured."

The number of insects and worms in some contact beds during certain seasons of the year is astonishing,—and there would seem to be little doubt that they play an important

---

[1] " It may be observed that the American chemists term the decomposition of nitrogenous matter ' putrefaction,' and of carbonaceous matter ' fermentation.' " *Author.*

part, after they have become established in the beds, in breaking up the larger solids, and so bringing them into a condition in which they are easily acted upon chemically, physically and bacterially.

Construction of contact beds. It is rarely the case that contact beds can be satisfactorily constructed by simple excavation in dense clay soils without the use of building materials. The method of construction by excavating the beds in heavy clay soil has, however, been successfully carried out at Burnley, where the contact beds extend over an area of some 24 acres ; in the vast majority of cases, however, the disadvantages of this system outweigh the saving in first cost. In some cases, leakages through the dividing embankments occur, rendering gauging of the bed capacities out of the question, and frequently necessitating the filling of several primary beds, or both primary and secondary beds simultaneously. Again, where space is valuable, concrete or brick walls take up much less area than embankments with a batter on both sides, and the smaller the bed units, the greater the waste of site area.

When contact beds are formed without bricks or concrete, the clay bottom is apt to become soft, and to work up into the contact material, besides damaging the underdrains ; rats and moles too are liable to cause leakage in dry weather, and in cold weather frost may bring about the same results, and it will often be found to be the case that leakages are most frequent in the immediate vicinity of the outlet chambers, which are bound to be made of building materials. A safer plan with clay soils is to cover the sides and bottom of the beds with a thin lining of sound Portland cement concrete.

Walls, floors and underdrainage. The walls and floors of contact beds may suitably be constructed of concrete or brickwork. With regard to the floors, there should be sufficient fall from inlet to outlet to admit of the beds being effectively run off and drained. The drainage should be such as to allow the beds to drain thoroughly and to admit of proper aeration before they are re-filled. As a general rule, a few lines of longitudinal drains are laid in each bed, or channels are formed in the concrete covered by flat perforated tiles, and coarse material is laid over the drains for a depth of six inches to nine inches. It would seem preferable, however, to form the entire floors of drainage tiles such as are now specially manufactured for use in percolating filters, and whenever funds admit, this course should be adopted. This method would of course result in a larger volume of partially purified liquid being run off at the first opening of the outlet valves, which might be of importance where only single contact is given, but where the liquid receives a second or third contact before finally passing away, this would not be of much moment.

When only a few lines of drains are provided, their size and distance apart will depend upon the size of the contact material, together with its depth and the volume treated per cube yard per 24 hours ; the finer the material the greater should be the number of drains provided, to ensure the empty-ing of the bed within a reasonable period. A few methods of forming underdrains for contact beds are shown in Fig. 42.

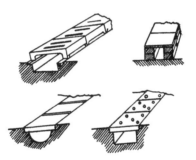

Fig. 42. Different types of underdrains.

It should, however, be borne in mind that the bulk of the work of purification by contact beds probably takes place when the bed is resting, nitrates being formed, and if the dis-tribution over the beds is good, these nitrates will assist in purifying the inflowing liquids, so that if the material is not coarse in grade, an appreciable degree of purification may be attained before the liquid reaches the floors and underdrains of the beds.

As a rough working guide it may be said that the depth of the underdrains plus the layer of coarse material immediately above them, should not exceed from $\frac{1}{5}$th to $\frac{1}{4}$th of the entire depth of the bed, thus ensuring that the first flush of liquid from the bed shall not exceed more than a small fraction of the entire liquid content of the bed.

To sum up, the main point to be borne in mind regarding floors and underdrains of contact beds, is that they must be constructed in such a manner as to permit of the liquid being drawn quickly and yet quietly from the beds, so that they may have the longest time practicable for resting. If the drawing off is too rapid, the result may be that the filtering material is disturbed, and if fine, some of it may be carried out of the beds, and caving in of the material will ultimately ensue.

Feed channels. As in the case of carriers for land treatment, feed channels should be so designed that they can be run completely dry when desirable. Further, it is useful, when satisfactory gaugings cannot well be made from the channel itself, to form a small chamber or basin at the commencement of the channel where gauging can be carried out, and this remark also applies to the feed channel of the secondary and tertiary beds, and the outlet channel of the tertiary bed. In certain cases it is advisable to interpose a small settling chamber or basin between the primary and secondary contact beds.

It is of importance to be able to gauge the flow of liquid from each individual contact bed independently from the rest, not only to ascertain its capacity from time to time, but also for the purpose of taking true average samples.

Inlet valves. Regarding inlet valves, the number of these will depend largely upon the size of the contact bed units; sluice valves or penstocks answer best. Disc valves are apt to become leaky in course of time ; iron and wooden hand sluices are not advisable, since more or less leakage generally takes place under and at the sides of the plates, and this leakage is increased when small pieces of gravel, coal, etc., become lodged in the bottom grooves in which the plates fit. A cross wall and penstock or sluice valve may be conveniently placed at the head of the inlet channel, so that positive measurements may be made of the capacity of the beds, which can be carried out as follows :—The channel is filled, the inlet valves to the bed having first been closed : when the channel is full, the sluice valve in the cross wall is closed, and the contents of the full channel drawn off into the bed, the process being repeated until the bed is filled up to a certain mark ; the capacity of the channel being known, and the number of times it was filled, the capacity of the bed can easily be worked out. It is often more convenient to provide this arrangement, than to construct the gauging chamber mentioned in the previous section.

Outlet valves. These can be similar to the inlet valves, and it is essential that they shall be capable of keeping free from any leakage when under a pressure of some four feet of water.

The number of outlet valves, as in the case of the inlets, will depend upon the size of the bed units, the size of contact material, and volume treated per cube yard per 24 hours.

Outlet valves should be placed, whenever practicable, in a position from which a sample from any individual bed can be drawn.

Contact materials. The essentials of a good contact material are that it shall be hard, durable, and possess a large surface area with a high percentage of voids when in position in the beds, further, that it shall be procurable at a moderate figure. When the material is broken up from the rough, it is important that it should break without much waste, and to a satisfactory cubical shape[1].

Very many materials have been employed at one time or another, such as clinkers, coke, coal, gravel, broken stone and brick, saggers, granite, quartzite, blast furnace slag, pan breeze, flints, etc.

The materials chiefly in use at the present day are hard furnace clinker and blast furnace coke, and when these are of the best they are probably as durable and efficient as any. The rougher and more irregular the surface of the material the better are the results obtained. Smooth beach gravel or

---

[1] Some materials break into flakes, which are certain to bind together closely in the beds, and lessen the interstices or voids.

shingle, for example, does not present nearly so great a surface area to the liquid to be purified as clinker or coke. This was found to be the case at Croydon, Birmingham, Hendon and elsewhere, and if a smooth material, such as gravel is used, a much larger total quantity of contact material will be required.

Burnt ballast has been used with success, but it requires very careful burning and screening, otherwise soft stuff is apt to creep in, and this speedily turns to a slurry.

Local circumstances must always play an important part in the selection of contact material, and if good gravel is found on the site of the proposed beds, it may be advisable to utilise this and to increase the total cubic content of the beds to make up for the lack of efficiency caused by the use of a smooth surfaced material.

The foregoing remarks concerning contact material apply with almost equal force to filtering material employed for percolating filters.

Careful experiments were carried out by Mr Creer, formerly City Engineer of York, on the relative merits of various materials for filtration purposes. A circular percolating filter seven feet eight inches deep was used for the experiment—four different materials—coke, clinker, slag, and broken bricks—of similar size in each case being used, the filter being filled in four sections or segments with the different material in each. The best results were obtained from the clinker segment, whilst almost similar effluents were obtained from the coke and slag segments, but not quite so good as the clinker segment; the effluent from the broken brick segment gave the lowest degree of purification; all four effluents were, however, of good quality.

Materials such as house cinders, unless a large local supply exists and the installation is a very small one, are quite unsuitable for contact material owing to their friable nature, and the deeper the bed, the greater is likely to be the disintegration which takes place.

Contact beds are often subjected to much walking on their surfaces, and this rapidly causes any non-durable matter to disintegrate and form "slurry." It must be borne in mind that there are wide variations in quality of clinkers, some being so soft as to be virtually useless, other qualities having too much lime in their composition, or other deleterious compounds. Hard, well-burnt destructor, boiler, or locomotive clinker, is generally the best, weighing in the rough from 17 cwt. to 20 cwt. per cubic yard. Such clinker, which was a drug in the market 20 years ago, has gone up considerably in price owing to the demand for it for contact and percolating filter installations, and good well-burnt clinker of about two inch gauge may cost anything from 2s. 6d. to 5s. per cubic yard free on rail. Since the contact material is by far the most costly item in a contact bed installation, it is very necessary to weigh all the factors before deciding upon any particular material. Some materials, such as saggars, owing to the limited thickness of the raw material, are best suited to filters or contact beds of fine material.

It should be noted here that roughness of material, especially in percolating filters, plays an important part in increasing the duration of contact, the unevenness of the material hindering the liquid from passing through the bed as rapidly as would occur with such material as smooth pebbles, gravel, etc., and this " duration of contact " also occurs to a limited extent when a contact bed is in process of being filled.

Grading of contact material. When contact beds first came into use, it was frequently the practice to grade the material into several sizes, but there appears to be little if any advantage in doing so, and the expense and labour incurred in grading are heavy. It has already been mentioned that rough material should be placed over the underdrains, and, in certain cases, where the tank settlement is not good fine[1] material may be used in a thin layer on the surface of the beds, or in the distribution channels, to arrest suspended matter passing away in the tank liquor, which would otherwise choke the bed. In the case of an entirely new plant, however, it will be found preferable to perfect the tank treatment and dispense with the fine material.

---

[1] When fine surfacing material is used an intermediate layer will be necessary between the coarse and fine material to prevent the fine material working into the coarser.

In any case, elaborate grading of the body of the contact material is unnecessary, and, as a matter of fact, unless the contact material is most carefully filled into the beds (and it is very difficult to get contractors to do this properly) after the rough stuff over the drains is in position, it will be found that the larger particles present generally roll down the face of the bank, and collect at or near the bottom of the beds.

Size of contact material. The finer the contact material, the larger is the combined surface area presented by all the particles, and other things being equal, the higher theoretically will be the purification obtained, owing to the intensified action on the sewage or tank liquor ; suspended matter being detained to a large extent, colloidal matter brought out of solution, and the duration of contact with the material lengthened. It is absolutely necessary, however, that air shall have free access to every part of a contact bed during the resting periods, and fine material is naturally more liable to clog than coarse, whilst contact beds composed of it take some time to fill, empty, and drain, and with very fine material capillary attraction tends to hold up the liquid in the material. There is therefore a limit to the degree of fineness which can safely be used in practice, this limit depending in great measure upon the quantity of suspended matter in the liquid that the beds are called upon to treat.

In the section dealing with washing of contact material, it will be seen that this is an expensive item, and with a liquid containing a given amount of suspended matter, the finer the material the more often, other things being equal, will washing be required. For this reason it is of importance that the size of the material should not be too small, and of late years the general tendency has been if anything to increase slightly the size of contact material in secondary beds, relying on final settlement of the effluent to remove solids which pass through the beds, and providing a tank liquor with a minimum of suspended solids for the beds to treat in the first place.

In America, where purification by means of contact beds has been rather consigned to the background, as in this country, the practice is to employ material of a rather coarser grade than is indicated theoretically, the main object being to avoid the heavy cost of frequent washing.

With regard to American practice it may be mentioned that the size of material recommended for the Plainfield contact material was about 1½ inch diameter, *i.e.* 1 inch to 2 inch.

If settling tanks were introduced between the various tiers of beds, as suggested in the section on settling of contact bed effluents, and a surface of fine material used on the beds, there is no question that much finer material could be employed for secondary and tertiary beds, but labour charges would be very greatly increased for attending to the surface of the beds, and removal and disposal of suspended matter.

Liquid capacity of contact beds. The capacity of a contact bed will vary within rather narrow limits according to the particular type of material employed, its size and form. Theoretically, the size of the material should make no difference to the liquid-holding capacity, but in practice it is found that it does affect the capacity to some extent, the liquid capacity of a bed filled with coarse or medium-sized material being greater than that of a bed filled with fine material.

Supposing an empty contact bed holds 100,000 gallons of liquid before the material is filled in: after the material has been placed in position, the liquid-holding capacity of the bed will drop to about 50,000 gallons; that is to say, the liquid content of a new contact bed of medium or coarse material will be about 50 per cent. of the empty bed or tank capacity; this will be the liquid capacity of the bed when first filled; after this first filling, however, settlement will occur, consolidating the material; and suspended matter entering the bed, capillary attraction, degradation of the material, and growth of spongy gelatinous matter on the material, will gradually reduce the capacity of the bed, and when it has become mature and in full working condition the capacity of 50 per cent. will be lowered to somewhere between 27 per cent. and 33 per cent. of the original water-holding capacity.

A cubic yard of empty tank will contain about 168·75 gallons of water, say 168 gallons; after the contact material is filled into the tank, this cubic yard will hold about 84 gallons, whilst when the cubic yard has got into working order, its water capacity will be reduced to about 30 per cent., say one-third of the original empty tank capacity (168 gallons), or, in round figures, 50 gallons, and this is the usual figure adopted in working practice.

The average working capacity of finer beds becomes somewhere about 40 per cent. of the empty tank capacity, since they usually receive less suspended matter than primary beds : it is, however, usual to take the capacity of primary, secondary and tertiary beds as being similar, thus allowing a margin of safety, so that one-third of the original empty tank capacity will be approximately the index of the liquid capacity of a contact bed filled with material.

Secondary beds composed of fine material might, as a matter of fact, be made smaller than primary beds, since with many installations the discharge of a primary bed is often insufficient to fill the corresponding secondary bed, and cases have occurred where two fillings of the primary contact bed have only just sufficed to fill the secondary bed ; this result, however, is generally due to the fact that the preliminary tank treatment is inefficient, or that the tanks need cleaning out oftener.

Size of contact bed units. This will depend upon a number of factors such as the configuration of the site, available fall, distribution, period of contact, etc.

For example, if the fall is such that contact beds only three feet deep can be put in, one and a half times the area will be required to obtain the same number of cubic yards as would be contained in beds four feet six inches deep ; further, more underdrains and outlets may be needed for the shallower beds. It is important to make the unit size of the beds as large as may be, without causing the beds to take an unduly long time to fill and empty, since division walls and extra valves and channels all cost money. Again, good distribution or the reverse will make a great deal of difference in the time taken to fill the bed. On an average, two hours contact and four hours rest, is a common cycle for contact beds, when the beds are filled three times daily. This means that the beds in dry weather will take one hour to fill and one hour to empty, or a total of two hours getting the sewage in and out of the bed, irrespective of the time it is left standing in the bed. If, therefore, the bed units are so designed that each one can be filled and emptied in from one to three hours three times a day, they will not be too large, but an increase in the volume treated per cube yard per 24 hours will mean that the number of fillings will have to be increased, and a decrease in capacity will have a like result. Since, however, in calculating the total number of cube yards of material, this total must be increased by 50 per cent.—to admit of the treatment of storm water up to three times the dry weather flow in wet weather—there will as a rule be margin enough to allow of cutting out and resting individual beds in dry weather.

The size of the works will largely affect the question of the size of the individual beds, and how many of the beds should be filled simultaneously. With a large works this is unavoidable, but in the case of small works it is generally convenient to send the whole of the sewage at any given time into the beds one after the other.

It is generally recognised that the largest economic area for contact bed units is about one acre ; beyond this size beds would take too long to fill and empty.

Depth of contact beds. This is a question which arises when the fall is ample, or when the sewage in any case must be pumped : otherwise it largely depends upon what the existing fall is. In connection with this point it may be observed that within certain limits, the depth of a contact bed (other things, such as size of material, etc., being equal) appears to make little difference to the efficiency of the contact material per cube yard ; but as has been already stated in the section upon underdrains, the coarse material at the bottom of the bed, together with the drains themselves, occupies from six inches to nine inches of the total depth of bed, and this particular stratum is probably less effective than the rest of the material. Hence it is not advisable that it should exceed from $\frac{1}{5}$th to $\frac{1}{4}$th of the entire depth of the material ; thus, taking the lower figures in each case, two feet six inches is indicated as about the minimum effective average depth for a contact bed, from surface level of material to invert of drains.

As a general rule it will be found that four feet or four feet six inches is a convenient depth for contact beds where sufficient fall exists ; in certain circumstances, however, where the fall is often extremely limited, as for example at seaside resorts on flat shores, a total depth including drains of as little as two feet six inches could be employed.

Distribution. This is a most important question in connection with contact beds, since it is required to fill them rapidly and at the same time quietly, and it is only by good and even distribution that the two things can be combined. If the distribution is good, the tank liquor will be evenly spread over the entire surface of the beds with very little smell, and not merely flushed on at one point, consequently the suspended solids will also be spread evenly over the surface of the beds, and kept at or near the surface, instead of being forced into the beds at one particular spot. Several methods of surface distribution are shown in Fig. 43.

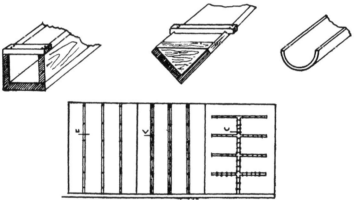

Fig. 43.   Different types of distribution.

At Manchester, shallow surface channels formed of fine clinkers are used.   At Burnley, a network of wooden troughs is employed, the troughs being partly buried in the surface of the beds, and excellent results have followed their use.

For small contact beds V-shaped wooden troughs or stoneware channel pipes may be used, and in some particular cases it may be advisable to place the distribution pipes just under the surface of the contact material.

When the flow of sewage is small and irregular, it is some-times of assistance to have a dosing tank, from which the beds can be charged in a reasonable time. Otherwise a bed may be slowly filling for hours, when the greater part of that time might be devoted to resting.

Dosing tanks consist of small tanks or chambers which fill up to a certain level with tank liquor, the capacity of the tank when such level is reached being sufficient to fill the bed ; the liquid is then discharged—usually by siphon—on to the beds. It may be observed that such dosing tanks require to be made capable of adjustment, so that when the original water-holding capacity of the beds becomes altered, they can be adjusted accordingly.

Filling and emptying of contact beds. It has been already mentioned, that the most usual method of working contact beds in this country, assuming three fillings a day, is to allot one hour to filling, two hours to standing full, one hour to emptying and four hours rest. It by no means follows, however, that this method is suitable to all kinds of tank liquors, and no rule can be formulated applicable to all cases. In certain instances, short contacts and long intervals of rest may be advisable ; for example, in the case of a strong sewage, it is worse than useless to permit the liquid to remain in the bed after the avail-able oxygen supply has been depleted, since the bulk of evidence goes to show that it is when contact beds are standing empty (or " resting ") that the various biological, chemical and phy-sical actions are at their height.

A point which is likely to occur in the case of new contact bed installations may be mentioned here. Whilst the house drains are being connected up to the sewers, the flow of sewage will be small and irregular, and insufficient in all probability to even fill one of the bed units. In such cases the bed should receive the same treatment as if it were really full ; *i.e.* the bed should not be allowed to take two or three days to fill but should be run off at once when its proper time arrives.

Recent practice, both in this country and in America, tends to giving much shorter contacts (say 15 to 30 minutes) than was usual when contact beds first came into use.

Automatic gear. Of recent years improvements have been made in automatic gear for filling and emptying contact beds, and, where the sewage works is a small one, the installation of filling and emptying gear reduces labour to a minimum and ensures regular working, but it must be clearly understood that at least one visit a day to the works by the man in charge is essential, in case anything should go wrong, and it is quite impossible to do away entirely with a certain amount of personal attention. Automatic gear is somewhat liable to get out of order, and is, as a rule, expensive to repair should any breakage occur.

With regard to large works, automatic gear is not so useful, as there are always men at hand to attend to the filling and emptying of the contact beds, and automatic gear in such cases would effect no saving in labour.

Most automatic gears are not adapted to variations in the sewage flow and its character, and to the gradual loss of capacity in the beds; and further, the drainings which continue after the bed has been discharged often collect at the bottom of the bed, and impair aeration during the resting period.

If automatic gear is used, it is absolutely essential that the beds should be constructed in a water-tight manner.

It is not proposed to give any figures of the many types of gear used at the present day, reference should be made for these to the various makers' catalogues.

Maturing or ripening of contact beds. It is important to note that contact beds in common with percolating filters, take some time to ripen before the material becomes coated with slimy growths, and before they begin to yield really satisfactory results. The period would seem to depend most of all upon temperature, together with the character of the sewage, time of year, mode of operation and other factors.

Contact beds treating sewages containing certain trade wastes, such as gas liquor, and acid wastes, take longer to mature than those dealing with a purely domestic sewage. It must be borne in mind that the contents of a contact bed changes from day to day after the first filling, fresh additions of suspended matter being carried on to the bed daily; some of this

TABLE XXVI. *Showing practicable rates of tr*

	Strong Sewage (Strength 160—230) absorbing 17–25 pts. per 100,000 of oxygen from $\frac{N}{8}$ permanganate in 4 hours at 27° C.					Average Sewage (Strength 100) from $\frac{N}{8}$ perma
Preliminary tank treatment		Strength of liquid to be treated by contact	Suspended solids in tank liquor in parts per 100,000	Rate of treatment per cubic yard in gallons per 24 hours	Number of (a) contacts „ „ (b) fillings per day	Preliminary tank treatment
Chemical precipitation with 2 hours quiescent settlement		90	2–5	43	(a) Double (b) $2\frac{1}{2}$	Chemical precipitatio with 2 hours quiescen settlement ..
Chemical precipitation with 8 hours continuous flow settlement ..		95–100	8	33	(a) Double (b) 2	Chemical precipitatio with 8 hours contin ous flow settlement
Quiescent settlement for 2 hours		100–105	10	27	(a) Triple[1] (b) 4	Quiescent settlement fo 2 hours .. ..
Continuous flow settlement for 15 hours ..		120	15–20	20	(a) Triple (b) 3	Continuous flow settl ment for 15 hours
Septic tank liquor ..		130	15–20	20	(a) Triple (b) 3	Septic tank liquor

[1] This rate of treatment per cube y

ent per cubic yard of various tank liquors.

ng 10-12 pts. per 100,000 of oxygen in 4 hours at 27° C.

Weak Sewage (Strength 60) absorbing 7-8 parts per 100,000 of oxygen from $\frac{N}{8}$ permanganate in 4 hours at 27° C.

...of liquor to be treated by contact	Suspended solids in tank liquor in parts per 100,000	Rate of treatment per cubic yard in gallons per 24 hours	No. of (a) contacts ,, (b) fillings per day	Preliminary tank treatment	Strength of liquor to be treated by contact	Suspended solids in tank liquor in parts per 100,000	Rate of treatment per cubic yard in gallons per 24 hours	Number of (a) contacts ,, (b) fillings per day
	1-4	100	(a) Single (b) 3	Chemical precipitation with 2 hours quiescent settlement	30	1-3	133	(a) Single[1] (b) 4
	3-6	53	(a) Double (b) 3	Chemical precipitation with 2 hours continuous flow settlement	30-35	2-5	133	(a) Single[1] (b) 4
	5-8	53	(a) Double (b) 3	Quiescent settlement for 2 hours	40	4-6	100	(a) Single (b) 3
	10-15	33	(a) Double (b) 2	Continuous flow settlement for 15 hours	45	7-8	66	(a) Double[1] (b) 4
	10-15	33	(a) Double (b) 2	Septic tank liquor	45	7-8	66	(a) Double[1] (b) 4

...ld not be doubled in wet weather.

is bound to reach the body of the material, and since it is not all decomposed, it tends to modify the nature of the material. As contact beds become mature, so the temperature of the body of the bed rises, by reason of the decomposition increasing, and this, assuming efficient underdrainage, causes diffusion of air throughout the beds.

It may be mentioned that during the experiments with percolating filters carried out by the Commission at Dorking, shallow filters of fine grade material were constructed, the material employed being the coarse material from the old deep percolating filters broken to fine grade, whilst tank liquor was employed to wash the material. The fine shallow filters constructed of this material yielded good effluents almost from the day they were set to work.

Limit of rates of treatment per cube yard. The rate at which tank liquor can be dealt with per cubic yard by contact beds depends upon the character and strength of the tank liquor, the suspended solids it contains, size of contact material, size and number of bed units, and also the type of effluent which is wanted to satisfy local conditions.

Table XXVI is compiled from statistics given in the Fifth Report of the Sewage Disposal Commission, and shows the rates of treatment per cube yard at which it is practicable to treat various tank liquors, together with system of contact, number of bed fillings, etc.

It is assumed in this table that both primary, secondary and tertiary beds are constructed of equal capacity. It should be noted that the figures given in the "rate of treatment" column, allow for dealing with sewage and storm water up to three times the dry weather flow; thus, to arrive at the total quantity of material needed for a particular volume of sewage—either strong, average or weak—the dry weather flow of sewage should be divided by the rate of treatment selected, and the result will be the total cubic content of contact medium required. When land is used for final treatment of the contact effluents, the rates of treatment given in the table might reasonably be reduced in certain circumstances.

In the greater number of cases met with in practice, double

contact will be needed, since single contact will only produce a good effluent when the sewage in question is weak, and after it has received good preliminary treatment.

For sewages of average strength, containing much suspended matter, double contact will be requisite to ensure a good effluent, and triple contact will be needed for strong sewages.

In America it is a general practice to treat daily some 600,000 gallons per acre of contact bed, four to five feet deep, which works out to about 93 gallons per cube yard with beds four feet deep, to 74 gallons per cube yard with five foot beds. Taking into account the weakness of most American sewages as compared with English, this is a somewhat lower rate of treatment than is usually adopted in this country for sewages of average strength.

Single, double and triple contact. There is occasionally some misconception as to the rate of treatment by double and triple contact, and as the matter is somewhat involved, a few words of explanation may be advisable.

It has already been shown that a cubic yard of medium or coarse material will hold about 50 gallons of liquid : with single contact then, and one filling a day, the rate of treatment must be 50 gallons per cube yard per day With double contact and one filling per day, twice the quantity of material used for single contact will be required, and therefore the rate of treatment will be decreased by half, being 25 gallons ($\frac{50}{2}$) per cube yard per day; similarly, with triple contact and one filling per day, three times the amount of contact material will be needed, and the rate of treatment will drop to about 17 gallons ($\frac{50}{3}$).

By increasing the number of daily fillings given to the beds, the volumes of liquid treated per cube yard are proportionately increased, as shown in the following tabular statement.

TABLE XXVII. *Showing rate of treatment per cube yard by single, double and triple contact.*

Rate of treatment per 24 hours in gallons per cube yard

	One filling per day	Two fillings per day	Three fillings per day	Four fillings per day
Single Contact	50	100	150	200
Double ,,	25	50	75	100
Triple ,	17	34	50	66

The expression two and a half fillings per day does not mean that a particular bed was filled twice, and then half-filled during the 24 hours, but that the bed was resting for part of the period over which the fillings were recorded : thus, this would occur in the case of a bed taking three fillings a day over a period of 12 days, including two days' rest : the total number of fillings in this case would be $3 \times (12 - 2) = 30$, and 30 divided by $12 = 2\frac{1}{2}$, which is the daily average number of fillings.

Loss of capacity in contact beds. This occurs sooner or later with all contact beds, and has been a serious stumbling-block to their more general adoption by towns. The finer the material, other things being equal, the more rapid is this loss of capacity.

For purposes of discussion, the dominant causes producing loss of capacity may be classified as follows :

Amount of suspended and colloidal matter present in the liquid treated in the beds.

Rate of treatment per cube yard.

Consolidation of contact material.

Disintegration of contact material.

Ineffective drainage and aeration.

Capillary action.

Want of rest.

Growth of organisms.

Amount of suspended and colloidal matter in liquid treated by beds. As would naturally be anticipated, when the suspended solids in the liquid treated on the beds, are not kept at the surface by fine material and removed at intervals, but gain access to the body of the bed, the loss of capacity is, roughly speaking, proportionate to the quantity and character of suspended solids it receives. It has long been an established fact that primary beds lose capacity far more rapidly than secondary beds, and conclusive evidence to this effect was given before the Sewage Disposal Commission. The reason is not far to seek, since primary beds receive the brunt of the work in the form of suspended solids, and probably in addition a certain amount of colloidal matter has been removed from the tank liquor in its passage through the primary bed.

The character of the suspended solids will influence the rate of clogging up ; for example, when they are of a slimy nature, it is difficult to put a contact bed out of action long enough to allow such matter to dry out.

It is said that precipitation liquor contains less colloidal matter than other tank liquors, and it may be observed that in the case of the Kingston-on-Thames contact beds, and the Roscoe experimental beds at Manchester, precipitation liquor containing very few suspended solids being treated by the beds in both instances, the capacity of the beds, after reaching an equilibrium, was retained for a long period.

Colloidal solids. There can be no question that a considerable loss of capacity results from the deposition of colloidal matter in the beds. Colloidal matter consists of exceedingly fine matter lying between matter in solution and matter in suspension, and it appears probable that it is originally derived in great measure from soap. After colloidal matter is brought into contact with mature contact or filtering medium, it comes into suspension, and a portion of it is therefore frequently held up in the bed.

If an effluent perfectly free from suspended matter but opalescent in tint, is left at rest for several days, quite a large amount of brown flocculent matter will be found to have settled at the foot of the bottle, whilst the opalescence has vanished or nearly so.

From what has been said it will be seen that it is often a waste of money to provide sand filters[1] some three feet deep to treat a contact or percolation effluent, because some of the colloidal matter may not come into suspension for hours after the effluent has left the sand bed, and very little more than mechanical straining takes place, which could just as easily be secured at far less outlay by sand straining filters nine inches or a foot in depth.

Rate of treatment per cube yard. The volume of liquid passed into a contact bed is bound to influence its capacity, since the greater the volume of liquid treated per cube yard of

[1] Such filters are sometimes wrongly worked in a water-logged condition, and then merely effect a mechanical straining.

contact material, the less time remains for the draining of the bed after emptying. This might not be of great importance in a new bed of medium to coarse-sized material, which had not become " filmed " with growth, but in the case of a matured contact bed, the material of which has become filmed or covered with gelatinous growths, it is often of considerable importance, especially if the bed is composed of fine material.

Further, it is clear that, other things being equal, the greater the rate of treatment per cube yard of contact material, the greater will be the amount of suspended matter passing on to the beds. For example, if a bed with one filling a day receives at each filling, say, one pound of suspended matter, then with three fillings it will receive three times as much.

Provided the preliminary tank treatment is efficient, contact beds can be worked for short periods at considerably higher rates per cube yard than the normal, but these periods of high rate of working should not recur too frequently.

Consolidation of contact material. This may result from a variety of causes, of which perhaps that most commonly met with is due to settlement of the bed, and this in turn is sometimes due to too great inequality of size of material, but often, particularly in the case of fine beds, to the motion caused amongst the material by the liquid entering the bed at each filling. It may be mentioned here that coke, owing to its buoyant nature, is apt to shift considerably from time to time, and, in the case of the large experimental contact beds used at Barking, the late Mr Santo Crimp employed a three inch surfacing of gravel to weight the coke down, and thus counteract its tendency to float. It should be remembered that in a contact bed some four or five feet deep there is a considerable weight on the lower layers of material, and some kinds of material, such as slag and clinker, cannot stand being constantly walked upon, and it is difficult to fork up the surface of beds when required. At Birmingham, Mr Watson has found that it takes the men more than twice the time to fork over the surface of a slag bed, as to deal with a bed of quartzite similarly.

In the Leeds experiments it was found that a contact bed composed of $\frac{1}{8}$ inch to $\frac{3}{8}$ inch furnace clinker, treating septic tank liquor, had its capacity reduced in less than six months from 29,500 gallons to 10,700 gallons, even although the material lying beneath the top two inches was still comparatively clean. After resting for six weeks, and turning over the material, the capacity was found to be 26,900 gallons. Similar results were observed during the treatment of precipitation liquor in a contact bed filled with five inch to one inch material. After a little over seven months work at three fillings a day, the capacity of the bed had fallen from 55,700 gallons to 21,600 gallons, and in this case also the material beneath the top few inches was found to be fairly clean, but much consolidated. The conclusion drawn from the experiments was that the loss of capacity in both cases was in great measure due to consolidation of rather fine material of uneven size.

Disintegration of contact material. This may result, as has already been stated, from the use of soft friable material, materials of unsuitable size, settlement of beds due to filling and emptying processes, walking on the surface of the beds, etc.

The amount of disintegration will vary according to the size and character of the material employed. When a bed comes to be washed, the amount of new screened material required to make the bed up to the original level gives a rough idea of the amount of disintegration which has occurred. It will, however, be somewhat less than this, since part of the old material on re-screening will go to waste, even if it is of the right size. If the section on washing of contact material be referred to (p. 242) it will be seen that the waste material, after about four years' use in the beds, amounts to about 25 per cent. on an average.

Ineffective drainage and aeration. Every effort should be made to secure free aeration and drainage, and contact beds would probably give better results if the floor of each bed were formed of aerating tiles after the manner of percolating filters : this has been actually done in several instances in American practice.

As regards aeration, if the beds are properly constructed of suitably-sized durable material, and with good underdrainage, the emptying and filling of the beds will, together with the action of the filmed matter, secure ample aeration and diffusion of gases.

The quicker a bed is drained the longer is the period available for rest, which is all-important.

Capillary action. This may result either from the use of too small a material, or, as more frequently happens, from this cause combined with the entry of suspended matter into the beds, causing clogging. When this occurs, the beds never become thoroughly drained off, and although an evaporation zone may exist for the first few inches of material downwards, the body of the bed will always be in a water-logged condition.

Want of rest. This will be discussed under the heading of resting of contact beds (p. 242).

Growth of organisms. If a contact bed is to perform its work efficiently, a certain amount of film or growth is necessary on the surface of the material, and the same remark applies to percolating filters. This film has been shown by Dr Dunbar, Dr Fowler and others, to possess the property of absorbing oxygen and liberating carbon dioxide to a marked degree.

As to the extent of the growths in contact filters, a good deal seems to depend upon the character of the sewage which is being treated. Domestic sewages containing much subsoil water appear to produce this jelly-like matter far more abundantly than strong domestic sewages or sewages containing trade refuse of certain kinds. Old brick sewers and manholes which admit large quantities of subsoil water, will often be found coated with a slimy gelatinous growth, frequently an inch or so in thickness.

A growth of quite another nature is sometimes to be found growing on the surface of contact beds in the form of algae closely resembling a miniature growth of *Ulva latissima*. Such a growth covered the beds at Harrow in the year 1913; the name of the alga being *Prasiola crispa*.

In the chapter upon percolating filters, suggestions are given for the removal of various growths from filters when they become excessive, by the use of various chemicals (p. 279).

Resting of contact beds. When the liquid content of a bed becomes materially reduced, the bed must be thrown out of action and allowed a period of rest, varying from a few days to as much as a fortnight, according to the condition of the bed. Care must be taken when giving rest, that the film on the material does not dry up in the body of the bed, otherwise a bad effluent will result; accordingly, rest should be given to the beds before they have become seriously clogged, since the greater the clogging, the longer will be the rest required to regain capacity. All outlet valves should be left open when a bed is drying, to facilitate the draining away of liquid imprisoned within the bed.

This gain of capacity consequent upon resting, it should be observed, is usually only temporary, and the regained capacity generally becomes less and less shortly after each successive rest, until it becomes essential to remove, wash, and replace the material.

At the Hampton Sewage Works, a primary bed commencing work with a liquid capacity of about 43,000 gallons, after being worked for about twelve months, had this figure reduced to some 8,600 gallons. After a fortnight's rest this figure had risen to about 13,000 gallons.

Time beds are out of use. A point which should be borne in mind when designing an installation, either of contact beds or percolating filters, is that the beds in both cases will be resting and therefore out of action for a good many days in the year. It would appear at first sight that the amount of time lost in this manner might be neglected, being so small, but if careful records are kept of bed fillings and restings for repairs, regaining of capacity, etc., it will be seen that the total time a bed is out of use in any one year is by no means negligible.

Washing contact material. This is an operation which sooner or later has to be carried out at most contact bed installations, and it should be noted that this expense rarely occurs with percolating filters.

As a general rule it is advisable to remove and wash the material when the water-holding capacity of the beds after proper resting periods fails to recover more than about 20 per

TABLE XXVIII. *Showing co*

Material washe

Place	Character of liquid treated by the beds	Average amount of suspended matter in liquid going on to beds. pts. per 100,000	Time beds had been in use	Nature and size of material	Quantity of material dealt with (cube yds.)
Burnley ..	Septic tank liquor	5–6	$3\frac{1}{2}$ yrs.	Clinker ($\frac{1}{8}''$ to $\frac{1}{2}''$)	3350
Manchester ..	Do.	5–6	4–5 yrs.	Clinker (medium coarse)	A very larg quantity
Birmingham..	Do.	—	4 yrs.	Clinker and coke (fairly coarse)	20,000
Averages	—	—	4 yrs.	—	—

Material wa:

Hampton ..	Crude sewage	48·5	2–4 yrs.	Clinker (medium to coarse)	260
S. Norwood ..	Screened ,,	not known	4 yrs.	Burnt ballast (medium to coarse)	1640
Beddington ..	Septic tank liquor		$3\frac{3}{4}$ yrs.	Flint and clinker (coarse)	15,377
Andover ..	,, ,,	$11\cdot10^5$	4 yrs.	Clinker ($\frac{1}{2}''$ size free from dust)	49C
Leeds ..	—	—	—	—	102C
Averages	—	—	about 4 yrs.	—	—

d by machinery.

Cost per cube yd., of operations, including making beds up to original level with new material, but excluding cost of washing plant and maintenance charges on same	Cost per acre 3 ft. deep, of washing operations, including making beds up to original level with new material, but excluding cost of washing plant and maintenance charges on same	Percentage of original material replaced in beds	Cost per cube yard of new material to make up to original level	Remarks
s. d.	£ s. d.			
1 0	242 0 0	60 %	—	—
1 6²	363 0 0	70 %–75 %	½"–2" 2s. 6d.–3s. over 2" 3s. –3s. 6d.¹	[1] Delivered in beds [2] Final disposal of rejected material not included in this figure
2 2½	534 0 0	80 %	6s. 6d.³	[3] New material—broken stones
1 6¾	380 0 0	71·25	—	

shed by hand.

2 6¾	620 0 0	Primary beds 75 % Secondary ,, 65 %	—	[3] Including cost of plant
1 6	363 0 0	—	—	
1 2½	292 0 0	No appreciable loss with flints	—	
2 4⁵	564 0 0⁴	—	—	[5] Based on the 3 sets of average samples taken in October, 1904
2 5	584 0 0	—	—	
2 0	£484 12 0	—	—	

cent. of its original water capacity. The washed material, if of good quality to start with, will perform its work all the better for the washing, since the bad material tends to become eliminated in the washing process. Further, the beds will not take nearly so long to mature as when new, and in hot weather they will commence to give good results shortly after being put to work again. If plenty of new material is at hand free of cost, as is sometimes the case with very small installations, it is occasionally more economical entirely to throw aside the old material and to replace all of it with new ; in this case, however, the beds will need to be matured in the usual way. The cost of washing naturally varies according to local conditions, and it must be noted that as a rule about 25 per cent. of the old material, largely owing to degradation, will need to be renewed. Table XXVIII., taken from the Fifth Report of the Sewage Disposal Commission, gives the cost of washing contact material at various places.

From this table it will be observed that the cost of washing large quantities of material by machinery averages 1s. 6¾d. (*i.e.* 1s. to 2s. 2½d.) per cube yard, or about £380 per acre three feet deep once every four years, or £95 yearly, and that washing becomes necessary on the average after four years' use. The period must of necessity depend upon several more or less variable factors, such as preliminary tank treatment, size and nature of material, method of working the beds, etc., but, apart from disintegration, the most important factor is the amount of suspended matter passing on to the beds, and it may therefore be said that the period for which the beds will last without washing will vary in inverse ratio to the amount of suspended solids retained in the beds.

Regarding the cost of washing contact material abroad, Fuller[1] mentions that at the Plainfield (U.S.A.) installation, the main body of contact material loses about 50 % of its original capacity after about 4 to 5 years' use, when it is found best to remove and clean the material. Under the conditions obtaining at Plainfield, this costs about 2s. 6d. per cubic yard.

Upward filling of contact beds. This has been tried in several instances, but it is a method which cannot be recommended

---

[1] *Sewage Disposal.*

with most tank liquors, although little smell is produced when the beds are filled in this manner. Any suspended matter which there may be in the tank liquor, settles on the floors and in the drains and lower strata of material, and it is very difficult to remove from such places. The distribution pipes are also difficult to reach for cleaning purposes. With downward filling a much better chance is offered of removing clogging suspended matter when occasion arises, or, the top 12 inches or so of material can be entirely removed, washed, and replaced. If there is really serious risk of smell during the filling of contact beds, the distribution pipes or troughs may be placed a few inches beneath the material : in this case the distributing channels will either have to be perforated pipes, open jointed pipes, or covered rectangular troughs perforated with large holes at intervals. In the majority of such particular cases where the sewage, by reason of its nature, is likely to cause smell, preliminary chemical precipitation would appear to be advisable, followed by distribution over the contact beds from the top downwards in the usual way.

Streaming of contact beds. This process consists in allowing the liquid to run or stream freely through the beds, and it has the effect of washing out considerable quantities of suspended solids from the beds, especially if the streaming is carried on in storm times. As a rule, when contact beds are streamed, the outlet valves are left open, the liquid passing through the beds; but they are sometimes constructed with an overflow at the foot of each bed, so that if a storm occurs at night time, when no attendant is present, the liquid in the primary beds, after filling them, passes by the overflows to the secondary beds.

It would appear that the purification obtained by streaming is mostly mechanical straining, and when the beds come to be used in the normal cycle, the lack of rest to the beds is apt to result in an indifferent effluent.

Sludge removed from surface of contact beds. The quantity of sludge removed by hand labour from the surface of contact beds, especially when it is retained by fine surface material, often amounts to a considerable item in the year's working, both in expense of removal and disposal.

At Hampton, Middlesex, for example, when the triple contact system was in use for the treatment of crude sewage, a quantity equivalent to about 350 tons of 90 per cent. wet sludge was removed annually from the surface of the primary beds.

At Plainfield, U.S.A. Fuller[1] states that the quantity of scum raked from the surface of the primary beds, amounted in 1909–10 to about ·5 cubic yard per million gallons of sewage treated, the sewage at Plainfield being subjected to preliminary treatment by screening and septic tanks before contact.

Settling of contact bed effluents.   Effluents from single and double contact beds generally contain rather large amounts of suspended solids, and it is important that these should be removed before the effluent leaves the works, since they are almost invariably putrescible.   Removal can be carried out in several ways, either by settling tanks[2] of the Dortmund type, by shallow straining or sand filters (cf. Chap. VIII, p. 274), or by land treatment.   In the former case a settling or "humus" tank having a capacity equal to about two hours' dry weather flow of sewage will usually be found sufficient.   With shallow straining filters nine inches to 12 inches in depth a high rate of filtration can be adopted—say 500 gallons per square yard, provided that the straining filters are duplicated, and that the surfaces are properly attended to.

Apart from the settling out of the suspended solids, a settling tank effects a most useful work, by equalising the discharges from contact beds.   When a contact bed discharge valve is first opened, the issuing liquid is almost invariably turbid and putrescible ; as the discharge continues, so the purity of the effluent being discharged increases until the finish, when the last drainings often reach a high degree of purification.   This is one of the greatest drawbacks to a contact bed installation, and it is most important that the integral parts of each bed discharge should be mixed and equalised.

When tertiary beds of fine material are employed, the suspended solids are generally small in amount and finely

[1] *Sewage Disposal.*
[2] A small dose of precipitant could be added, as was done by Mr Newton at Accrington, where a small addition of alumino-ferric to the unsettled effluent, before entering the effluent settling tanks, brought about good results.

divided, and if it is deemed necessary to remove them, sand filtration effects a better removal than simple settlement, and filtration can proceed at a high rate per yard super, since only mechanical straining out of the solids is sought.   It would seem advisable in the case of triple contact to interpose settling or humus tanks between the three tiers of beds where sufficient space can be spared for the purpose ; this would save the labour required for removing solids from time to time from the surface of the fine tertiary beds.   Concerning the design of effluent settling tanks, the rectangular tank with conical bottom, designed by Mr J. D. Watson, has given good results at Birmingham with percolating filter effluents, and seems to be as suitable as any form.   The amount of suspended matter removed from contact effluents by settlement is a variable amount ; very approximately about five cwt. of dry solids may be expected per 1,000,000 gallons of effluent.

It may be noted here that the suspended solids, issuing in the effluent from percolating filters, require treatment for their removal in a similar manner to contact bed effluents.

Artificial aeration of contact bed effluents. Contact bed effluents are frequently deficient in aeration, and if the levels admit of it, a series of steps in the effluent channel, causing a miniature cascade at each step, will be found very beneficial. Other methods which can be applied, but which are somewhat costly, are different forms of air lift worked by compressed air.

Flies and worms on contact beds. As a general rule contact beds may be said to be free from swarms of flies and other insects, and in this respect they offer a marked contrast to percolating filters, which during certain seasons of the year swarm with insect life.   Insects resembling *Podura aquatica* occur freely on the surface of contact beds, but these are not noxious insects.   Worms of various species often form the greater portion of the higher forms of life found in contact beds, but a dose of some trade waste, such as gas liquor, will drive them out on to the surface material.

During the normal working of a contact bed, these worms will be found mainly in the upper surface of the material, where they live amongst the peaty-like matter which accumulates there in course of time. It would appear doubtful whether as a whole these worms are habitually in contact with the liquor in the beds, or whether the burrows they form in the exceedingly fine humus ever become saturated, unless the contact is unusually prolonged[1]. When the bed is empty and resting, especially at night time, the worms probably leave their haunts for a short distance to feed upon vegetable matter after the manner of the common lobworm, and at such times, if matter injurious to worms was present in the beds, they would get the full benefit of it. It seems quite possible that the burrows formed by the worms may be of some assistance in holding up oxygen in contact beds, and also in rendering organic debris assimilable by smaller forms of larval life, and also by microbes.

Smell from contact beds. On the whole, given proper management, it may be said that the treatment of sewage in contact beds is remarkably free from smell once the sewage is in the beds, and with upward filling of the beds there is still less. When septic tank liquor is being treated there is apt to be smell from the feed channels, and also from the primary beds when they are discharging, but this can be greatly lessened by providing movable covers to the channels, so that as little as possible of the liquid is exposed to the air. Frequently, it will be found that when contact beds are first put in operation smell arises, but as the beds become mature it gradually diminishes. There can be no doubt that contact beds are less liable to cause nuisance from smell than percolating filters, where almost every particle of the tank liquor is freely exposed to the air.

When an exceedingly strong liquid is being treated in the vicinity of houses, it is sometimes advisable to treat it in the first instance by means of contact beds to eliminate risk of nuisance from smell, afterwards subjecting the effluent to treatment by percolating filters, in order to ensure a proper degree of oxidation.

---

[1] If the contact is a prolonged one, worms rise in numbers to the surface of the beds, and lie on the material which is above the water level.

Contact bed effluent temperatures. It may be interesting to give a diagram (Fig. 44) showing the mean monthly temperatures of atmosphere and effluent taken over a period of one year from contact beds at Hartley Wintney. It will be seen that the effluent during the colder months of the year is several degrees warmer than the temperature of the air. The diagram should be compared with the one given on page 204, having reference to land effluents, and also with that on page 286, where air and effluent temperatures are given relating to a percolating filter installation (Buxton).

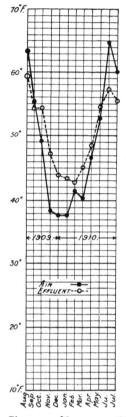

Fig. 44. Mean monthly temperatures of air and contact bed effluent at Hartley Wintney.

Cost of contact beds. The cost of contact beds depends upon a number of local circumstances, any one of which may affect the cost considerably, quite apart from the great variety in the general design of beds, and price of the ironwork used for inlet and outlet valves, system of underdrainage, etc. Again, if automatic filling and emptying gear is used, the variety in type and cost is endless. The cost of the contact medium will be the chief item, and if constructed on suitable "side-lying" ground, and good durable material can be obtained locally at a reasonable price, and gravel suitable for concrete obtained on the site, contact beds constructed in such circumstances may cost over a third less than where the local conditions are unfavourable in these respects. Again, the depth of beds and the size of the installation are important factors, small installations costing proportionately more than large areas of contact beds. No standard figures of cost, therefore, can be given, since these must vary with each installation, it may be said, however, that in all but a very few cases, where conditions are specially favourable, a contact bed installation to treat, say, 50,000 gallons of sewage per 24 hours, will cost considerably more than a percolating filter plant capable of dealing with a similar flow, both as regards initial capital outlay, and also in respect of working expenses, which latter will be touched upon shortly.

As a very approximate guide it may be observed that the cost of constructing contact beds may vary from 15s. to 25s. per cubic yard inclusive, according to local conditions, as against about 12s. to 20s. in the case of percolating filters.

At Hampton, the original installation consisted of triple contact beds, treating in 1904 a·daily flow of about 180,000 gallons of crude sewage derived from a population of 6500. The works consisted of three tiers of beds, having a total area of 3373 yards and a cubic content of 4195 yards, the beds in each tier being four feet deep, the floors and walls being constructed of cement concrete.

The underdrainage in each case consisted of 16 lines of three inch agricultural pipes connected up to a main drain at the foot of each bed. The primary bed material consisted of boiler furnace clinker over one inch, ·the average size being four inches in diameter. The secondary material was similar in character, but ranged in size from ¼ inch to one inch, whilst the tertiary bed material was composed of clinker under ¼ inch including dust. The material cost 2s. 6d. per cube yard on the works, and 6s. to 7s. 6d. in position in the beds.

Distribution was effected in the case of the secondary beds mainly by half pipes laid herring-bone fashion, whilst in the case of the tertiary beds it was carried out by means of grips cut in the fine material : there was no distribution in the case of the primary beds.

The total capital outlay on the works was as follows :

	£	s.	d.
Land	3500	0	0
Buildings	2296	3	3
Contact beds	2970	2	7
Engine boilers, ejectors, air receivers and condensers	7302	16	1
Total £16069		1	11

As regards American practice, Fuller[1] gives the cost of contact beds as being from about £3000 to £7000 per acre, the cost depending upon amount of excavation, size and design of filter units, and cost in place of contact material. Where false bottoms are used and the beds are about 5 feet deep, arranged as primary and secondary beds and with at least three complete sets of units, the ordinary cost is stated to be about £7000 per acre.

Cost of working contact beds. The question of the initial cost of contact beds can scarcely be dissociated from the cost of working them, maintenance and loan charges, etc. Here again, working charges are as a rule heavier than would be the case with percolating filters, this being largely due to heavy charges incurred by washing of the contact material from time to time. Again, it will often be found that where the cost of running contact beds taken by itself appears to be unusually low, the figures of the cost for the preliminary process are high, and that the cost of sludge disposal is higher than usual; in other words, the capacity of the contact beds has been maintained by efficient and costly tank treatment, the washing of contact material having been avoided thereby. In any case, where comparisons are made between the cost of various processes, the figures compared should, if practicable, be based on an average of several years, and it is of great importance in comparing any processes to pay particular attention to the strength of the liquid treated, and the quality of the effluent produced. In many cases where the cost of working contact beds has been heavy, the beds have been altered to percolating filters, the cross walls of several units having been removed and travelling distributors installed.

The figures of cost in the case of the Manchester sewage works (contact beds) may be given as typical of a very large works: it must, however, be recollected that the Manchester sewage is not a strong one.

The following figures give the average for five years ending March, 1913 :

						Cost per millon gallons (exclusive of interest and repayment of loan)	
						s.	d.
Sludge	..	..	..	..	..	11	4·9
Filtration ..	..	..	..	..	..	17	7·7
General expenses		..	..	..	..	9	5·4
Coal	..	..	..	..	..	1	9·3
			Total	£2	0		3·3[2]

Cost per head of population, pence 10·7

[1] *Sewage Disposal.*
[2] For the year ending March 26, 1924, the cost was £3 19s. 2.4d.

The average annual cost per head of population for·maintenance, including interest and repayment of loan for the same period, was 1s. 10d. (calculated at five per cent. on total capital outlay to date)

In terms of per million gallons this would be equivalent to £4. 2s. 10d.

The writer is indebted to Dr Fowler for the foregoing figures relating to Manchester.

At Exeter—septic tanks and single contact—the cost of treating the sewage in 1905, excluding the cost of subsequent land treatment, based on the dry weather flow, amounted to about £3 per million gallons of sewage, the total cost per head of the population draining to the works being about 10½d. These figures are inclusive of loan charges in respect of capital outlay on works.

At Hampton, Middlesex, the total cost for the year 1904 of treating the sewage per million gallons by triple contact, inclusive of loan charges in respect of capital outlay, and based on the actual quantity treated, was about £8, the cost per head being about 1s. 8d.

At Plainfield, U.S.A., Fuller[1] states that the total cost of maintenance for the year 1910 was about £680, which, with an average daily flow of 1·7 million gallons American, gives a cost of about 22s. per million gallons of sewage treated.

Single contact beds treating septic tank liquor can be seen at Exeter ; double contact of septic tank liquor at Burnley, Manchester, Andover, and Berkhamsted; triple contact of septic tank liquor at Sawbridgeworth.

BIBLIOGRAPHY.

Dunbar. *Principles of Sewage Treatment.* Griffin and Co., Ltd., London (1910).

Fuller, G. W. *Sewage Disposal.* McGraw-Hill Book Company, London and New York (1913).

Kershaw, G. B. *Modern Methods of Sewage Purification,* chap. XIII. Griffin and Co., Ltd., London (1911).

Leeds, City of. *Report on Experiments on Sewage Disposal,* by Col. T. W. Harding and Mr W. H. Harrison. Jowett and Sowry, Leeds (1905).

[1] *Sewage Disposal.*

Massachusetts State Board of Health   *Fortieth Annual Report.* Brown
    and Potter, Boston (1909).
Royal Commission on Sewage Disposal. *Fifth Report*, Appendix III to
    Fifth Report ; *Eighth Report*, Appendix I. Wyman and Co., Fetter
    Lane, London.
Venable. *Sewage Treatment.* John Wiley and Co.   New York.
York, City of. *Report to the Sewage Committee on Sewage Purification
    experiments at Naburn Disposal Works.* York (1901).

CHAPTER VIII

PERCOLATING FILTERS

Description of percolating filters.   In the case of percolating
or continuous filters, the liquid to be treated is usually applied
continuously to the filter (leaving out of the question for the
present resting periods and intermittent filtration), and passes
through and from the filter continuously, whereas in the case
of contact beds, as has already been shown, the liquid is held
up in the beds for a certain period before it is discharged.   It
is not to be understood from this that there is no period of
contact with percolating filters ; there is such a period, and it
will be discussed later, but the liquid in a percolating filter is
continually moving downwards by gravity, whereas in a contact
bed it is virtually at rest.

There is also another marked difference between percolating
filters and contact beds : with the former, the supply of air is
practically constant, whereas with the latter, aeration only
occurs during the resting of the bed.   It follows from this
that a sewage liquor stands a better chance of thorough oxidation, other things being equal, by being sprinkled in a fine
spray, as is usually the case, over the surface of a percolating
filter, and trickling slowly through the filter with ample aeration, than held up in contact material, where, when a strong
liquid is being treated, the imprisoned oxygen in the bed is
often rapidly exhausted, and where in any case the supply of
oxygen is limited.

Experiments with percolating filters were made in America at the Lawrence experimental station as long ago as 1889; the development of the percolating filter, however, and its successful use on a practical basis, has been largely due to English sanitarians.

About 1891, Mr J. Corbett at Salford constructed percolating filters, and Mr Scott Moncrieff brought out his process. Later on, about 1897, Col. Ducat constructed his covered-in filter at Hendon, and in 1898, Messrs Whittaker and Bryant built the Accrington filters.

Preliminary treatment before filtration. The observations made regarding tank treatment of the sewage antecedent to contact bed treatment, apply with equal force to filtration through percolating filters. Whilst no hard and fast rule can be laid down as to the precise degree to which suspended solids should be removed before filtration, it may be said that the finer the filtering material used, the better should be the clarification of the tank liquor, otherwise clogging will ensue. On the other hand there are cases where percolating filters of coarse material are advisable, with subsequent settlement of the filtered effluent.

When the final purification process is taken into account, there is not a great deal of difference between the costs of the various tank processes, and both preliminary and subsequent treatment must be considered conjointly. Local conditions, *e.g.* likelihood of ease or the reverse of disposing of the sludge, must decide this. In certain circumstances, although there might be a brisk demand for sludge in the neighbourhood, frequent sludging operations and the risk of smell which they sometimes involve when carelessly carried out, might render it preferable to produce a tank liquor heavily charged with suspended matter, to treat this upon coarse percolating filters, and to remove the suspended matter *after* filtration, instead of *before* it, in an unobjectionable state, by means of settling tanks or straining filters. The question of the extent to which suspended solids should be removed before filtration is also intimately connected with the character of the sewage and the rate of filtration per cube yard.

Different kinds of percolating filter. Setting aside differences in the method of distribution, and based on the size of material, there may be said to be, roughly speaking, three classes of continuous or percolating filters, and they are classified as follows in the Fifth Report of the Sewage Disposal Commission.

" (1) Percolating filters constructed of material coarse enough (say, over 2½ inches in diameter) not only to give free access of air to its interior but also to allow the suspended matter in the liquid free passage through the whole depth of the filter.....

" (2) Percolating filters constructed of medium-sized material (say, ½ inch in diameter) which temporarily retards the passage of suspended matter through the filter, while allowing free access of air to the interior.

" (3) Percolating filters constructed of very fine material."

The Commissioners further observe that in filters of medium-sized material the suspended solids are held back for some time in the upper layers of the material, this stratum of the filter in consequence receiving a larger proportion of oxidisable suspended matter than the central or lower strata. When much suspended matter is being treated, filters of this type tend to clog in the top few inches of the material, thus preventing proper distribution. With percolating filters of very fine material, suspended matter is kept back on the surface, preventing free access of air to the interior, unless the filter is constructed with banks of material at intervals above the general surface level.

After sewage has been applied to fine material filters for some little time, the surface of the sand or fine clinker becomes covered with a matting of suspended matter, necessitating either the drying off of the filter, when the scum can be scraped or raked off, or the washing of the filter by upward flow.

Filters constructed of fine material require frequent rests.

Intermittent filters. With some types of filter, such as filters composed of very fine material, the supply of liquid to the filter must necessarily be given in intermittent flushes. In certain cases, however, where the flow of sewage is irregular, the flow during its minimum period would not be sufficient to cause moving distributors to work properly, if the liquid were permitted to flow directly from the tanks to the filters. Consequently, methods must be devised to store up the liquid in a chamber, until a sufficient volume has accumulated to cause the distributor to start at once and remain in action for some minutes. There are many devices for bringing this about, one of the types most commonly met with taking the form of a dosing tank or chamber, which just holds the requisite volume of liquid, an automatic siphon coming into action when the liquid in the tank reaches a certain height, discharging the contents of the tank in a flush to the distributor. Fig. 45 gives a plan and section of a small dosing tank.

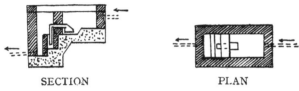

SECTION   PLAN

Fig. 45.   Dosing tank.

With certain types of siphon the amount of liquid discharged from the tank can be varied at will within certain limits.

Filters fed by the method just described are intermittent in action, the filter resting whilst the tank is filling up, and working for a few minutes at a time whilst the tank is discharging its contents. As a rule, the volume of liquid treated per cube yard by this means varies a good deal throughout the 24 hours—unless the supply of liquid to the tank can be throttled down satisfactorily—since the siphon may discharge say, every eight minutes for 40 minutes, and then, owing to an increase in sewage flow, the siphon may discharge every five minutes. The main difficulty, however, is to prevent the liquid dribbling from the distributor arms on one particular part of the bed during small flows of sewage, and the siphon chamber gets rid of this objection.

Another point which may be mentioned in connection with

intermittent distribution, is that freezing is perhaps not so liable to occur during severe cold.

Aeration of percolating filters. The generally accepted view as to the aeration of filters is that the air essential for aerating purposes is carried down through the filter by the flow of the sewage, and in the case of filters with solid brick or concrete walls this must necessarily be so.

Fine material filters, as would naturally be expected, require careful working and resting if the body of the filter is to remain well aerated for any length of time, and in the case of very fine material, such as sand, aeration would appear to be best brought about by flushing the liquid rapidly some inches in depth over the entire surface of the bed, since the sinking of this body of liquid through the bed would probably draw the air after it in the manner of a piston.

Since the efficiency of percolating filters depends entirely upon a free and unrestricted air supply, it is of the utmost importance that good aeration should receive every attention.

Blowing air through a filter artificially has been suggested and tried, but if a filter is properly constructed with good underdrainage, and, further, if it is not overworked and receives good attention, there is no need for any additional air supply.

Duration of contact in percolating filters. This depends upon the size, condition and depth of the material, and also upon the rate of treatment per cube yard.

Although liquid applied to a percolating filter appears to pass out as effluent in five minutes or even less, that liquid passing out is not necessarily the same as the liquid applied to the filter, *i.e.* it has become modified in many ways ; part of the suspended solids originally in it may not leave the filter for months, and similarly, a certain part of the liquid itself may not pass out of the filter for some hours.

This may be understood if a sponge is taken as representing a percolating filter, and small doses of solutions of different strengths, of say, one, two, five and seven dripped on to the top surface of the sponge ; the liquid, however, dripping from the under surface of the sponge will not come out in solutions having strengths of one, two, five and seven, but a mixture of the various liquids.

In like manner, the *average* duration of contact in a perco-lating filter is usually several hours, as may be realised by reference to experiments carried out by the Sewage Disposal Commission at Ilford and Dorking to elucidate this point.

Ilford experiments. A strong solution of salt was added to the septic tank liquor as it passed on to the two filters, samples of the effluent being drawn at frequent intervals, until nearly all the salt had worked out of the filters, in this particular case a period of about 19 hours.

The chlorine in each sample was then determined. It was fully realised with this experiment that the passage of a salt solution through a filter would not be precisely similar to the passage of a sewage liquor, the impurities in which are partly in true solution, partly colloidal, and partly in suspension, and it was assumed that sewage impurities were held up in a filter for a longer time than a salt solution, whose passage through a filter may be regarded for practical purposes as purely physical.

The result showed that the figures for the two filters were almost similar throughout the experiment, but that during the first hour a rather greater proportion of salt came through the deep filter, although at the very beginning the salt issued quicker from the shallow filter. The figures obtained are shown in Fig. 46, and the experiments as a whole suggested that, with good distribution and ample aeration, the degree of purification effected by a percolating filter depends upon the length of time during which the liquor is in contact with the material, or, strictly speaking, upon the proportion of highly purified sewage in the effluent (*i.e.* sewage which has taken some hours to pass through the filter) to the proportion of sewage which has passed through more rapidly by a more direct route.

Salt experiments were also carried out at Dorking, and they served to demonstrate in a striking manner the close relationship between the duration of contact and the quality of the effluent.

258

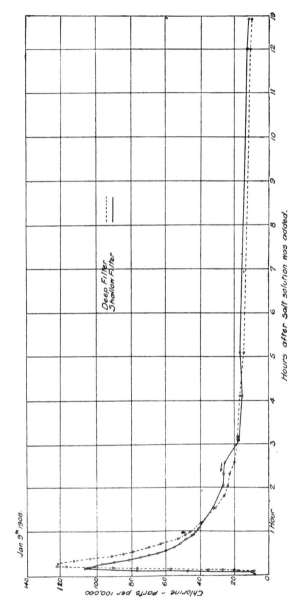

Fig. 46. Curves showing the rates of filtration through two coarse percolating filters of different depths at Ilford as tested quantitatively with a solution of salt.

Shape of filters. As regards the shape of the filters, this will be governed by the shape of the site. Circular filters are perhaps more frequently met with than any other shape, but octagonal filters are in use. The waste area in octagonal filters consists of the area contained between the retaining walls and a circle traced by the ends of the distributors, together with the small rectangle enclosed by four filters where the installation is a large one. Rectangular filters require special types of travelling distributors which are expensive to install in the first instance and usually require more head to work, but they are useful where rectangular contact beds are converted into per-colating filters.

Size of filters. This depends a good deal upon the type of distribution employed. There are now in this country distribu-tors in use revolving over 200 feet in diameter on the sprinkling system. With the flush system, as carried out at the Chorley sewage works, the filter units must be small, not only to ensure that the flush covers the whole of the surface of the bed, but also because with this type of filter frequent scraping or washing of the top material is essential, and it would not do to throw too large a proportion of the beds out of use at any one time.

In any case, save in the smallest of installations, there should not be less than three units to allow for resting and repairs. When stationary distributors are used, such as tipping troughs, jets, or trays, the size of the filter units is not very material, since any desired portion can be cut out and rested when necessary.

As regards American practice, the sprinkler nozzle or jet appears to be the favourite form of distributor; and in this case, the unit size of the filters is a matter of convenience, dependent largely upon site considerations.

Depth of percolating filters. This is a question which depends upon rather a large number of factors, e.g. levels, nature of tank liquor and the suspended solids it contains, size and character of material, rate of filtration, and method of distribution. The length of contact of the liquid with the filtering material will decide the purification which will be effected, and this depends mainly upon the size of the material, the rate of the treatment, and the nature of the distribution.

In the majority of instances, percolating filters in this country have been made as deep as the levels would allow without pumping, and shallow filters have only been put in where there was little fall. There is no doubt that this practice has been a sound one, but it was not recognised some years ago that the same purification will be obtained from a cubic yard of coarse material, whether arranged in the form of a deep or shallow filter, providing the rate of treatment per cube yard is the same in either case.

As long ago as 1897, Mr C. J. Whittaker carried out experiments at Accrington to ascertain the depth of filtering material required for the purification of a particular septic tank liquor. He compared the results given by two filters of coarse material, respectively six and nine feet deep, but it should be noted that both filters received the same quantity of liquid *per square yard*, and not per cube yard. The nine-foot filter gave a better purification and nitrification than the six-foot filter.

Many other experiments were carried out by various people, all of them, however, working the filters (of different depths and therefore of varying cubic content) at equal rates of treatment *per square yard*, and naturally, under these conditions, the deeper the filter the better was the purification which resulted. There do not appear, however, to have been any experiments at that time concerning the treatment of sewage or tank liquor on filters of varying depths at equal rates of filtration *per cube yard*, and therefore the Sewage Disposal Commission initiated some experiments at Ilford and Horfield to ascertain whether it is better to arrange a given quantity of filtering material in the form of a deep or a shallow filter.

Horfield experiments. In the Horfield experiments (1904–1905) two filters were used, respectively seven feet five inches and three feet deep, the material being coarse clinker, both filters treating precipitation liquor at about the same rate *per cube yard* per day for a period of ten months. Distribution was effected by means of Stoddart trays.

The results obtained showed the effluent from the deeper filter to be slightly the better of the two ; they also demonstrated that wherever possible, with coarse material, a deep

filter is preferable to a shallow one, particularly where a strong
liquid is being treated, owing to any faults in distribution
affecting the shallow filter to a greater extent than the coarse.

Further experiments at Ilford lasted from June, 1907, to
January, 1908, the septic tank liquor being treated at a rate
of 125 gallons *per cube yard* per day.

The results obtained showed that slightly greater oxidation
was obtained from the deep filter; this, however, might have
been due to the fact that imperfect distribution affected the
purification to a greater extent in the shallow than in the deep
filter. The conclusions arrived at were that within somewhat
wide limits of depth, assuming sufficient aeration and good
distribution, the same degree of purification could be obtained
from a cube yard of coarse material, whether arranged as a
shallow or a deep filter.

It is important to note that with very deep percolating
filters working normally at a high rate of treatment per cube
yard, it would not be practicable in many cases to double the
rate of treatment without ponding the surface of the filter,
unless the filtering material were very coarse and free from
growths. About six feet is perhaps the average depth of most
of the percolating filter installations in this country.

From an engineering point of view it makes for economy of
construction if the beds are made as deep as practicable, having
regard to limiting rates of filtration per cube yard, since the
disposition of the material largely affects the cost of flooring,
drains, distribution, etc., and a filter containing 1000 cube yards
of material arranged six feet deep is a very different matter
from a filter having a similar cubic content but arranged three
feet deep.

Regarding the depth of percolating filters in use in other countries, the
Baltimore filters are eight feet six inches deep to the top of the underdrains,
whilst the Columbus and Reading filters are five feet deep.

Fuller[1] states that in the great majority of designs for percolating filter
installations in America, the depth of the main body of material has been
about six feet, but that of late years there has been some tendency to increase
slightly upon this depth.

[1] *Sewage Disposal*, Fuller. McGraw-Hill Book Company, New York and
London (1912).

Double filtration. As a general rule, it will be found advisable, from considerations of economy, when the fall admits of it, to utilise a given volume of filtering material as deep percolating filters, rather than two tiers of percolating filters of medium depth. Certainly rather better aeration would result from the disposition of a given quantity of filtering material in two filters three feet deep, but the suspended matter from the primary filters would be received on the surface of the secondary filters, and would be apt to choke them, unless a settling tank were interposed between the two sets of filters. The deeper the filter, the greater the likelihood of any inequalities of distribution being equalised, whereas, in the case of shallow filters, any lack of uniformity in distribution soon manifests itself in the effluent. Double filtration, it may be mentioned, is carried out at Newcastle-under-Lyne, Kenilworth, Chester and elsewhere.

Owing practically to twice the amount of flooring, under-drains, walls, distribution, etc., being required with double filtration, the initial cost alone of this method of purification is not an inducement for its adoption by local authorities ; in the case of exceptionally strong liquors, however, double filtration might be serviceable.

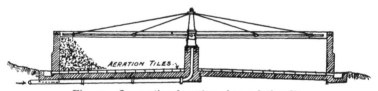

Fig. 47.   Conventional section of percolating filter.

Construction. It is quite important that all floors and walls of percolating filters should be constructed in a sound and durable manner. Holes dug in the ground and boarded may answer for a short time for experimental filters, but they are not to be recommended for even the smallest works, and the popular fallacy that they result in economy is apt to be somewhat rudely dispelled after a short lapse of time. Fig. 47 shows a conventional section of a circular percolating filter.

Floors. Portland cement concrete (six to one) may usefully be employed for floors of filters, with the surface properly brought up and smoothed, any irregularities of surface tending to hold back suspended matter. It should be fully recognised that the construction of percolating filter floors (including the underdrains) is of prime importance, and free outlets for suspended matter, and also for aeration purposes, are absolutely essential.

The floors of filters should be given a slope or fall towards the effluent channel, to enable the effluent and suspended matter to drain off effectively. In some cases it is convenient to make the filter floor slope to the centre of the filter, but in most cases it will be found advisable to slope the floors from the centre of the filter to an effluent channel running round the circumference. Much depends upon the size of the filter units and their shape, underdrainage, etc., as to the fall which can be given. In this country, slopes of about 1 in 100 to 1 in 40 have been used with satisfactory results.

Walls. These may be constructed of brickwork or Portland cement concrete, and as it is not now considered necessary to provide side aeration, the walls can be built solid.

It is not, as a rule, economical to omit walls[1] to filters and let the material lie at its natural angle of repose, since the extra flooring, material and effluent channel often cost more than the retaining wall. If it is desired to compromise, the wall can be partly carried up, as shown in Fig. 48, and the exposed sides of the material battered, large selected pieces of clinker being packed against the material which stands round the clinker walls. Rubble walls in districts where stone is cheap, when well put together, are durable and economical, but workmen used to

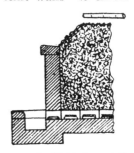

Fig. 48. Battering of filtering material at circumference of filter.

this special class of work are sometimes difficult to obtain. With regard to the

---

[1] When walls are omitted, insects can gain access to the filtering material much more easily.

bricks used for percolating filter walls, nothing is better than Staffordshire blue bricks, red Accrington engineering bricks also answering well. Second quality blue bricks can be used to effect economy; ordinary bricks such as Fletton do not stand well and are very liable to perish, split and disintegrate in continued frosty weather.

In certain windy exposed situations, it is sometimes advantageous with small filters to carry the retaining wall some 18 inches above the surface level of the filtering material, to neutralise to some extent the tendency of heavy winds to blow the spray from the distributors, or cause it to overdose a particular part of the filter. If this is done, access holes should be provided in the walls for rodding out the distributor arms when necessary.

It is perhaps scarcely necessary to say that all the brickwork should be built with Portland cement mortar. Should it be desired to provide openings in the filter walls for sampling and taking of temperatures at various depths, this can easily be provided for by leaving openings in the walls at the desired intervals and laying lines of four-inch stoneware pipes leading from them.

It may be of interest to observe that the Columbus percolating filters (U.S.A.) were constructed with watertight walls, to allow of using the filters alternately as contact beds, if severe weather interfered with the ordinary method of working.

Underdrains. The underdrainage system of percolating filters should, wherever reasonably practicable, take the form of a complete false floor, and the larger the filter units, the greater the force with which this statement applies.

When coarse filtering material is employed, suspended matter very soon begins to work out through the filter to the floor, and unless means are provided for carrying off this matter as fast as it comes through the filter clogging will result, with consequent falling off in the quality of the effluent due to impaired aeration, and later on ponding on the surface of the filter and faulty distribution.

Even in the case of filters constructed of medium-sized

material, solids will in course of time work through and out of the filter, and the provision of a stratum of coarse material at the bottom of the filter will not entirely obviate ultimate clogging ; further, should this large material become by any means disintegrated, and it is peculiarly liable to become so, free drainage and aeration at once begin to be impeded.

Different kinds of false floor. Most false floors are formed by specially made hard vitrified stoneware tiles, such as the Stiff, or the Mansfield tile (Fig. 49), resting upon short feet and thus raising the whole body of the filtering material some inches above the concrete floor. An alternative method of forming a false floor by means of channels and perforated cover tiles is shown in Figs. 50 and 51.

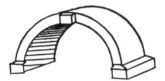

Fig. 49.   The Mansfield tile.

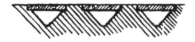
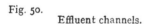
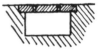

Fig. 50.   Fig. 51.

Effluent channels.

Where fine material is used, it is necessary to use a layer of somewhat coarser material between the surface of the tiles and the fine material, otherwise this would fall or be washed through the slots or openings in the tiles ; similarly, a layer of coarse material should be interposed between the tiles and medium-sized material.

It is usual to carry the tiles of the false floor (or aeration tiles as they are sometimes called) right through the retaining walls of the filter units up to the effluent channel, and specially heavy " purpose-made " tiles can be obtained for taking the weight of the retaining wall.

Whatever the system of underdrains employed, the main point is to keep the base of the filter as open as possible : if this is done, there will not be much wrong with the filter as regards underdrainage.

In American practice, nearly all the percolating filter installations appear to have been provided with false floors, amongst others, Columbus, Atlanta, Batavia, Baltimore, North Plainfield, etc.

Effluent channels. These may be suitably formed in Portland cement concrete rendered, or concrete faced with blue bricks, or stoneware half-pipes. As has already been pointed out under the section which deals with floors, the effluent channel is usually most conveniently formed round the circumference or margin of each filter, when these are circular or octagonal in plan. With rectangular filters the effluent channel is usually best placed at the end of the filters, or down the centre, if the filters are in two ranks.

Gauging facilities should be provided, and means of sampling the effluent from each filter unit. If the gauging cannot be suitably arranged after the filtration of the effluent, provision should be made for it in the feed channels, before the tank liquor leaves them for the cast-iron pipes supplying the distributors.

Sampling and inspection chambers. In the case of fairly large installations small access chambers can be provided in the material of the bed itself, or the distributor well can be so devised that samples of various kinds may be drawn at different depths, and the condition of the material noted, from the surface of the filter down to the underdrains.

At Wakefield[1], where a new installation of percolating filters has recently been installed, an inspection chamber has been provided in the filtering material itself by the city surveyor, and in the walls of the chamber at various depths are sliding trays containing filtering material, so that samples of effluent, growths, larvae, etc., can be withdrawn at the depth of the various trays for purposes of analysis or inspection.

[1] *Trade Waste Waters*, by H. MacClean Wilson and H. T. Calvert. Griffin and Co., Ltd., London (1913).

Filtering materials. What has been already said concerning contact material in the preceding chapter applies equally to filtering material for percolating filters. Durability, large and rough surface[1] area are the chief desiderata for filtering media. Clinker is perhaps more generally used than other materials, but large quantities of quartzite have been used by Mr Watson at Birmingham with satisfactory results.

The particular kind of material to be employed will depend upon the class of filter it is proposed to utilise, *i.e.* whether of (1) coarse material, (2) medium-sized material, or (3) fine material. For fine material filters, sand, clinker, and coal have been used with good results, and sand can usually be obtained without much difficulty. It is most essential that the material used in fine grade filters should not be liable to disintegration.

Size of material. This is a very important question and much depends upon it. The size of the material will in the first place vary according to the type of filter used, and also according to the kind of liquid to be treated and the suspended solids which that liquid contains. The degree of purification brought about by a percolating filter, assuming sufficient aeration, varies with the *average* length of time occupied by the tank liquor in passing through the filter (in other words, the duration of contact already referred to); consequently the size of material exercises a marked influence, other things being equal, on the quality of effluent produced.

There are, however, limits to the size which can be used in practice, dependent mainly upon the quantity and nature of the suspended solids contained in the liquor treated. Generally speaking, the practice of the last few years has tended in the

[1] The Massachusetts State Board of Health (40th *Annual Report* (1909), pp. 412, 413) carried out experiments on the different action of rough and smooth materials. Coke and glass beads of the size of a pea were used, the depth of each filter being five feet.

Nitrification commenced in the coke filter within the first month, whereas in the glass bead filter it did not become established for over two months; moreover, the effluent from the bead filter never contained more than 50 per cent. of the nitrates in the coke effluent, nor was it ever of so satisfactory a quality.

direction of producing better tank liquors as regards suspended
matter, and encouraging the free passage of suspended solids
through the filter, to be subsequently removed by settlement
or straining. The size of coarse percolating filter material has
been if anything slightly reduced, but not sufficiently so to hold
back solids, whilst there is a general tendency to employ rather
larger " medium-sized " and " fine " materials than formerly,
and the same trend is noticeable in American practice, an
average size for material there appearing to be $1\frac{1}{2}$ inches to
2 inches diameter.

Grading of filtering material. Grading of material, in the
common acceptance of the term, is not necessary with percolating filters, beyond the ordinary coarse layer of material just
over the underdrains, which is usually placed there for the
same reasons as with contact beds; but with filters of fine
material, such as sand, it is necessary to interpose medium-
sized material between the body of the sand and the underdrains. In order to prevent the sand becoming gradually
washed away, the writer has found a 3 inch layer of $\frac{1}{2}$ inch
to $\frac{3}{4}$ inch material immediately over the underdrains, followed
by a 3 inch layer of $\frac{1}{4}$ inch to $\frac{1}{8}$ inch material suitable as a
substratum in the case of filters of fine river sand; the
coarser material assists in aerating the sand, which, owing to
its capillarity, is difficult to drain, and requires all the assistance
that can be given, both for aeration and drainage purposes.

Fine material has not been very much used for the surfaces
of percolating filters, as it entails much labour in scraping and
keeping clean, but a layer of peat fibre forms a good distributor,
whilst straining out suspended matter. It should be mentioned
that fine surface material answered very well in the case of a
filter at Prestolee, but the sewage there was exceptionally weak.

Distribution. This can be effected in several ways which
will be described. The chief point is to distribute the liquid
uniformly all over the surface of the filter; since, if this is done,
each portion of the filter will receive a similar dose of liquid,
and therefore the rate of filtration will be even, and the duration
of contact of the liquid with the filtering material a maximum
for the particular rate of treatment adopted.

Most distribution devices can be classified under three headings, viz. :

(1) Revolving distributors for circular filters, working for the most part on the Barker's mill principle, but some driven by power and others again working after the fashion of a water-wheel.

(2) Travelling distributors for rectangular filters, both power driven, and also actuated by the head of sewage on the distributor.

(3) Stationary or fixed distributors such as jets, nozzles (with or without spreaders or dash plates), tipping troughs, fixed troughs, perforated trays, fine surface material, perforated pipes, etc., worked by head of sewage on the distributors ; these methods admit of intermittent or continuous distribution.

The chief requirements of a mechanical distributor are uniform distribution at high and low rates of flow, freedom from choking, simplicity, durability, and power of working under low speed ; a good distributor should also be unappreciably affected by extremes of temperature, and the component parts should be simple and easily accessible for cleaning purposes.

Moving distributors. In this country preference is usually given to the rotary form of distributor with perforated arms, at all events in the case of small to medium-sized works, but in most cases sufficient fall cannot be spared for distributing devices requiring a head of several feet. Of automatic mechanical distributors, the rotary distributor and the travelling distributor are the most efficient as regards uniform distribution : rotary distributors have, however, certain drawbacks such as liability to be affected by wind and frost, choking of holes when perforated arms are used, and frequent attention requisite to clean them.

Rotary distributors which distribute the sewage liquid through holes in the arms, are likely to cause a very bad smell when septic tank liquors containing brewery refuse are being distributed, but they are nothing like so bad in this respect as the jet or nozzle system. Revolving distributors in frosty weather are apt to stop, owing to formation of icicles, if placed lower than about four inches from the surface of the bed.

Travelling distributors do not appear to have found much favour in America, although they have been used experimentally at Lawrence and Baltimore : this may be ascribed to apprehensions of " zero " weather in some of the states, which would presumably call for covering in of the filters.

Travelling distributors driven by power do not cause very much smell as a rule, and are not liable to stoppage by frost, but they are unfortunately expensive to install in the first instance, and the running costs are high. It is of primary importance that both cost and maintenance should be as low as possible compatible with efficiency. The siphon feed channels of rectangular distributors on long beds should be supplied with several inlets, and not only at one end of the channel.

Stationary distributors. These take many forms, one form being that in which the sewage is discharged from a store tank into a network of perforated pipes lying on the surface of the filter.

The Stoddart trays consist of galvanised iron sheets, perforated in the concave and convex sections, the former perforations being filled in with nails about $\frac{3}{4}$ inch long. These trays arc fed from a channel or channels at one or both ends of the tray or series of trays, the liquid to be distributed rising in the concave section until it overflows through the holes in the convex section whence it runs down to the nail points depending from the underside of the trays. These trays require very careful levelling ; it is understood that covers can be provided for use in frosty weather, and also for the purpose of keeping down smell.

Distribution by means of a fine layer of material on the surface of the filter has been carried out at several places, *e.g.* Prestolee, and at Chorley in the case of the fine sand filters; the material takes the place of the usual mechanical distributor. Dr Fowler has used fibrous peat for the distribution of raw sewage with success.

It will be realised that this form of distribution would not be well adapted for filters composed entirely of medium-sized or coarse material, and it would not be advisable to apply tank liquors containing very much suspended matter to fine surfaced filters, owing to the expense entailed by constant surface cleaning.

Jets or nozzles have been used with satisfactory results, notably by Mr J. D. Watson at Birmingham, but they require a head of several feet to work satisfactorily, and need a good deal of attention for cleaning purposes. The distribution is inferior to that obtained by moving distributors, and it is therefore inadvisable to use them for shallow filters ; distribution is best when the holes for the jets are as small as can be used without choking. The liquid dealt with at Birmingham is septic tank liquor containing about eight parts per 100,000 of suspended matter, and the attendance of one man (night and day) is required to clean the nozzles for each 1½ acres of filter. The constant walking over the surface of the beds—especially in cases where the liquid to be filtered contained much suspended matter—would in the case of clinker or similar material cause disintegration and choking, but the majority of the filters at the Birmingham installation are composed of quartzite, a very hard and durable material and easily forked over when necessary. Jets are useful, since they can be applied to filters of irregular shape. One of the main objections to the jet and perforated tray forms of distribution is that the spray from the jets and drips from the trays are nearly always falling upon the same area of bed.

In America, the jet, or sprinkler nozzle as it is there termed, is regarded as the best type of distributor for the conditions met with in the States. The first form used appears to have been the nozzle devised by Mr Gregory for the Columbus installation, but many other types are in use, such as the Weand nozzle at Reading, and the Taylor nozzle at Kings Park.

Fuller[1] observes, that at Reading about 10 per cent. of the nozzles on an average require cleaning once a day, and that with about 250 nozzles per acre one man can without difficulty attend to some three acres or more : it is to be noted, however, that American sewages admit of the use of larger nozzle orifices than could be used with the stronger sewages of this country ; further, the intermittent working allows of a higher rate of application for the time being than would be permissible with continuous distribution.

That clogging of nozzles has been a serious matter, however, at times, even with somewhat dilute sewages, is shown by the fact that at Columbus and Baltimore, fine screens have been interposed between the tanks and filters.

The spacing of jets on percolating filters requires some care in setting out, and loss of head absorbed by friction in the distributing pipes must be carefully taken into account.

[1] *Sewage Disposal*, Fuller. McGraw-Hill Book Co., New York and London (1912).

With regard to jets spaced on the outside of the filter, it is desirable that these should not spray on to the wall of the filter or into the effluent channel should there be no retaining walls. Special nozzles are made for such situations, so devised as to throw only a half spray.

In America, special attention has been directed to means for varying the head on nozzles, so as to obtain better distribution as regards uniformity : in the majority of instances this has been achieved by dosing tanks, in conjunction with siphons, whilst a device consisting of a butterfly valve, suggested by Mr E. P. Stearns, has also been employed. An ingenious method, consisting of a taper dosing tank resembling the bottom half of the Birmingham separator tank, has also been used at Reading.

A somewhat unusual method of distribution was designed by Professors Winslow and Phelps at the Massachusetts Institute of Technology, by which the sewage flows along pipes raised above the filtering material ; the pipes are perforated at intervals, and the sewage falls from these openings upon concave discs termed dash-plates, which cause the sewage liquor to separate into small globules. Fuller states that the system is in operation in Mount Vernon, N.Y., but that in northern climates it necessitates a filter house, whilst it is not suitable for a varying head of sewage.

Tipping troughs have given good results in several cases, and they are more especially suited to small installations. They consist of troughs balanced on pivots at each end, the trough being so centred on the pivot that when it is full it capsizes, upsets the liquid and returns to its original position. By means of a suitable division plate running down the centre of the trough, and dividing it into two compartments, a tipping trough can be made double-acting, tipping the liquid out first one side and then the other. One advantage of tipping troughs is that they will work at any rate of flow, and, further, it is unlikely that, failing regular attention, more than one or two troughs would fail to tip and return properly ; on the other hand, distribution by tipping troughs is by no means good, and they are therefore only suited to rather deep filters. Unless they are carefully centred and hung, a good deal of attention is needed to see that the troughs return to their original position after tipping, which is their particular failing. Severe frost would be liable to throw tipping troughs out of action, and they should therefore only be used in covered filters, in localities where severe weather is likely to be experienced.

It will be seen from what has been said that the particular type of distributor to be adopted in any particular case will

TABLE XXIX. *Giving practicable rates of treatme*

	Strong sewages Absorbing 17-25 parts of oxygen per 100,000 from strong permanganate in 4 hours at 80° F.			Average s Absorbing 10-12 parts of strong permanganate
	Suspended solids in tank liquor pts. per 100,000	Coarse deep filters	Fine shallow filters	
Preliminary tank treatment		Rates of filtration in gallons per cube yard per 24 hours		Preliminary tank treatment
(1) Precipitation and 2 hours' quiescent settlement ..	2–5	100	66	(1) Precipitation and 2 hours' quiescent settlement ..
(2) 8 hours' continuous flow precipitation	8	66	50	(2) 8 hours' continuous flow precipitation .. ..
(3) 2 hours' quiescent settlement	10	50	22	(3) 2 hours' quiescent settlement .. .. ..
(4) 15 hours' continuous flow settlement	15–20	33	16	(4) 15 hours' continuous flow settlement .. ..
(5) Septic tank	15–20	33	16	(5) Septic tank .. ..

	Strong sewages absorbing 7-8 parts of oxygen per 100,000 from... 4 hours at 80° F.		Weak sewages — Absorbing 7-8 parts of oxygen per 100,000 from strong permanganate in 4 hours at 80° F.		
		Coarse deep filters	Fine shallow filters	Preliminary tank treatment	Coarse deep filters	Fine shallow filters
Suspended solids in tank liquor pts. per 100,000	Rate of filtration in gallons per cube yard per 24 hours		Suspended solids in tank liquor pts. per 100,000	Rate of filtration in gallons per cube yard per 24 hours	
1–4	133	133	(1) Precipitation and 2 hours' quiescent settlement ..	1–3	(133–200)	200
3–6	100	66–100	(2) 8 hours' continuous flow precipitation	2–5	133–200	167–200
5–8	100	66	(3) 2 hours' quiescent settlement	4–6	133	133
10–15	66	20–33	(4) 15 hours' continuous flow settlement	7–8	100	100
10–15	66	20–33	(5) Septic tank	7–8	100	100

depend upon a large number of factors, of which the chief ones will usually be the suspended matter in the liquid to be dealt with, and depth of filter which can be obtained.

In the designing of sewage purification works, possibly more so than in any other branch of engineering, the design of one part of the process will be found to be intimately connected with another part, and that the many factors have to be considered conjointly by the engineer responsible for the design of the works, and not dealt with separately one by one.

Rate of filtration per cube yard. The rate at which a particular tank liquor can be treated depends upon a number of factors, such as strength of liquid, suspended matter contained in liquid, size of material, etc. ; the most important of all, in the case of ordinary domestic sewages, is the suspended matter which the liquid contains. With some excessively strong liquids derived from special trades and industries, dilution of the original liquid with water may be advisable before filtration. This course was adopted with the distillery "pot ale" before filtration, and was also adopted by the author in the case of a sewage derived from some 500 pigs, where the ammoniacal nitrogen was about 10 times as high as that found in a strong domestic sewage.

Table XXIX, compiled from data contained in the Fifth Report of the Sewage Disposal Commission, gives some particulars regarding rates of filtration of various liquids per cube yard per 24 hours, in the case of coarse deep and fine shallow filters respectively, the effluent produced in each case being satisfactory. It should be noted that the figures given are the rates of filtration when the whole area of filters is in use, i.e. during wet weather, and these figures divided into the dry weather flow of sewage will give the total number of cube yards of filtering material required, allowing for treating up to three times the average dry weather flow during wet weather. In certain cases where land treatment is used after percolating filters, increased rates of filtration might be adopted.

It should be observed that in the case of very deep percolating filters—say 7 feet to 12 feet deep—there are mechanical difficulties in the way of filtering more than a certain quantity of liquid *per yard super*, even when the material is medium-sized. For example, taking a filter 12 feet deep and having a cubic content of four yards ; assuming the average rate of filtration in dry weather to be 200 gallons *per cube yard*, this would be equivalent to 800 gallons per yard super in the instance quoted, and if three times the dry weather flow were to be dealt with in wet weather, this would mean treating at a rate of no less than 2400 gallons per square yard.

In America, percolating filters six feet deep can apparently be worked regularly at a rate of about 200 gallons per cube yard, and without clogging when the material is not smaller than one inch diameter, but American sewages on an average are more dilute than European sewages, owing to the larger quantity of water used.

Settlement of percolating filter effluents. Unless very fine material filters are used, it will be found that large quantities of suspended solids pass away in the effluent, especially during the spring " flush-out," and, unless the effluent is passed over land before reaching the river or stream, some form of settlement or final straining will be necessary. At Birmingham, Mr Watson uses the Birmingham separator tank, square in plan and with a hopper-shaped bottom, which answers its purpose well. Shallow straining filters are also used ; whether of sand or other fine material, it is not necessary to make these more than say 12 inches to 15 inches deep in all, and the rate of filtration can be about 500 gallons per square yard per 24 hours. A plan and section of some small sand filters for straining out suspended matter are shown in Fig. 52, and a plan and section of an effluent settling tank in Fig. 53. Purification is not aimed at during this part of the process, but only mechanical straining.

At Caterham, in Surrey, sand filtration is used after the percolating filters, to remove the suspended matter. When tanks are used, a two hours' flow is a reasonable time for settling out the solids, which, although more " worked out " and therefore less putrescible than the solids from contact beds, are nevertheless putrescible and will in the majority of cases require removal ; roughly speaking, about 10 cwt. of dry solids may be looked for per million gallons of effluent tanked.

In American practice, final settling basins appear to be provided in most cases, admitting of two to three hours' settlement of the filter effluent.

The final settlement of both contact bed and percolating filter effluents—especially the former—is a matter which is likely to come to the front if a general standard for suspended

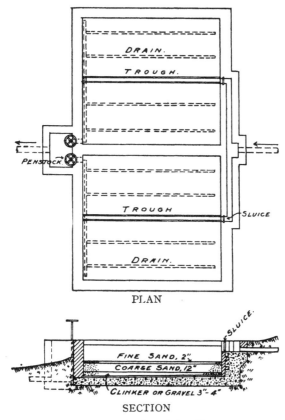

PLAN

SECTION

Fig. 52.   Sand straining filters.

solids is adopted in this country.   In the case of contact bed effluents, anyone can take a sample of effluent just after the outlet valves are opened on almost any works in the country, and feel fairly sure that it will not conform to a standard of say three parts of suspended solids per 100,000 and two parts oxygen taken up from water in five days, and if such chance samples are to be admitted as evidence of pollution, the equalisation as regards quality of effluents by means of settling or

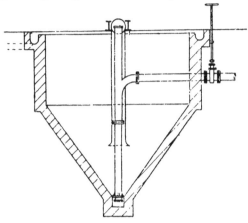

SECTION

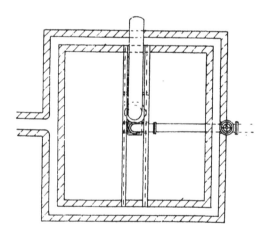

PLAN

Fig. 53. Effluent settling tank;

equalisation tanks will have to be considered ; such a plan, however admirable from an academic point of view, is not likely to be received with favour by communities who already have spent large sums upon sewage purification, and who would view with alarm any suggestion of full tank treatment not only as a preliminary but also as a final process, with contact beds or percolating filters sandwiched in between.

Land effluents, given good land and management, are almost free from suspended solids, and in this respect are superior to effluents from any artificial processes. Even land effluents, however, vary in quality throughout the day, even when purely domestic sewage is being treated, and it is possible to draw a series of six samples of effluent resulting from land treatment, which may differ considerably in quality. With artificial processes the differences are still greater, and any storage of the effluent producing an equalising effect is beneficial.

Clogging of filters. Unless means are taken to prevent it, filters made of medium-sized and fine materials are apt to become clogged in course of time by the suspended matter which enters them, and also by a certain amount of disintegration of material, and by gelatinous growths. This clogging is most apt to occur during the cooler months of the year. Filters constructed of coarse material, which allows the suspended matter to pass through freely, do not often choke or clog by reason of suspended matter, but they are more affected by growths than filters of fine material, and these growths may in course of time cause ponding and choking.

With medium and fairly coarse material a good deal of the suspended matter can sometimes be washed through the filter by means of flushing with a hose, or by simply holding the distributor in one position for a few minutes, repeating the operation all over the surface of the bed ; it should be stated, however, that this method is apt to upset the working of the filter for some little time.

Forking the top 12 to 18 inches of the filtering material is effective if the choking has only taken place superficially, but in bad cases it may be advisable to remove the top layer of material, wash it, and replace it.

The question of choking of filters by gelatinous growths will be dealt with in a later section.

In many cases choking is the direct result of overworking

the filter, and rests should be tried before anything further is attempted. The surface layers of fine materials are especially liable to become clogged, and unless this is taken in time it will gradually affect the whole depth of the bed.

Sand filters, if rested for a short time and the surfaces kept clean by scraping or washing, should not become clogged.

Renewal of filtering material. It is very seldom that filtering material needs renewal in the case of percolating filters, except with filters composed of very fine material, where frequent cleaning of the surface gradually removes a certain quantity, which has to be replaced. Coarse material, if of good durable quality in the first instance, will last for years without any sensible deterioration. At Horfield, Bristol, the material of a coarse percolating filter which had been in use for some five years was as good as new at the end of that period, when the filter was pulled down.

Washing of top material, on the other hand, has been found advisable in several cases. At the Little Drayton sewage works, the top material of a Ducat filter was removed after about $3\frac{1}{2}$ years' working, washed, and replaced.

All things considered, maintenance charges for renewal and washing are not likely to be material as regards filters of medium-sized to coarse material, and in the case of fine material filters the material scraped off the surface of the filters can often be used again after exposure to the weather.

Ponding on surface of filter. This is due to clogging by slimy growths, or improper increase in rate of treatment per cube yard. The subject is touched upon in the sections upon clogging and growths, and these should be referred to together with the remedies outlined in those sections, and also in the section upon removal of organic growths by various chemicals (p. 280).

Resting of filters. All percolating filters require resting sooner or later, and it may be laid down as a general rule that filters of very fine material can only be worked for limited periods without resting, since solids accumulate upon the surface of the filters and quickly obstruct filtration, so that resting periods, during which the surface of the filter can be scraped or washed, follow as a natural corollary to the use of very fine material filters, and it may be observed in passing that to obtain the maximum of work out of a given quantity of fine material it should be arranged if practicable in the form of a shallow rather than a deep filter. Similarly, it would be best on theoretical grounds to construct filters of medium-sized material in shallow rather than deep form, if first-class distribution could only be relied upon. Unfortunately, this cannot be taken for granted. Resting is extremely beneficial in the case of coarse material percolating filters which have become slightly clogged.

Growths on percolating filters. These usually make their appearance during the months of winter or early spring, and take the form of slimy gelatinous growths which grow on the surface of percolating filters of medium-sized or fairly coarse material. They do not appear to affect fine material filters to anything like the same extent as coarse, the chief reason for this being possibly due to the fact that the fine material shifts slightly when receiving the distributed liquor. Sometimes these growths are slight and remain so, but more often they extend until they seriously interfere with the proper working of the filter, causing ponding on the surface, preventing free aeration, and consequently bringing about a falling off in the character of the effluent. In addition, where distribution is effected with jets or rotary distributors having perforations in the arms, these growths soon choke up the holes, causing inefficient distribution : in many cases a long streamer of growth can be seen depending from each perforation.

The writer has noticed that these growths seem to be especially prevalent where the sewage is a domestic one containing large quantities of subsoil water. Light, too, appears to be essential to their well-being.

Dorking experiments on destruction of growths. The Sewage Disposal Commission gave considerable attention to the question of growths, and experiments on this question were carried out at the testing station at Dorking.

A percolating filter at this installation treating septic tank liquor became covered with a large quantity of gelatinous growth, causing local ponding in the track of the distributor jets. On March 16th, 1907, the filter was rested for 24 hours in dry weather, and the surface of the filter divided up into eight equal segments of 1·6 square yards each. Seven of these segments were treated with various reagents, the eighth segment being used as a " control."

The chemicals employed were as follows :

1. Powdered quicklime.
2. Bleaching powder.
3. 20 per cent. solution of " chloros."
4. 20 per cent. solution of copper sulphate.
5. 20 per cent. solution of ferrous sulphate.
6. 20 per cent. solution of caustic soda.
7. 20 per cent. solution of sulphuric acid.

As regards the lime and bleaching powder, a fine surface layer was used on two of the segments, the remaining five each being treated with a litre of each solution applied with a brush; the filter was then allowed to rest for 24 hours. At the expiration of this time, the only segment showing any marked destruction of the growth was the one treated with caustic soda. On re-starting the filter the same day, large quantities of coarse brown suspended solids came away in the effluent at first, but after a lapse of 24 hours the quantity had fallen from 20 to 30 parts per 100,000 to about six parts, and the working of the filter was not seriously impaired. On April 22nd, local ponding began to show again, and two gallons of 20 per cent. solution of caustic soda was applied to the entire surface of the filter, which was then rested for 24 hours.

On examining the filter the following morning, the surface of the material was seen to be covered with a white deposit of carbonate of soda, and when the filter was re-started a great quantity of dark brown solids came away in the effluent, and a considerable quantity continued to come away for about a week. The working of the filter was not seriously upset, and there was no fall in the figure for oxidised nitrogen two hours after the re-starting of the filter. The caustic soda solution was found to have completely cleared the top surface of clinker of the growth, but some still adhered to the protected surface underneath. The ponding was entirely cured, and no further growth made its appearance for several months: it was estimated that three similar applications of soda would be necessary on the Dorking filter to keep the growth down during the winter and spring months. The cost of the treatment in-clusive of labour was heavy, being about $2\frac{1}{2}d$. per square yard.

Growths are usually more abundant in channels carrying dilute sewage liquors than in those carrying strong sewage liquors, particularly if the liquid is free from suspended solids.

It may be noted that at Leeds, Col. Harding and Mr Harrison found it possible to keep down growths on a coarse material filter by using an intermittent sprinkler instead of a continuous one.

Nuisance from smell. It cannot be gainsaid that where the character of the liquid to be treated is naturally offensive, and is applied direct to the filters either by moving distributors or stationary jets, percolating filters are more likely to cause nuisance from smell than any other method of filtration.

A moment's consideration will show that this must of necessity be so, since the liquid is broken up into a fine spray whilst being spread over the surface of the filter, and a very large superficial area of finely divided liquid is exposed to the air and often carried some considerable distance. This results in infinitely small particles of liquid bring brought into contact with the mucous membrane of the nose. Smell is recognised by infinitely small particles or globules of a particular substance being brought into contact with the organs of smell. It follows, therefore, that when a particular smell is noticed, minute particles of the substance causing the smell have been carried to the membrane of the nose, which registers the smell, and it also follows from this that if a smell can be detected at a distance of one mile, that particles have also been con-veyed through that same distance of space.

The tipping trough and flush system of feeding continuous filters do not give rise to much nuisance as a rule, but unfor-tunately in the former case the distribution is not nearly so effective as is the case with a spraying distributor, and the flush system is only adapted to filters of very fine material, such as sand, where the liquid is discharged by a dosing tank and siphon on to the surface of the bed, slowly sinking through it.

The only remedy against nuisance from smell in the case of large installations of percolating filters fed by spraying methods, is either to have the filters constructed in an isolated site, or to subject the tank liquor to some deodorising process before distribution on the filters.

It may be taken for granted that where sewage contains brewery refuse in any quantity there will be considerable smell arising from its treatment, unless steps are taken to counteract it during the preliminary process, e.g. by precipitation by lime, which, together with bleaching powder, appears so far to be the best known method of treatment.

It should be noted that smell and nuisance from smell are by no means the same thing, and "nuisance" is a word very difficult of interpretation. For instance, smell may be noticeable 20 yards away from a trench which is being filled with sludge, but that is not necessarily a nuisance from smell ; if, however, a strong smell is evident to the inhabitants of houses say 200 yards off, they might be said to experience nuisance from smell, the extent of the nuisance depending upon the degree of smell, frequency of occurrence, and its total duration in any one day.

All sewage works are from their nature apt to smell somewhat at certain seasons and in certain conditions of weather, but a mere temporary local smell would appear to be quite distinct from nuisance from smell.

Spring flush-out of solids. It is found to be the case that percolating filter effluents, as the weather begins to get warmer, contain abnormal quantities of suspended solids, due to the movement of the insect life within the filter. Percolating filters form homes for enormous numbers of larvae of different species, in addition to many varieties of worms and insects. The small midges (*Psychodidae*, or moth flies) undergo their transformation by thousands in filters, the larvae feeding upon the vegetable debris, and the insect *Achorutes purpurescens*[1] multiplies under like conditions. There can be no doubt that these higher forms of life assist considerably both in breaking

---

[1] Some confusion appears to exist between *Podura aquatica* and *Achorutes purpurescens*, the latter being far more frequently met with on sewage works.

up and assimilating organic matter, and also at certain seasons of the year they help the peaty-like matter to move through the filter. As a general rule, the suspended solids entering a filter in the tank liquor, should be about equal to the solids contained in the effluent leaving the filter.

It may be noted that contact beds do not show this spring flush-out of solids to anything like the same extent as percolating filters, since conditions for larval life are not so favourable in contact beds as in continuous filters composed of coarse and medium-sized material. The temperatures in the interior of percolating filters are ideal for furthering insect life in the larval stage, and the temperature increases towards the centre of the filter; it seems probable that when the temperature of the filter rises in the spring, the larvae gradually move towards the outside of the filter, prior to emergence in the perfect insect stage.

Insects on percolating filters. This question is one of interest in connection with percolating filters, these often forming breeding receptacles for myriads of insects of various species. As a general rule, however, it will be found that the vast bulk of insect life belongs to the genus *Psychoda*, or small midge-like flies, together with gnats of various kinds and a small fly known as *Limosina pumilio*, Zett. Quite apart from the question of infection being carried by these insects, they may occur in such vast numbers as to be a nuisance to the dwellers of houses in the vicinity, sticking to clothes, food, lamps, etc., and, in bad cases, occurring in such numbers as to make breathing without swallowing them a difficult matter.

I am indebted to Mr J. C. Kershaw, F.Z.S., for the following notes concerning *purpurescens*.

Over 95 % of many hundred *Collembola* taken at random from the S. Norwood sewage farm were *Achorutes purpurescens* Lubbock, fam. *Poduridae*. These *aptera* feed upon green algae, humus from contact beds and percolating filters, the fungi *Carchesium Lachmanni* and *Sphaerotilus natans*, also feeding voraciously on damp blotting paper, even when supplied with plenty of the foregoing foods. Sometimes they devour dead bodies of their own kind. The eggs are laid in haphazard heaps in damp places on the filter, amongst the filtering material, and on the coping-walls near this material. They hatch in about ten days. Several females will sometimes lay in the same heap, and accordingly the number of eggs in a batch varies from ten or twenty, to several hundreds.

The two kinds of midge most frequently met with on sewage works are referable to the *Psychodidae*, the specific insects being *Psychoda sexpunctata* and *Psychoda Phalaenoides*. These insects undergo similar metamorphoses to lepidoptera in the damp filtering material, *viz.* : (1) ovum, (2) larva, (3) pupa, and (4) imago or perfect insect. The two insects may generally be found in all four stages in the external material (if there are no retaining walls) of coarse percolating filters, and apparently the period of oviposition is an extended one. Fine material filters do not appear to possess much attraction for the insects. The food of the larvae consists of any kind of decaying vegetable matter, and damp humid surroundings appear to be essential to their well-being.

The duration of life of the perfect insect does not appear to have been ascertained. The pupa is provided with excrescences or bristles somewhat similar to those found on *Sesiid* pupae, and apparently they serve the same purpose, *i.e.* to assist the pupa to travel towards the outside of the material just prior to emergence.

Several instances have occurred where men working on sewage works have complained of bites from flies, which often produced intense irritation, and in some cases acute inflammation, usually after a lapse of several hours, but it would appear difficult to ascertain whether the irritant poison was mainly introduced through the agency of the insect at the time of settling on the skin, or subsequently by the finger nails of the victim whilst trying to allay the irritation.

In the case of the English *Psychodidae*[1], the poison cannot be introduced by the mouth parts, as these are not capable of inflicting any damage, but it may easily come about by the minute hairs with which these particular insects are abundantly provided, after the manner of the hairs of urticating larvae, *e.g. Liparis chrysorrhea* and *Liparis auriflua*.

Doubtless the modern percolating filter, by reason of its warm equable internal temperature and the damp material of

---

[1] *Phlebotomus papatasi,* an Indian species of the genus *Phlebotomus* (family *Psychodidae*) carries virus of the disease known as "sandfly fever": only the female of this species bites.

which it is composed, forms a capital asylum for the life processes of various insects, offering a maximum of protection
against hostile living agencies in the form of birds, spiders,
etc.

Sewage appears to possess a fascination for insects as well as
animal life, and several butterflies, *e.g. Lycaena argiolus, Apatura
iris,* and the *Pierids,* have a predilection for it, whilst on the
continent sewage is employed by lepidopterists to attract
noctuid moths.

As regards remedies for excessive insect life, it would seem
feasible to destroy it in the imaginal stage by periodical fumi-
gation with some heavy poisonous gas, such as carbon bisul-
phide. Again, kerosene or some similar liquid might be
applied sparingly to the filter.

House martins, swallows, flycatchers, and the three com-
moner species of wagtail destroy enormous quantities of midges,
and possibly in the near future it may be the engineer's lot
to provide suitable niches around percolating filters so as to
encourage the martins to build there.

Percolating filter effluent temperatures. During the York
experiments[1], careful records were taken daily about 9 a.m.
The observations extended from January 9th, 1901, to May 1st
of the same year : temperature records were taken of atmosphere, sewage, air contained in filter, and filter effluent.

It is interesting to note that the average temperature of
the filter taken 3 feet into the filter, from January 9th to
February 19th, 1901, was 41° F. ; at 13 feet into the filter it
was 42·9° F. ; whilst at 29½ feet into the filter it was 43·7° F.

The average temperature of the sewage during the above
period taken at 9 a.m. and 9 p.m. was 42·9° F., the atmosphere
34·8° F., and the filter effluent 39·9° F.

On January 9th, with an atmospheric temperature of
23° F., the average filter temperatures were :

3 feet into filter 42·2° F.

13   „   „   42·7° F.

29½   „   „   43·9° F.

[1] City of York. *Report to the Sewerage Committee on Sewage Purification
Experiments at the Naburn Disposal Works.* Yorkshire Gazette Co. York (1901).

The sewage on January 9th was 45° F., the septic tank liquor 41° F., and the filter effluent 42° F.

Fig. 54 gives the mean monthly air and percolating filter effluent temperatures at the Buxton sewage works taken daily over a period of one year. These temperatures may usefully be compared with those of the land and contact bed effluents given on page 204 and page 248 respectively.

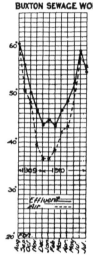

Fig. 54. Mean monthly temperatures of air and percolating filter effluent

Cost of percolating filters. The cost of percolating filters will vary according to the local conditions, the type of filters, and also the suspended matter contained in the tank liquor, and no prices can be given which would be generally applicable. Taking the question of suspended solids alone, this may influence the ultimate cost of the filters very largely; for example, if a tank liquor contains no more than say three to five parts of suspended solids per 100,000, and the tank liquor is of about average strength, it can be treated at a much greater rate per cube yard of filtering material than a tank liquor similar as regards strength but containing say 10 to 12 parts of suspended solids per 100,000. From this it will be seen that the particular preliminary process adopted may influence the cost of the filters very considerably. As a rough guide it may be said that a cost of about 18s. per cube yard of filter, including distribution, etc., is perhaps an average figure at the present day in this country.

The cost of the Accrington filter installation, consisting in 1904 of 14 filters, having a total cubic content of 12,934 yards and varying in depth from seven feet to nine feet three inches, was £9000. The cost per cube yard of the filtering material in position in the beds varied from 3s. 7½d. per cube yard for clinker to 10s. 6d. for coke.

At Prestolee, the total cost of the installation, including

closed septic tank and filters, was £398. The filters, three in number, were constructed with brick walls and concrete bottom, and filled with (bottom of filter upwards) one foot of rough cinders, three feet of mixed cinders, and one foot at the top of cinders ¼ inch to ⅛ inch diameter. The total cubic content of the three filters was 395·5 yards, the filtering material being obtained locally at a cost of 3s. 3d. per cube yard; the cost per cube yard finished and in position in the beds being 6s. 9d.

Fuller gives the cost of percolating filters in America at from £6000 to £10,000 per acre of effective area, the cost depending upon local conditions as to cost of stone, amount and character of excavation or embankment, depth of bed, etc.

These figures do not include cost of outfall sewer, land, settling tanks, screens, buildings, etc., which naturally vary with different installations.

Cost of working percolating filters. There can be little question that where a good effluent has to be produced from a strong sewage, a percolating filter installation is the cheapest present day method of purifying sewage ; as to the actual cost of working, this will depend largely upon the original design of the scheme. If the size of material, for example, is too fine, endless labour and expense will be incurred in keeping the surface of the filters clean, whereas if the works have been designed correctly and detail properly attended to, each part of the purification process will dovetail into the other parts and labour will be reduced to a minimum. Much of what has already been said regarding the cost of working contact beds applies also to percolating filters.

With correctly designed works, the cost of maintenance charges for treating a sewage of average strength by percolating filters should be, and moreover is, considerably cheaper than by means of contact beds ; and, other things being equal, this must be so, since double the quantity of liquid can be effectively treated per cube yard of material in the former case, owing to the facilities for continuous aeration in the percolating filter ; moreover, a better effluent is produced, and also one of more even quality than an effluent from a double contact bed installation. Initial cost is generally less than in the case of double contact beds, and therefore annual loan charges are less ; less site area is requisite as a rule, and the rate of treatment per cube yard of filtering material can be varied within wider limits than could be obtained with double contact beds. When the sewage is weak, and has first been well precipitated and given quiescent settlement, single contact will produce a satisfactory effluent, and the relative costs of the two processes become more nearly similar, but even in such cases the continuous filter would be the cheaper, all things considered, and the effluent produced by it is more uniform in quality, better aerated, and more stable than a contact effluent.

At Chorley, the cost of treatment for the year 1904 was about £3. 4s. 0d. per million gallons, the cost per head of the population being about 1s. The sewage at Chorley is under average strength.

It should be carefully borne in mind that the above operating costs are based upon the dry weather flow of sewage in each case, since at few installations is any record kept of the quantity of sewage treated in wet weather. If the extra volume treated in wet weather were included, the above figures would undergo a material diminution.

It may be questioned whether the cost per million gallons taken by itself is a reliable index, unless both the character of the sewage and the quality of the effluent produced, together with local conditions, are taken into account. Assuming for the sake of argument two cities, each having a population of 300,000, the one (A) dealing with a weak sewage, and the other (B) treating a very strong sewage ; further, that the effluent produced by A is of moderate quality, whilst that produced by B is good. The dry weather sewage flow per head from city A will necessarily be a high one—let it be taken at 40 gallons per head ; similarly let the sewage flow per head at city B be taken at 30 gallons per head. Leaving storm water out of the question for the moment, the relative volumes of sewage dealt with during the year by the two cities will be : A 4380 million gallons, and B 3285 million gallons. Take the annual cost of treating the sewage to be similar in each case, say about £13,000. Judged on the basis of cost per million gallons alone, A produces a moderate effluent from a dilute sewage at a cost of about £3 per million, whilst B produces a good effluent from a strong sewage at a cost of about £4. From this it will be seen that comparisons between different works may be very misleading, unless the full facts are known. The same degree of purity of effluent may not be required in the case of A as with B: again, if A is in a rainy district and B in a dry one, and storm water is included in the calculation, the costs of treatment at the two cities will differ by a still larger amount. Nothing, however, is more certain than that were A required to purify down to the same standard as B, the cost of treatment per million gallons would increase very considerably, whilst if the sewage of A were as strong as in the case of B, the increase in cost of treatment per million gallons would be still greater.

Turning to American percolating installations, Fuller notes that for the year 1910 the Columbus plant cost altogether about £1975, $9876.66, for working charges, about £1483 being for regular salaries, and about £200 for unusual repairs and extensions.

It is to be noted that the volume of sewage dealt with for that year amounted to 4598 million gallons, giving for working and maintenance charges a total of 9s. 10d. per million gallons.

In the case of Birmingham a good effluent is produced from an exceptionally strong sewage with a four-hours' oxygen absorption figure of not far off 30 parts per 100,000. The cost of treatment at Birmingham is about £3. 4s. 2d.[1] per million gallons, and about 10d. per head of population, but it must be recollected that the effluent in this particular case has to be a good one, since in dry weather it enters a river of practically the same volume as the effluent. It would be manifestly erroneous to compare the Birmingham figures of cost of treatment with those, say, of Chorley, where the sewage is less than half as strong, and the rainfall of the district higher than at Birmingham.

BIBLIOGRAPHY.

Cambridge Natural History Series, vol. v. Macmillan and Co., London (1895).

Carpenter, G. H. *Insects, their Structure and Life.* Dent and Co., London (1899).

Dunbar, Professor. *Principles of Sewage Treatment*, translated by H. T. Calvert. Griffin and Co., Ltd., London (1908).

Eaton. Monograph. *Ent. Mag.*, XXIX. and XXX. (1893, 1894). Supplement, *op. cit.*

Entomological Society of London. *Trans.* (1895).

Fuller, G. W. *Sewage Disposal.* McGraw-Hill Book Co., London and New York (1912).

Geer, Charles de. *Memoirs*, Vol. VII. L'Imprimerie de Pierre Hesseburg (1778).

India, Report on Sanitary Condition of, Vol. XLIV. (1910–1911). Wyman and Sons, Fetter Lane, London.

Kershaw, G. B. *Modern Methods of Sewage Purification*, chap. XIV. Griffin and Co., Ltd., London (1911).

Leeds, City of. *Experiments on Sewage Disposal*, by Col. T. W. Harding and Mr W. H. Harrison. Jowett and Sowry, Leeds (1905).

Lubbock, Sir J. *Trans. Linn. Soc.* (1867).

—— Monograph. Published by Ray. Soc. (1873).

Massachusetts State Board of Health, *40th Annual Report.* Brown and Potter, Boston (1909).

Miall. *Aquatic Insects.* Macmillan and Co., London (1903).

Royal Commission on Sewage Disposal. *Fifth Report.* Appendix III to *Fifth Report.* Wyman and Sons, Fetter Lane, London.

Wilson, H. M., and Calvert, H. T. *Trade Wastes.* Griffin and Co., Ltd., London (1913).

York, City of. *Report to the Sewerage Committee on Sewage Purification Experiments at Naburn Disposal Works.* York (1901).

CHAPTER IX

STERILISATION

In this country at all events it has been considered that the burden of supplying pure water to a community should rest upon the shoulders of the Water Company, and this would seem to be the fairest way of looking at the matter. This view was held by the Sewage Disposal Commission in their Fifth Report, some extracts from which on the subject of sterilisation will presently be quoted. As the Commission point out, rivers are exposed to pollutions other than sewage, a fact which will be apparent to anyone who considers the matter, and it seems unfair on the face of it that towns and villages on a particular river from which water for potable purposes is drawn for a particular community, should be called upon to purify their sewage to a far greater extent than would be warranted in the case of a river not so used. In the event of the river being eventually abandoned as a drinking-water source, who is to indemnify the authorities who have been put to this extra expense for sewage purification works ? If an arrangement between the Water Company and the various authorities on the river were come to, under which the company reinbursed these authorities for extra purification works and maintenance in excess of what would ordinarily be needed, that would be quite another matter.

It would seem reasonable that if an authority is discharging an effluent into a river which does not interfere with the ordinary amenities of that river, they should be deemed to have carried out their duty satisfactorily ; that an effluent suited to local circumstances should be the first consideration, and that the ratepayers should not be burdened with the cost of providing drinking water for other communities in which they have no interest. Supposing sterilisation to be insisted upon: during storms, not only would very many times the ordinary dry weather rate of flow have to be sterilised, and quickly sterilised, but elsewhere in the town storm overflows would in all probability be discharging storm water directly to the same river receiving the sterilised effluent.

Extracts from the Fifth Report of the Sewage Disposal Commission. The Sewage Disposal Commission say :

" We observe that previous Commissions have reported that, of all the processes which were proposed for the purification of sewage, or of water polluted by excrementitious matter, there is not one which is sufficiently effective to warrant the use, for dietetic purposes, of water which has been so contaminated, and the 1868 Commission stated that, in their opinion, ' rivers which had received sewage, even if that sewage had been purified before its discharge, were not safe sources of potable water.' We, therefore, conclude that the framers of the Rivers Pollution Prevention Act, 1876, did not contemplate that local authorities should be required so to deal with their sewage that the rivers into which the purified sewage flowed might be regarded as safe sources of water supply, in cases in which the water was not to be filtered before distribution.

" In our opinion, much the same position must be taken up to-day. Although the methods available for the purification of sewage are more numerous than when the 1868 Commission reported, our examination of a very large number of effluents from sewage farms, and from artificial filters of various kinds, shows that, although such effluents may be very good as judged by chemical and physical tests, they are generally liable to contain large numbers of micro-organisms of intestinal derivation, and that if such organisms are to be destroyed, or eliminated, the effluents must be subjected to some treatment additional to that which is ordinarily employed.

" We have carried out some experiments for the purpose of ascertaining the practicability of certain of the methods which have been suggested for the removal or destruction of these micro-organisms. These experiments, which are described in Dr Houston's report, Appendix IV, have shown that, while it would be practicable to render sewage effluents fairly pure, bacteriologically, the cost of the necessary additional treatment would be serious.

" Moreover, a false sense of security would be obtained by the adoption of such further treatment unless, at the same time, storm overflows on sewers were abolished.

" In the great majority of towns, sewers are provided with storm overflows, by which, in times of storm, large quantities of sewage are discharged into the rivers or streams untreated. Such discharges, we find, are frequently more impure, bacteriologically, than the normal crude sewage.

" In the opinion of some engineering witnesses whom we have called before us, it would generally be impracticable to dispense with storm overflows, but assuming, as an engineering possibility, that they could generally be dispensed with, it is quite clear that the necessary enlargement of the sewers would involve a very large outlay. In some towns, if there were no storm overflows, the effect of a storm would be to cause the flow in the sewers to be very many times the normal rate for a short period.

" By constructing a separate system of sewers for storm water, the effect of storms on the other sewers would no doubt be greatly lessened, but if bacterial purity is to be required in the case of all discharges from sewers, it would be necessary to provide a second plant for the treatment of the liquids flowing in the storm water sewers, as these liquids are often exceedingly impure.

" The amount of liquid which would be brought down by such separate sewers would vary, according to local conditions, but during the course of a year it would probably be at least half as much as the volume carried by the other set of sewers.

" In our opinion, the cost of reconstructing the sewers so as to allow of the abolition of storm overflows, together with the cost of providing and maintaining purification plant which could be relied on at all times to render the total refuse waters of a town both chemically and bacteriologically pure, would in most cases be practically prohibitive ; and further, even if this additional burden were placed on local authorities, the water of rivers would generally still require to be treated before it could be safely distributed for drinking purposes.

*   *   *   *   *

" Apart from the question of drinking waters, we find no evidence to show that the mere presence of organisms of a noxious character in a river constitutes a danger to public health or destroys the amenities of the river. Generally speaking, therefore, we do not consider that in the present state of knowledge, we should be justified in recommending that it should be the duty of a local authority to treat its sewage so that it should be bacteriologically pure."

From the extracts just given, it will be gathered that the Commission held strong views to the effect that sterilisation would be of little value as applied to the dry weather flow of sewage alone.

Report on sterilisation by Dr Houston. Dr Houston's report, referred to by the Commission (Appendix IV, Fifth Report), is mainly devoted to the question of sterilisation of sewage effluents by means of chloros (sodium hypochlorite), and in an addendum to the report are given the experiments from which the conclusions are arrived at.

Dr Houston at the commencement of this report, quotes from one of his previous reports to the Commission (Second Report, pp. 27–28), as follows :

" Next, as regards the complete or partial sterilisation of the effluents by chemical substances. By complete sterilisation is meant the absolute destruction of all microbes, sporing and non-sporing. By partial sterilisation, the death of all bacteria present as bacilli (or in coccus form) is implied, but not the death of the spores of bacteria. And for a reason presently to be explained, it is of advantage to limit this a little further by saying that this partial sterilisation may be judged to be sufficient if *B. Coli* is destroyed.

" This destruction is important, because the difficulty of killing spores is very great, whereas bacilli (and cocci) are much more easily destroyed. Thus the thermal death point of *B. Coli* is about 60–65° C., of some spores actually 120° C. And the same striking difference holds good in the main as regards chemical antiseptic substances. It is evident, then, that the difference in cost between the complete and partial sterilisation of an effluent would be a very material difference, and it may be questioned if the additional freedom from danger resulting from complete sterilisation would merit the extra expenditure.

" The number of spores of aerobic and anaerobic bacteria in sewage would seem to be about 100–1000 per cc. in the case of a total bacterial flora of 1–10 million or more. So that the spores form a relatively small proportion of the total germs in sewage. Of pathogenic spores, habitually or occasionally present in sewage, *B. Enteritidis sporogenes*, tetanus, malignant oedema and anthrax must be considered. Are we to consider that the risk of these and other sewage spores remaining in an effluent which is being discharged into a potable river is so grave that complete sterilisation is necessary ? In the present state of knowledge this can hardly be said, and having regard to the almost insuperable difficulties attending complete sterilisation of effluents, to insist upon it would seem to be impracticable...."

The experiments with chloros carried out by Dr Houston showed the importance of prolonged contact of the liquid to be sterilised with the sterilising agent, as economising the dose employed. Other methods of sterilisation are also mentioned and the probable working costs given in each case. They are as follows :

1. *Heat.* 65° C. is sufficient to ensure partial sterilisation. Probably a working cost ranging from £1 to £10 per 100,000 gallons; probably nearer the latter than the former figure.

2. *Ozone.* Working cost £1 to £10 per million gallons. £1 to £5 per million gallons probably a safe estimate, but perhaps wiser to calculate cost at from £2. 10s. 0d. to £5. Initial outlay and depreciation of plant important factors.

3. *Filtration.* Results obtained by filtration through sand relatively good, but actually unsatisfactory, *i.e.* the percentage reduction often remarkable, but the actual numbers of bacteria remaining in effluent still too high.

4. *Chloros* (sodium hypochlorite).

Dr Houston's conclusions regarding the use of this sterilising agent are:

1. " The amount required to sterilise a sewage effluent obviously depends on the quality of the sewage effluent and the duration of contact. Questions of light and temperature should also be taken into consideration.

2. " Assuming 10 hours' contact and a non-putrescible sewage effluent yielding to the four hours' permanganate and the albuminoid nitrogen tests less than one part and ·1 part per 100,000 parts, respectively, and containing less than three parts of suspended matter, it may be said that the proportion of chloros (containing 10 per cent. available chlorine) required for the destruction of *B. Coli* (in 1 cc. of effluent) varies from

$$\left.\begin{array}{c} 1 \text{ to } 100,000 \\ \text{to} \\ 1 \text{ to } 10,000 \end{array}\right\} \quad \begin{array}{l} \text{but between 1 to 50,000} \\ \text{and 1 to 25,000 would} \\ \text{probably suffice.} \end{array}$$

" The cost at 1s. a gallon would thus mean extreme prices of from 10s. to £5 per million gallons, but probably the cost would be from £1 to £2 ; nevertheless, I think that under specially favourable conditions the cost should not exceed £1 per million gallons."

3. " If the duration of contact was shortened to one hour it is probable that the dose would have to be increased to about one in 10,000, entailing a cost of £5 per million gallons."

4. " If the duration of contact was only six minutes, the approximate dose required would probably be about one to 2,500, at a cost of £20 per million gallons."

5. " As regards questions of practicability, a working cost per million gallons of less than £1 is, I think, practicable ; a cost of from £1 to £10 can hardly be entertained seriously unless it does not greatly exceed this former sum, or unless the conditions are so exceptional as to merit a large expenditure ; and a cost of over £10 appears to be, in any case, out of the question."

6. " The sterilisation (as regards *B. Coli*) of a well-clarified, well-oxidised, and otherwise well-purified sewage effluent is thus not an impracticable measure, assuming tank accommodation of at least one hour, but preferably 10 hours."

" Careful experiments have been carried out with fish, and the results lead me to conclude that no danger to fish life is to be apprehended, provided the dose of chloros is not greatly in excess of what is actually required for sterilisation purposes, and the duration of contact is sufficiently long to exhaust most of the active part of the material."

In the event of an epidemic, it might be found possible and even advisable to sterilise a sewage effluent for a certain period, but even in such a case, storm overflows, owing to the solids they discharge, would offer an almost insuperable difficulty ; it may be mentioned, however, that at Cologne, where the sewage passes through very fine screens and a settlement basin, it is insisted upon by the Imperial Board of Health that the sewage shall be disinfected when demanded.

Sterilisation in America. In America a good deal of attention has been devoted to the sterilisation, or " disinfection " as it is termed, of sewage effluents, and numerous experiments have been carried out by various sanitarians, of which those conducted by Mr E. P. Phelps will be alluded to presently.

Mr G. W. Fuller[1] mentions one of the first attempts at sterilisation as being at the Red Bank sewage works, N.Y., the primary object being to protect the shellfish layings ; the process, consisting of hypochlorite treatment of septic tank effluent, has been in use intermittently since October, 1906.

In December, 1910, Messrs Hering and Fuller recommended the use of hypochlorite treatment for the New Brunswick sewage, the object in this case also being to protect shellfish layings.

At Baltimore, Md., it was decided finally to adopt hypochlorite treatment if necessary, for the protection of oyster layings in Chesapeake Bay.

At New Bedford, Mass., hypochlorite treatment has been strongly recommended by Messrs Sidgwick and Phelps, owing to risk of pollution of shellfish.

Mr Fuller states that the hypochlorite treatment has been recommended at many places where there is risk of shellfish pollution, *viz.* Providence, R.I., Stratford, Conn., New Brunswick and Riverton, N.J., whilst sterilisation of the Reading filter effluent has been suggested with a view to providing a further safeguard as to the quality of the water supply of Philadelphia, which is partly derived from the Schuylkill River, some 30 miles below Reading. In most instances, however, it is not clear whether disinfection is to be continuous, or only intermittent, and further, whether storm water is to be dealt with.

Mr Phelps' Report.   Turning to the Report[2] on *The Disinfection of Sewage and Sewage Filter Effluents*, by Mr E. B. Phelps.

Mr Phelps, after treating of the advisability of sterilisation in certain cases, enumerates the various methods and chemicals which have been proposed from time to time for sterilisation, and discusses them in the following order :

1. Heat.
2. Lime.
3. Acids.
4. Ozone
5. Chlorine and its compounds.
    (a) Chlorine gas.
    (b) Hypochlorites, or oxychlorides.
    (c) Electrolytic chlorine process.

6. Copper and its compounds.
7. Miscellaneous.
    (a) Permanganates.
    (b) " Amines " process.
    (c) Sodium benzoate and other organic compounds.

Experiments carried out at various places with most of the above substances are quoted, and results given in tabular form, together with extremely useful comments thereon.   Summarising the various disinfection methods, Mr Phelps observes that of the substances which have been sufficiently experimented with, chlorine compounds and copper salts alone appear applicable to the sewage problem, and further, that a detailed study of results from the point of view of cost, leaves no room for doubt that the efficiency of chlorine is much greater than that of copper.   He also points out that chlorine in the form of bleaching powder, being to some extent a by-product, is very cheap.

The particular experimental investigations cited in Mr Phelps' Report in connection with the disinfection of sewage and sewage effluents, were carried out at the Massachusetts Institute of Technology at Boston, at the

---

[1] *Sewage Disposal*, Fuller.   McGraw-Hill Book Co., New York and London (1912).

[2] Water Supply Paper 229.   Washington (1910).

sewage disposal works at Red Bank, N.J., and also at the Walbrook testing plant at Baltimore.

It may be useful to give the scope of the investigations at each of the above places, since it is impossible, owing to lack of space, to do more than give extracts from the Conclusion at the end of Mr Phelps' report: the whole report should be read by those who are interested in the subject.

At Boston the experiments comprised :

(1)   Preliminary experiments with chloride of lime.

(2)   Studies of the comparative efficiencies of chloride of lime, sulphate of copper, and sodium benzoate.

(3)   Small-scale experiments to determine the comparative efficiencies of free chlorine, commercial hypochlorites, electrolytic hypochlorites, and the hypochlorites of several bases.

(4)   Studies of the comparative effect of hypochlorites on the typhoid and colon bacilli.

(5)   Routine disinfection of 5000 gallons a day of trickling filter effluent with chloride of lime, and

(6)   Disinfection of crude sewage with chloride of lime in 700-gallon tests.

At Red Bank, N.J., disinfection of septic sewage by chloride of lime was tried, and at Baltimore the disinfection of trickling filter effluent, with a similar sterilising agent, was experimented upon.

Cost of disinfection.   Mr Phelps, in his Conclusion, states that trickling filter effluents similar to those experimented upon could be satisfactorily disinfected by three parts per million of available chlorine in the form of bleaching powder, the removal of bacteria in the effluent averaging over 95 per cent., whilst the cost of disinfection ranges from 4s. 2d. to 6s. 3d. per million gallons of effluent, depending chiefly upon the size of the plant.   Effluents of higher degrees of purity can be disinfected at still lower cost, whilst five parts per million represents the probable maximum amount of chlorine required for trickling filter effluents of poorer quality.   It is important to add here that Mr Phelps observes that the results obtained with the specified amounts of disinfectant do not of course amount to complete sterilisation, but they may reasonably be called " practical disinfection."   Considerable additional cost is required to improve them but slightly.

The disinfection of crude sewage was found to require from 5 to 10 parts per million of available chlorine, the cost being from 6s. 3d. to 14s. 7d. per million gallons.

The disinfection of septic sewage required from 10 to 15 parts per million of available chlorine.   It may be noted that commercial bleaching powder generally contains about 33 per cent. of available chlorine.

It should be borne in mind that American sewages are as a rule much weaker than English and European sewages, and that what may be economically practicable with a liquid containing little suspended matter, may not be feasible with a strong liquid containing much organic matter.

BIBLIOGRAPHY.

Houston, Dr A. C. *Report on Sterilisation.* Appendix IV to *Fifth Report of Royal Commission on Sewage Disposal* (1910).

Kershaw, G. B. *Modern Methods of Sewage Purification*, chap. XVI. Griffin and Co., Ltd., London (1911).

Phelps, E. B. *The Disinfection of Sewage and Sewage Filter Effluents.* Water Supply Paper 229. Washington (1909).

Royal Commission on Sewage Disposal. *Fifth Report.* Appendix IV. Wyman and Co., London (1908).

CHAPTER X

TRADE WASTES

It would be quite impossible within the limits of a few pages to deal with all the wastes comprised in this subject, and the treatment of trade wastes themselves scarcely comes under the heading of sewage purification or disposal. The subject has been dealt with in such textbooks as Mr W. Naylor's *Trade Wastes*[1] and Messrs Wilson and Calvert's *Trade Waste Waters*[1], and reference may be made to these books for detailed information. Certain trade wastes, however, such as brewery, tannery, fellmongers, dairy wastes, etc., etc., are of frequent occurrence in or near both large and small towns throughout the country, and it is believed that it will be useful to deal very shortly with these particular trades, since they are frequently carried on where there is no means of access to a sewer, and pollution of rivers or streams sometimes occurs, often because the trader, naturally enough, does not wish to embark on a scheme of purification which may turn out a failure, and as a rule local authorities have not the requisite knowledge to assist him in the design of such works. Another fruitful cause of unwillingness to put down works, is to be found in the fact that the trader has no guarantee as to where his outlay on purification works will end ; *i.e.* whether he will not be told in a year or so's time, " You must do something more,"

[1] Griffin and Co., Ltd., London. *Trade Wastes* (1902); *Trade Waste Waters* (1913).

without being given, however, any indication as to *how* the works—which should have been properly designed in the first instance—may be improved.

Trade wastes may consist of solids or liquids ; as a general rule, however, the bulk of trade wastes is in liquid form, consisting of water used for trade purposes, and carrying various impurities both in solution and suspension.

The fact must not be lost sight of, that solids in the form of heaps of chemical refuse may, through the agency of rainwater, become most serious sources of pollution, either continuous or intermittent.

Trade wastes differ materially from sewage liquors, in that they do not for the most part contain disease-causing microbes[1]. On the other hand, some of them may contain poisonous substances injurious to cattle and fish. Again, clean hot water, such as condenser water, may be the indirect cause of trouble in a stream by causing waterweeds to die off and putrefy, and in some cases, where the stream is small, by destroying fish life.

Equable flow of trade wastes to sewers desirable. Where the trade liquors are admitted to town sewers, it makes a very great deal of difference to the working of the sewage purification plant whether the trade wastes are let off evenly throughout the greater part of the day, or, as is more frequently the case, in sudden rushes at any time of day, and in the case of a small sewage works, these sudden heavy flows of waste are particularly difficult to deal with, especially if precipitants are employed. If, on the other hand, the wastes are let off as they should be from a tank, equably throughout the 24 hours, or at all events spread over as long a period as practicable, the difficulty of dealing with it at the sewage works will be very greatly lessened.

It should be observed that the discharge of trade effluents into rivers or streams is usually limited to 12 hours out of the 24, whereas the discharge of sewage effluents is almost invariably spread over the 24 hours ; hence with similar total daily volumes

---

[1] Waste liquors from tanneries and fellmongers' yards may, as is well known, contain the spores and bacilli of anthrax.

of effluent from (*A*) a manufactory, and (*B*) a sewage works, the dilution given by any river or stream will in the case of *A* be only one-half that of *B*.

Paper manufacture. There are many branches of paper making, including the manufacture of high-class writing and drawing papers, newspaper, brown paper, wall paper, blotting paper, etc. Brown paper is usually made from peat, old sacking, rope, tarpaulin, etc. ; high-class papers from esparto grass and cotton or linen rags, with sometimes a little wood pulp. Wood pulp imported from Canada, Norway and Sweden is chiefly used for newspapers; both "mechanical" and "chemical[1]" wood pulps are employed.

The nature and volume of the waste liquids produced at various mills vary considerably according to the kind of raw material used, and the amplitude or otherwise of the water supply. Many of the waste liquids produced are exceedingly alkaline and polluting, in particular those derived from the kiers, especially where esparto is used, rags not requiring so strong a solution of soda.

Other waste liquors are the washings and water from the washing and breaking engine, the bleach waters and machine water.

The amount of sludge produced at paper mills is very large, and in the case of mills making inferior grades of paper it is usually pressed and tipped, or used to fill up waste land. In some cases, however, as with wood pulp, the pulp has a value, and it is either re-used or sold for making inferior paper.

Selective settlement in specially devised tanks does not appear to have been tried with waste liquids from paper making, *i.e.* the regulating of the velocities throughout the tanks so that the suspended solids are separately settled out according to their several specific gravities. In cases where a particular portion of the suspended matter in a waste liquid is valuable, and differs as regards specific gravity from other matters which are worthless or of less value, this method of recovery might prove of use.

---

[1] " Chemical " wood pulp does not require bleaching.

Well-designed settling tanks of ample capacity, and capable of being worked on the chemical precipitation method, will as a rule produce from the mixed waste liquids a tank liquor containing a low quantity of suspended solids, it being assumed that the strong alkaline kier[1] liquors are treated separately by a recovery process. This tank liquor can in many cases be discharged direct to the river ; in certain cases, however, the tank effluent may need filtration. Alumino-ferric appears to be the best precipitant to employ. In any case, if the tanks are to be effective, they *must* be kept regularly cleaned out. A storage tank is needed to equalise the various waste liquors, and a sludge draining lagoon to receive the sludge from the settling tanks, whilst in some instances where the sludge cannot be tipped, or utilised for making brown papers, a filter pressing plant will be required. Up to the present time, no economically practicable means appears to exist of dealing with the kier liquors by biological filters, where they are not strong enough to make a recovery process pay.

Messrs Crossley Brothers kindly carried out some experiments for the writer on gasifying esparto sludge. The sludge was taken from the tips in the wet state and dried, when it formed pieces about one inch to two inches long by about $\frac{1}{4}$ inch to $\frac{1}{2}$ inch in thickness.

In this state it was found easy to gasify in a producer, although the ash amounted to 14 per cent. ; the consumption of dried sludge per B.H.P. per hour being estimated at from 2 to 3 lbs. The consumption of dried sludge as burnt under a boiler was calculated to be from 8 to 10 lbs. per B.H.P. per hour, and it would have required a special boiler constructed with enlarged grate area, and possibly coal would have had to have been burnt with it, in which case it might have had an actual negative value burnt under a steam boiler.

Refuse from fellmongers' yards. The fellmonger's business consists in the removal of the wool from sheep and lamb skins, thus preparing them for the tanner. The liquid wastes produced by a fellmonger are objectionable, both on account of their

---

[1] " Kiers " or iron boilers.

highly polluting nature, and also when discharged into small sewers by reason of the silting up in the sewers caused by the lime and fibre. Frequently the "limes" employed in fell-mongering are used for long periods, and are permitted to get very foul, to the detriment of the skins. The volume of waste liquids produced in the fellmongering business is not large, an average quantity from a medium-sized yard being perhaps some 10,000 gallons weekly ; it varies, of course, according to the number of pelts on hand. The liquid wastes are amenable to biological treatment, and would appear to be best dealt with by mixing in settling tanks of adequate capacity, the resulting tank liquor being treated by deep percolating filters, or by means of filtration through suitable land, where this can be obtained. In either case the rate of filtration per cube yard of filtering material or per acre of land must be low, by reason of the strength of the liquid.

Tanning. There are many tanning processes in general use, the tanning substances used being oak bark, mimosa and other barks, Sicilian sumac, alum, oil, bichromate of potash, etc. The waste liquors produced in a tannery are much larger in volume than those resulting from fellmongering, the total volume from an ordinary tannery amounting to from 5000 to 10,000 gallons daily. Of this quantity, the liquids from the lime pits and the pures or bates are excessively polluting, and in addition to this, there is always a quantity of polluting liquid reaching the drains of the tannery, resulting from the handling of the dripping skins on the floors. As regards treatment of tannery waste liquids, they are amenable to precipitation in tanks, followed by either land treatment (where this can be obtained) or percolating filters, but, owing to the strength of the liquid, a low rate of treatment must be adopted per acre or per cube yard of filtering material.

The lime and tan liquors tend to precipitate one another when mixed, but it is generally necessary to use either lime or alumino-ferric in addition.

The Crossley process for utilisation of spent tan. The particular spent tan gas plant to be described is one devised by Messrs Crossley Brothers, Limited, Manchester and London, and consists in utilising the spent tan for power purposes. The plant is the largest in the world working on spent tan, and consists of two generators, one of 300 h.p. and a larger one of 400 h.p. The smaller generator is used for power only, and the larger one for supplying gas for gas firing steam boilers ; the pipes are so arranged that the larger plant can, if necessary, be used for driving a gas engine. The plant is run continuously from Monday morning to Saturday night without any stoppage, and is run on spent tan solely. A photograph of the plant is shown on Fig. 55.

Description of process. The spent tan is first passed through calender rolls, which brings down the moisture to 50 per cent. A special gas generator is used, so that a very deep layer of tan is built up without using any coal, the gas produced being clarified so as to distil the tar and cool it for use in driving purposes.

Since the gas produced depends almost entirely upon the combustion of the carbon in the fuel in the presence of moisture or steam, it is not necessary to transmit heat to an external surface.

Moisture driven off by heat in the lower portion of the fuel bed is condensed in the colder upper portion of the bed, automatically increasing the weight of the upper portion, thus preventing any pulling over by the suction of the engine or exhauster. It is consequently possible to give say 3 to 4 lbs. of spent tan about 70 cubic feet of producer gas at 130 B.T.U. per cubic foot, or 1 B.H.P. from a gas engine. This 70 cubic feet of gas when applied to a suitable boiler, gives an evaporation of 7 lbs. of water at 212° F.

If the gas produced is only used for firing on other boilers for steam raising, it is unnecessary to pass it through the cooler or cleaner, the sensible heat in the gas thus being utilised ; it is, however, essential to clean and cool it when used for the gas engine for driving. When the plant is used for both steam raising and power, the gas producer is treated as a separate unit, but the pipes are so arranged as to admit of this producer supplying the gas engine also.

The fire grates are of Messrs Crossley's patent stepped type,

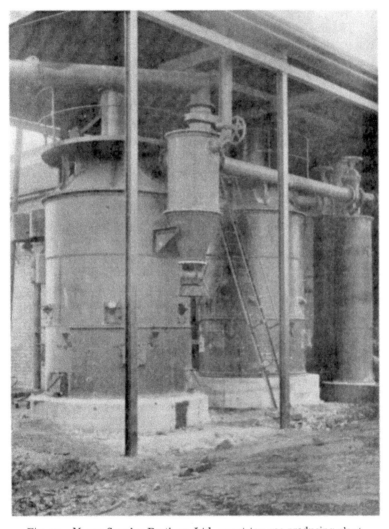

Fig. 55. Messrs Crossley Brothers, Ltd., spent tan gas producing plant.

and so arranged as to afford every facility for the removal of ash or clinker, without interfering with the quality of the gas, and the particular feature of this grate is that no good fuel can fall away.

The gas produced is controlled automatically to the use of the works, the operator's work consisting mainly in seeing that the fuel is supplied to the producer ; the fire can be examined without disturbance to the quality of the gas, and if an elevator is used for lifting the material to the top of the producer, the amount of labour is only a fraction of that required for feeding an ordinary boiler under similar conditions.

Brewery wastes. These wastes are probably more frequently met with than any other, and they often cause considerable difficulty when mixed with domestic sewage unless special precautions are taken in the purification process, whilst, in cases where a sewer does not exist, serious pollution of the local stream often happens, and masses of fungus are fostered in the bed of the stream by the waste liquids. Fortunately in such cases suitable land is sometimes available for the purification of the waste liquids.

Frequently malting and brewing are carried on by the same firm and at the same place, and the steep waters from malting are, contrary to popular notions, very polluting.

Brewing operations require large quantities of water, a large part of which is used for rinsing and cleansing vessels and floors, since all waste liquids must be removed from the brewery premises with as little delay as possible, to prevent detriment to the beer.

The waste liquors are mainly derived from the mash tuns, underbacks, coppers, hopbacks, yeastbacks and fermenting vessels ; the water from the refrigerators and attemperators is generally pure water, and does not need purification. In addition, a large amount of pollution is derived from beer spilt on the floors, and especially from cask and bottle washing, soda or calcium bisulphite being often used for these processes, whilst steam and boiling water are employed, producing a liquid of high temperature, and containing spent hops and stale beer. Sulphuric acid is often used for cleaning out vessels.

The total volume of liquid waste from breweries varies in particular cases, and also according to the season of the year, but as a general rule, where refrigerator and attemperating water is mixed with the wastes, the total quantity of waste liquids will be from two to five times the volume of beer brewed.

The mixed liquids from a brewery are of a very polluting character, and they very soon decompose and become acid, the acidity being caused mainly by the formation of lactic acid. At Burton-on-Trent, where about 60 per cent. of the sewage consists of brewery waste, lime has been used for many years to neutralise this acidity, and to lessen nuisance from smell. The dose of lime is an extremely heavy one. For preliminary treatment of brewery waste, there is probably no better method at present than chemical precipitation in tanks, using a heavy dose of lime. For final purification, land, if it can be obtained of suitable quality, offers as good a chance of purification as any, given first-class distribution, but deep percolating filters can be used, working at a low rate per cube yard.

Mixing a small quantity of domestic sewage with brewery refuse and passing both through a septic tank has been suggested and tried, but a septic tank in conjunction with brewery refuse is often the very best means of creating a serious nuisance ; ordinary sewage might, however, be mixed with the brewery liquids in a precipitation tank.

Contact beds, it may be observed, are not so suitable for the treatment of brewery wastes as percolating filters, and triple contact is generally needed to produce a good effluent, but if percolating filters are used, the liquor applied to the filters should be a precipitation tank liquor.

Dairy wastes. During the past 20 years, considerable attention has been paid to this industry, especially in Ireland, and there are now many large concerns scattered over the countryside, devoted to the production of cream, butter and cheese, and the number seems likely to increase. That the industry is an important one in Ireland, may be gleaned from the fact that in 1912, butter to the value of no less than four million pounds was exported. Dairying projects in Ireland, which number some 800, exclusive of butter factories, may be classified as follows :

1. Creameries.
2. Cream-separating depôts.
3. Butter factories.

The butter factories are most of them situated in towns, and it is at the creameries and cream-separating stations situated in country districts that the disposal or purificaton of the waste liquors is a troublesome matter.

The waste liquids produced are very rich in organic matter and difficult to purify.

At cream-separating depôts the milk is brought in by farmers to the depôt, where it is weighed and strained, and after being heated to from 120° to 195° it is conveyed to the separators. The cream is cooled and placed in cans to be conveyed to the churning station, whilst the separated milk is cooled and returned to the farmers proportionately to the milk delivered, for feeding pigs and calves.

At creameries, in addition to the work detailed above, the cream, after separation, is cooled, soured, and churned when at the right temperature. When the butter has come, the buttermilk is run off and conveyed to a tank, from which it is taken by the farmers supplying the milk. The butter is then washed from one to three times, being subsequently salted and worked on a butter worker.

In cheese-making rennet is added to the milk in vats when at a proper temperature, and when the curd is firm enough it is cut into equal-sized cubes by a special curd knife, to allow the whey to separate out. The vats are usually jacketed and can be heated if desired to obtain further separation of the whey. The curd is finally salted and pressed. The whey is generally returned to the farmers.

The waste liquids produced may perhaps be divided into two classes, *i.e.* (1) non-polluting, and (2) polluting.

1. Under this heading comes the clean water used for cooling the milk, cream and separated milk, water from refrigerating machine, and sometimes rainwater from the roofs of

the premises ; these can be discharged without any treatment, as they virtually consist of clean water.

2. The polluting liquids are derived from washings from various machines, *e.g.* separators, coolers, churns, butter workers, tanks and vats, rinsings of milk cans, washing of floors, etc.

All these liquids are more or less polluting, the worst being the first washings from the churning of the butter and the whey from cheese-making. In appearance, the waste from a creamery resembles milky water, and it contains fat, casein, albumen, milk sugar and lactic acid, becoming highly putrefactive.

The volumes of waste liquids produced varies according to circumstances and time of year: generally speaking it is from one-third to five-sixths the volume of the raw milk entering the depôt. June, July and August are the "flush" months in a creamery. There has been a good deal of litigation between farmers and creameries, the farmers alleging that their cattle have been poisoned or damaged by the creamery wastes entering the streams from which they drink. So far, however, there seems to have been no proved case where cattle have actually suffered damage from the above cause, and it seems more likely that the creameries are regarded as fair game by neighbouring farmers. Still, quite apart from the question of damage to cattle, creamery refuse turned into a small stream in its crude state is objectionable by reason of the appearance it gives to the water, and in hot weather it may cause bad smells.

The most suitable method of purification is by means of land, where this can be obtained of suitable quality, and the waste should receive preliminary treatment by passing it through a bank of peat fibre, the peat being removed at intervals and used for manure. It can then be treated at the rate of some 2000 to 4000 gallons per acre if the distribution is properly attended to.

In cases where an artificial process is called for, good precipitation with sulphate or persulphate of iron and lime in tanks holding about a two days' supply of refuse will leave an almost clear liquid, but the dose of precipitant must be a rather heavy one, and it is imperative that the tanks shall be kept frequently cleaned out and properly attended to. The resulting tank liquor can be treated upon deep percolating filters. It seems advisable to remove as quickly as possible the solids, which form the chief difficulty in dealing with this refuse, rather than to pass it through a septic tank of large capacity in the attempt to break up all the solids.

The difficulty is in getting proper attention given to regular cleaning out of the tanks when precipitation is used. The cost of the precipitant need not be high, since the total daily volumes of liquid from a dairy are not large, and with a dairy turning out one million gallons of waste annually, a dose of 15 grains per gallon would only use up about one ton of precipitant yearly. It may be mentioned that casein can be made into excellent imitation ivory for knife handles, pianoforte keys, etc., whilst separated milk enters into the composition of several insecticides.

Piggery sewage. The liquids derived from large piggeries are exceedingly rich in ammonia, being often ten times as strong in this respect as average domestic sewages.

In Ireland piggeries are sometimes worked in conjunction with creameries, and herds of as many as 600 pigs are kept. The amount of urine produced by each pig averages about $\frac{3}{4}$ gallon per 24 hours, but to this must be added about $2\frac{1}{2}$ to 3 gallons used for washing-down purposes in addition to rainwater, apart from the pig faeces, which latter, how-ever, should be collected at frequent intervals and sold for manure. From a herd of, say, 300 pigs kept in sties, an average flow per 24 hours of some 1000 gallons of an exceedingly strong ammoniacal sewage may be anticipated, the purification of which is a difficult matter. In many cases the local conditions obtaining—such as a large body of diluting water—do not call for a high degree of purification. With a sewage of such strength, contact beds are not suitable, and deep percolating filters of medium-sized material, followed by shallow sand straining filters, will produce a highly oxidised effluent. The preliminary treatment should be precipitation with lime in settling tanks constructed in duplicate, and each capable of holding about 1½ days' flow of sewage. The greater proportion of the sewage will be produced during the daytime, say 12 hours, and in order that the filter should not be overdosed, it is advisable that the precipitation tanks shall be designed on the quiescent flow method, the tank liquor being drawn off by means of floating arms, when the feed to the filter can be spread over the greater part of the 24 hours.

In cases where the flow of sewage is very small and irregular, a small dosing chamber and automatic siphon are useful for feeding the filter distributor at intervals. If this is not done there will at times be an insufficient flow to keep the distributor rotating, and the liquid will dribble from the arms on to the filter at one spot, causing a bad effluent.

Coal washing. This process is concerned with the removal of dust and impurities from the coal by water. This water after use is black and dirty, containing much coal dust, dirt and fine coal, and its discharge into a stream in this condition causes considerable injury. In some cases, the water, after being used for coal washing, is settled in tanks and re-used for washing, and good results can be obtained in this way if the tanks are properly attended to and promptly cleaned out when necessary. At some collieries the wash water is passed into pits or lagoons excavated in waste shale heaps, and allowed to percolate away, good results being obtained.

Spent gas liquor. This waste is derived from the distillation of ammoniacal liquor produced by manufacturing coal gas or coke, and when entering the sewers in any quantity it frequently occasions great difficulty in the treatment of the sewage, and when it enters streams, decimates fish life, besides being destructive of all vegetation.

Spent gas liquor in its crude state consumes an enormous quantity of oxygen. So far, no economically practicable process can be said to have been found suitable for its treatment in the case of a small works, and in the case of large coke ovens, the waste liquor is either pumped on to waste heaps, or diluted and used for quenching coke.

A process has been devised by Mr J. Radcliffe for treating

gas liquor so that its discharge into sewers is not attended by injurious results as regards the subsequent purification of the sewage at the sewage works.   This process is shown in plan and section on Fig. 56, the waste gases remaining after the absorption of the ammonia being used to purify the waste liquid.

The plant can be added to any sulphate plant, and being constructed of cast iron and brickwork, depreciation charges are small, whilst any attention needed can be supplied by the sulphate operator, no special skilled knowledge being required.

The waste gases are usually taken after they have given up a portion of their heat in the liquor heater, but instead of then passing to the condenser, the gases enter the plant by the pipe at E, passing away to the condenser through the outlet at the summit of the purification column.

The waste liquor enters the plant from the ammonia liquor still at A.   The lime settling tank is shown at B, whilst C is an accumulation or variation allowance tank for the cleared liquor, where it is pumped to the purification plant entering at D.   This consists of a contact plant somewhat similar as regards construction to liquor still.

Whilst the liquor is falling to E the waste gases passing in the opposite direction act upon it.   The purification plant in reality consists of two separate columns ; i.e. between D–E and E–H, there is no connection for gases, since the liquid must pass through the upper seal-pot, and although the waste liquor passes down the whole of the column, the waste gases only pass through from D–E, and the air and steam only through E-H.

The liquor leaving the upper part passes through the seal-pot, re-enters the plant at F, and passes down and away through the seal-pot G.

At H a current of air is injected, passing upwards and away at I through J, and away at K.

The liquor leaving G passes to a tank M and filter tanks N, downwards through one and upwards through the other, when the treatment is complete.

A small volume of air is added to the waste gases passing from E to D by means of a pipe from H (not shown).

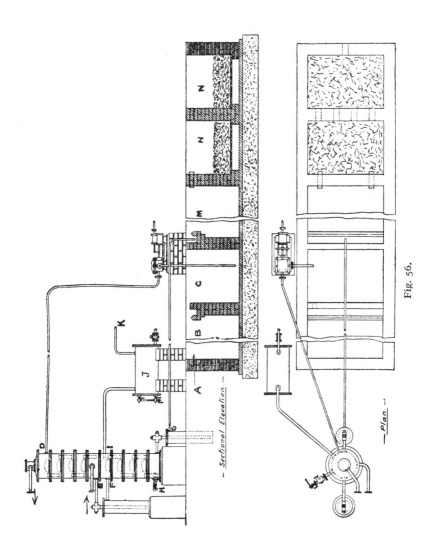

— Sectional Elevation —

— Plan —

Fig. 56.

The treatment carried out in the upper part of the apparatus precipitates free lime in solution, decomposing phenylate and cresylate of lime and cyanogen compounds, together with soluble organic matter in solution. If desired[1] (though not necessary as a rule), a more complete removal of cyanogen compounds can be effected by substituting for the upper seal-pot a continuous settling tank for the removal of carbonate of lime and adding continuously to the liquid a small quantity of strong acid.

The stream of air and steam passing from H carries off the gaseous and vaporisable impurities set free in the upper portion of the apparatus, including any sulphuretted hydrogen and pyridine from the devil-water. This leaves at I, whilst J accumulates any condensate, and at K the vapours are either led to a fire and destroyed or otherwise treated for recovery.

It should be observed that no nuisance arises from the working of the plant, and it is stated that there is a reduction in the oxygen absorbed figure of upwards of 75 per cent., whilst there are no costs for purification materials other than a small amount of steam and coke.

Coke oven plants can utilise the whole of the purified effluent for works purposes; it may also be used for quenching the coke without discolouring it or damaging it in any way.

Otto-Hilgenstock coke oven process. In this process the gases with practically all their tar contents are taken from the hydraulic mains and led straight into the sulphate house, where they are subjected to a strong spray of tar, the whole object of the tar spray being to take out the tar quantitatively at a temperature above the dew point of the gases, collecting the very fine particles of tar from the gas and depositing them in a tank or drum underneath. After passing through the tar extractor, the gases are pumped straight through the saturator by exhausters.

---

[1] At the Rushden gas works, in order to secure the maximum purification, the carbonate of lime is precipitated as described above, and arrangements made for its settlement. The sulphuric acid is added in quantity according to the law of equivalents to decompose the sulphocyanides, the sulphate of lime is settled out and the liquid passes to the purification still as before.

The saturator consists of a lead vessel containing sulphuric acid, with a dip pipe, sealed in sulphuric acid, the whole of the oven gases being subjected to cleansing by the sulphuric acid ; the saturator is so worked that there is a continuous overflow, and it is circulated so that just an occasional froth is taken off, the salt being continuously ejected, the saturators being so shaped that the salt falls to the bottom and is ejected mechanically with steam.

The gases on leaving the saturator pass on direct to ovens. The plant is an extremely simple one and several installations are in course of erection in this country.

At Oldbury considerable trouble was caused by the large volumes (8 per cent. at times) of wastes discharged from chemical works engaged in the recovery of ammonia from gas liquor. The sewage at Oldbury is treated by means of open septic tanks and triple contact beds[1]. As little as ·5 per cent. gas liquor in a domestic sewage has been known to cause difficulty at times in its treatment.

At Malvern, where the sewage is treated by means of settling tanks and percolating filters, the addition to the sewage of gas liquor caused trouble, which, however, ceased when the gas company constructed large precipitation tanks, and strained the gas liquor through a filter of fine stone chippings.

BIBLIOGRAPHY.

Bowles. *Septic Treatment of Creamery Sewage. Engineering Record*, Vol. LXIV. p. 419 (1911).

Dunbar and Calvert. *Principles of Sewage Treatment.* Griffin and Co., Ltd., London (1908).

Hubner. *Cantor Lectures*, Society of Arts. London (1913).

Journal of Department of Agriculture and Technical Instruction for Ireland, Vol. IV. No. 3 (1904). A. Thom and Co., Ltd., Dublin.

Kayser, Ed. *Microbiologie Agricole.* J. B. Baillière et fils, Paris (1911).

Kershaw, G. B. *Modern Methods of Sewage Purification*, chap. xv. Griffin and Co., Ltd., London (1911).

Kimberley, A. E. *Report on the Treatment of Creamery Refuse. Engineering Record*, Jan. 8th, 1910, p. 50.

---

[1] Percolating filters would certainly seem better adapted to the treatment of sewage containing substances requiring good oxidation, and it is not clear why contact beds were selected.

Massachusetts State Board of Health. 40*th Annual Report*, pp. 359–361. Brown and Potter, Washington (1909).

Naylor, W. *Trade Wastes*. Griffin and Co., Ltd., London (1902).

Rivers Pollution Commission (1868). *First and Fourth Reports*.

Royal Commission on Sewage Disposal (1898). *Fifth Report. Sixth Report. Seventh Report*, Vol. III.

Royal Sanitary Institute. *Journal*, Nov. (1912).

Tillmans and Taylor. *Water Purification and Sewage Disposal*. Constable and Co., London (1913).

The Gas World, Jan. 27th, 1908.

The Iron and Coal Trades Review (1911), Vol. LXXXIII.

The Leather World, No. 124, Vol. V. No. 20, May 15th, 1913. 90, Tooley Street, London, S.E.

Wilson, H. M., and Calvert, H. T. *Trade Waste Waters*. Griffin and Co., Ltd., London (1913).

CHAPTER XI

ACTIVATED SLUDGE PROCESSES, SLUDGE DIGESTION, ETC.

Briefly described, the activated sludge process[1] consists in circulating in a grit-settled sewage, the finer suspended matter which it contains, for a given period, the distributing or mixing agent being an air supply. Before the suspended matter is in a condition necessary to effect the required purification, it is essential that it should first of all undergo a process of ripening, which has the effect of rendering the suspended matter highly active in various forms of microscopic life; hence the name "activated sludge." After an appropriate period of thorough intermingling of activated sludge and sewage, during which

[1] In the "Definitions of Terms used in sewerage and sewage disposal practice," suggested by the Sanitary Engineering Section, American Public Health Association, the Activated Sludge Process is defined as "the agitation of a mixture of sewage with about 15 per cent. or more of its volume of biologically active liquid sludge in the presence of ample atmospheric oxygen, for a sufficient period of time at least to coagulate a large proportion of the colloidal substances, followed by sedimentation adequate for the subsidence of the sludge flocculi; the activated sludge having been previously produced by aeration of successive portions of sewage and adequate aeration by itself or in contact with sewage."

time it is important that the velocity of movement should be sufficient to prevent deposition of the sludge, the sewage with its load of activated sludge is settled, and the effluent passes away to the river or stream, no further treatment being necessary, and it may be observed that the activated sludge process is remarkably efficient in the removal of colloidal and suspended matter.

The circulation of the sewage is carried out in an aeration tank, the sewage gradually and continuously passing from this tank to a settlement tank or tanks. A portion of the sludge which settles in these last tanks is returned to the aeration tank, the remainder being run away for sludge disposal.

Formerly it was customary to aerate the sewage; cut off the air supply; allow time for settlement, and decant the clear liquor, this being known as the "fill and draw" method: it involves considerable loss of fall, and the continuous flow plan is now usually adopted.

It will be noticed that, whereas with a percolating filter installation, the sewage or tank liquor is passed through filtering material which has become coated with a gelatinous envelope of organisms—this effecting the real purification—so, in the case of the activated sludge and agitation processes, the finer suspended matter or sludge, with its attached organisms, is kept circulating throughout the sewage liquor: in other words, the moving activated sludge takes the place of the quiescent filtering material in the percolating filter.

In the same way that a percolating filter requires time to become coated with the requisite gelatinous coating, so, with the activated sludge process, a certain time is required in the first place for the sludge to become "activated," as it has been termed, and the deposits from contact beds or percolating filters are often used for producing or building up activated sludge in the first instance.

The time taken to ripen or activate sludge, depends upon the character of the sewage or waste liquor which is being dealt with; intractable wastes taking longer to produce a thoroughly activated sludge than an ordinary domestic sewage of average strength.

With regard to the ratio of the volume of sludge to sewage kept in circulation with the sewage, the optimum percentage has been found to vary considerably with different sewages. Probably 25 per cent. would be an average figure, although much larger and smaller volumes have been successfully used with different sewages. In certain cases it is necessary to re-aerate the sludge, before its return to the aeration tank, in order to keep it thoroughly active.

The volume of air used, again, per unit volume of sewage, varies considerably, according to the strength and nature of the liquor treated: it is also affected by the depth of the tank.

For a domestic sewage of average strength, from 1 to 1·5 cubic feet of air per gallon of sewage would probably be needed. The quantity of air required could seemingly be reduced by the extension of the aeration period, in the same way that a dose of chlorine in the case of sterilising a water supply can be reduced, if the period of contact be lengthened.

Activated sludge is very light and bulky, and it may contain from about 97 per cent. to 99·5 per cent. of moisture. The effect of this high moisture content may be realised, when it is considered that a reduction of from 99·5 to 99 per cent. of water, would result in reducing the volume of sludge by one-half. The sludge does not readily part with its moisture, and in this respect it compares unfavourably with ordinary sewage sludges; it contains, however, considerably more nitrogen than ordinary sludges, and it is remarkably free from odours.

In the light of present knowledge, the two methods of dealing with this sludge which appear likely to be most successful are drying in thin layers on specially constructed bed, and irrigation through pipes on land.

With regard to this latter method, little appears to be known concerning the friction of sludge in mains, and Mr Wm. Clifford, A.M.Inst.C.E., the manager of the Wolverhampton Sewage Works, has devoted considerable thought to this subject.

It may be of interest in this connection to observe that the American Society of Civil Engineers, realising the dearth of information on this subject, appointed a Committee on Feb. 23rd, 1923, to inquire into the matter.

The initial work which suggested the development of the Activated Sludge process, had its origin in the earlier experiments carried out by H. W. Clark, at the Lawrence Experiment Station of the Massachusetts State Board of Health, as a preliminary process to filtration. The actual development of the process, however, as a practicable means of oxidising sewage without filters, is due to Dr Edward Ardern and Mr William T. Lockett, to whom Dr Gilbert Fowler communicated the results obtained by Clark, and who worked out the process through all its stages at Davyhulme, and reference should be made to the original paper by these workers, entitled "Experiments on the Oxidation of sewage without the aid of filters" (*Society of Chemical Industry. Jour.* vol. XXXIII. 1914).

The Davyhulme experiments, commencing on a laboratory scale, showed that Manchester sewage could be made to yield a good effluent, by aerating it in contact with the lighter suspended matter for a period of from six to nine hours.

These experiments led to further work upon a larger scale, with improved methods of applying the air blast, diffuser tiles being used instead of perforated pipes, improvements which had the effect of reducing the time required for aeration to four hours.

Working scale units followed, and there are now several large installations at work on this system, both in this country and abroad.

Coming to existing treatment works; a description of the latest activated sludge unit at the Withington sewage works, constructed under the supervision and direction of Dr Ardern, will be of interest.

WITHINGTON ACTIVATED SLUDGE UNIT.

This plant is designed to treat a dry weather flow of one million gallons per 24 hours, and storm water up to three million gallons.

The aeration tank measures 180 feet by 60 feet wide, overall, divided longitudinally, thus forming two independent aeration chambers, placed one on each side of a central common channel for the return and re-aeration of sludge.

Each aeration chamber is 177 feet long by 20 feet wide, with a capacity of 145,000 gallons. Two longitudinal walls, with suitably placed portholes, divide each chamber, providing an aeration channel 530 feet long by 6 feet 3 inches average width, and about 7 feet deep to water level.

Cross baffle walls, each with 1 foot 6 inches by 2 feet openings, fitted with deflectors, are provided at an average interval of 35 feet, along the entire length of the aeration channels.

The sludge return and re-aeration channel has a capacity of about 35,000 gallons. It is 160 feet long by 6 feet average width below water level, by 5 feet 6 inches deep to water level, and it is also provided with cross baffle walls.

Aeration is effected by lines of diffusers placed alongside the inclined footings of the divisional walls on one side only of the channels.

The diffusers measure three feet by 4½ inches overall, their total area being approximately one-seventeenth of the aeration tank area.

The ratio of actual diffuser area to total tank area is approximately 1 : 23.

Overhead air pipes are provided, air being admitted to these diffusers by a series of down pipes, one to each diffuser.

Valves are arranged on the air mains, so that the tank may be sectionised so far as air supply is concerned. In addition, each down pipe is fitted with a needle and orifice for securing uniform air distribution.

The settlement tank is a deep pyramidal one, with four pockets, 36 feet by 36 feet by 21 feet 4 inches deep from water level to the apex of the pyramids. A 24 inch pipe, conveying the mixed liquor, passes from the aeration tank outlet to a central distributing chamber. This chamber communicates with four Clifford inlets, arranged over the centre of the pyramidal pockets.

Deposited sludge is discharged by hydrostatic head through 6 inch pipes into a small central sludge channel, communicating with the re-aeration channel, by a 15 inch pipe.

The sewage enters the plant through a small mixing chamber, into which the return activated sludge is discharged, and thence passes to the aeration chambers: the mixed liquid ultimately discharges over sills into a narrow lateral channel, before passing to the settlement tank.

The sludge returning from the settlement tank, after traversing the length of the re-aeration channel, is lifted by the combined effect of two air lifts, working in series, into the mixing chamber previously referred to.

The mixing chamber and narrow shallow lateral channel are common to both aeration chambers, and the arrangement is such that if necessary, the flow to one or other of the aeration channels may be stopped, or either aeration chamber may be emptied, without placing the whole plant out of commission.

The effluent leaves the settlement tank over a periphery sill, and passes through a measurement chamber, before discharging into the main effluent carrier.

The surplus sludge is removed through a valve in the floor of the re-aeration channel, and passes through a 6 inch pipe to the general sludge well, where, if required, it may be densified before being lifted by compressed air, and delivered through the existing sludge pipe track into trenches on the land area.

Provision has been made for an ample supply of air, both for the old and new units, by the installation of two new type air compressors, each capable of compressing approximately 700 cubic feet of free air per minute.

These compressors are each driven by 30 H.P. electric motors.

Meters are provided for measuring the electrical units consumed, and the volume of air employed.

The plant occupies a total area of approximately 1450 square yards: aeration chambers (overall) 1200 square yards, and settlement tank and measurement pond, 250 square yards.

The construction and equipment of this unit was completed in August, 1923.

The author is indebted to Dr Ardern for the foregoing particulars.

AIR-BLOWN ACTIVATED SLUDGE PROCESS.

The Sewage Treatment Works designed for the Hale Urban District Council by Messrs John Taylor & Sons, and at present under construction, may be instanced as a good example of the air-blown activated sludge process.

The population served by these works is about 7500, and the sewage is a domestic one, of slightly below average strength: it contains no trade wastes.

The dry weather flow of sewage is 327,000 gallons per 24 hours, and the sewerage system is combined. Flows up to six times the dry weather flow of sewage will be brought to the works in wet weather, half of this will be fully treated; the balance being passed through storm water tanks.

On arrival at the works, the sewage will be screened and passed through detritus chambers. Following the detritus chambers will be a mixing chamber, immediately preceding the aeration tanks. The aeration tanks will be four in number, with a combined capacity of 104,000 gallons, and they are designed to be worked on the continuous flow plan. The dry weather detention period including the returned sludge will be about 6 hours. Air will be supplied by means of one compressor driven by a 25 B.H.P. motor, and one compressor driven by a 15 B.H.P. motor; both compressors and motors being provided in duplicate.

The air blast will be diffused through the liquor by plate diffusers, and the consumption of free air used per gallon of sewage will, it is estimated, be about one cubic foot per gallon of sewage. After leaving the aeration tanks, the liquid will pass to settlement tanks, two in number, having a total capacity of 66,000 gallons. Two re-aeration tanks will be provided, with a combined capacity of 26,000 gallons. Returned sludge, amounting in volume to about 25 per cent. of the incoming sewage will be sent from these tanks to the mixing chamber previously mentioned; the surplus sludge will be run off to sludge drying beds, having a superficial area of about 6000 yards, and constructed of ashes. The liquor draining from these beds will be pumped to the inlet channel leading to the mixing chamber.

G

F

A

AERATION TANKS

Nº 1.   Nº 2.   Nº 1

MAIN INLET CHANNEL

15 INLET SEWER

SETT

Nº 1

WOODEN GUARD

CLIFFORD INLET

SLUICE VALVE

SLUDGE VALVE

INLET CHANNEL

15 PENSTOCK   15 PENSTOCK   18 PENSTOCK

PATHWAY

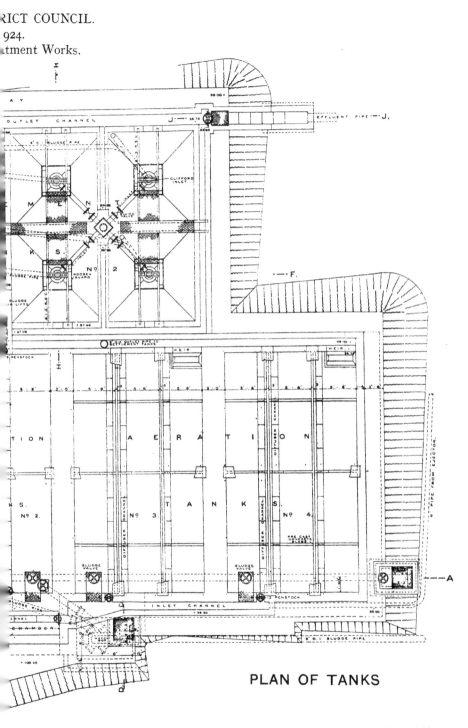

PLAN OF TANKS

Reproduced by courtesy of John Taylor & Sons, Civil Engineers, Caxton House, Westminster, S.W. 1.

The settlement tanks will provide about four hours settlement including the returned sludge, on the continuous method, the effluent finally passing to the river Bollin. The plan of the general layout follows, showing the arrangement of the works.

The author is indebted to Messrs John Taylor & Sons for the foregoing details of these works, and for permission to reproduce the general plan shown on Fig. 57.

Other interesting works on this system are being constructed at Reading, Hertford and elsewhere.

THE SHEFFIELD BIO-AERATION PROCESS.

At Sheffield, in 1912, certain experiments were begun by Mr John Haworth, F.I.C., the General Manager of the Sheffield Corporation Sewage Works. About this time a paper was published by Messrs Ardern and Lockett, relating to aeration of sewage and "activation" of sludge.

Some of the tanks used in the Sheffield experiments were suitably equipped for aeration, and they had been utilised for various aeration experiments. They were then adapted to the lines suggested by Messrs Ardern and Lockett.

On account of difficulties which arose, Mr Haworth conceived the idea of separating the two generally accepted main functions of the air supply—that is to say, the provision of oxygen for biological purposes and also for agitation—by utilising mechanical agitation without air for the mixing; change of surface produced by the stirring action supplying the necessary atmospheric oxygen for biological purposes.

In 1916, a tank of about 800 gallons capacity was fitted up with a paddle stirrer, and it was worked for 5 years at three fillings a day, on the fill and draw method.

The sewage treated, it should be mentioned was an industrial one, containing at times a large proportion of iron liquor, soap, etc.: these sometimes necessitated extended periods of treatment. Larger scale experiments followed the small one.

In 1919, with the object of obtaining information and data respecting the application of the process on a large scale installation on the continuous flow plan, a large installation was put in hand, and it was completed in 1920.

This plant consists of:

> Aeration Tank,
> Three retention chambers,
> Three settling Tanks,
> Gauging Chamber,
> Motor House.

Fig. 58 shows a general plan and sections of the installation. The aeration tank is 201 feet 6 inches by 75 feet 10½ inches by 4 feet deep to water line, the capacity being 354,400 gallons. Thin division walls separate the tank into 18 channels, each 4 feet wide, with a transverse channel 2 feet 3 inches wide, by 6 feet deep at the end adjoining the retention chambers. The channels are rounded at their ends, and connected so as to form one continuous channel 3544 feet long.

The transverse channel was made deeper than the longitudinal one to admit of retention chambers of increased size.

The floor of the tank is level. Two sewage inlets are provided, one of them being fitted with a float regulating valve.

Eighteen paddle wheels are placed across the centre of the tank, and these agitate and circulate the sewage.

The outlet from the tank consists of a weir wall running the full length of the transverse channel, and forming one side of the retention chambers.

The paddle wheels in the aeration tank effect rapid surface changing of content, agitating and circulating the sewage round and round the channels. Rate of outflow from tank is governed by rate of inflow of sewage.

The retention chambers are triangular in section, and are 4 feet 3 inches wide by 4 feet 8 inches deep. Opposite to the inflow weir is formed the weir over which the liquid flows into the channel feeding the settling tanks.

In the bottom of the vertical wall, openings are provided through which any sludge settling in the retention chambers may return to the aeration tank.

The function of the retention chambers is to diminish

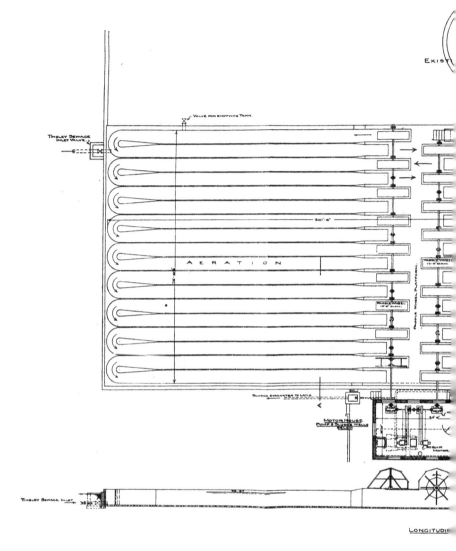

EXIST

VALVE FOR EMPTYING TANK.

TINSLEY SEWAGE
INLET VALVE.

A E R A T I O N

201'-6"

SLUDGE EVACUATED TO LAND

MOTOR HOUSE.
PUMP & SLUDGE WALLS
BELOW

PADDLE WHEEL
15'-0" DIAM.

PADDLE WHEEL PLATFORM.

PADDLE WHEEL
10'-0" DIAM.

250 B.H.P.
MOTOR

24"

TINSLEY SEWAGE INLET

LONGITUDI

SECTION A-A.

SECTION B-B

CITY OF SHEFFIELD - SEWAGE DISPOSAL WORKS.
BIO-AERATION PLANT.
SCALE OF FEET.

INCHES 12 0   10   20   30   40   50   60   70   80   90   100 FEET

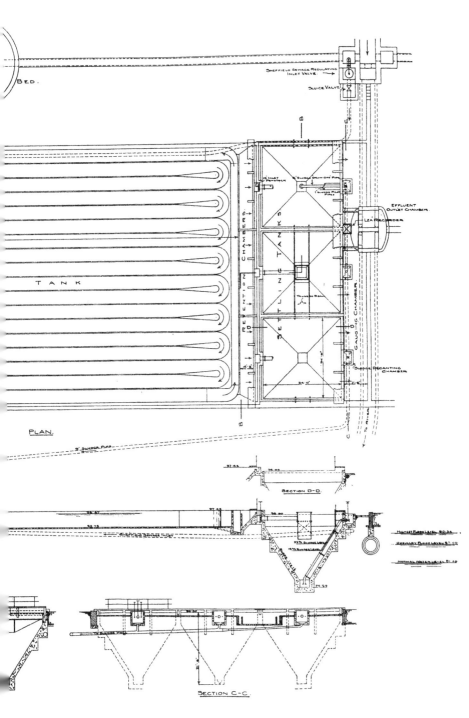

PLAN.

SECTION D-D.

SECTION C-C.

Reproduced by courtesy of John Haworth, F.I.C., General Manager, Corporation Sewage Works, Sheffield.

velocity of flow, and therefore obtain partial settlement of the liquor before reaching the settling tanks, thereby reducing the amount of sludge reaching the settling tanks and consequently requiring pumping, and also reducing the volume of inert sludge.

The settling tanks are three in number, and of the pyramidal Dortmund type, with sides sloping 1 to 1½. Each tank measures 24 feet square by 21 feet 6 inches deep, and they have a total capacity of 102,600 gallons.

The liquid enters each tank by a 12 inch penstock and pipe, connected up to a bottomless vertical box, 4 feet square inside, and submerged in the liquid for seven feet of its depth. The four sides of each tank form the weir over which the effluent passes, either to the collecting channels, or direct to the gauging chamber. Sludge from the settling tank is raised by water pressure through 6 inch pipes into small sludge chambers, in which are fixed the control valves. Two small pilot pipes with valves, in each of these small chambers, show the level of the sludge in each tank.

From the sludge chambers the sludge gravitates to the sludge well below the motor house, where it is pumped back to the aeration tank, entering the channel furthest from the Motor House: a Lea Recorder meters the volume of sludge pumped. Surplus sludge can be sent to the land by a bye-pass valve and chamber placed on the sludge return main.

The Motor House is 24 feet long by 16 feet wide, containing two 20 B.H.P. motors, belt-connected to worm reduction gears, which in turn drive the two shafts on which the paddle wheels are geared. One motor is a standby.

Each motor is equipped with a liquid starter. The sludge and pump wells are placed under the Motor House.

Two 4 inch centrifugal pumps are installed, directly coupled to 7 B.H.P. motors: these motors are controlled, either by a float in the sludge well and an automatic relay switch, or by hand.

The sludge well has a capacity at invert level of inlet pipe of 2500 gallons.

The electric supply current is 3-phase alternating, 50 cycles per second, 440 volts.

The paddle wheels are 10 feet in diameter, by 2 feet 6 inches wide, weighing about 6 cwt. apiece. Each wheel is provided with eight arms, every arm presenting a blade surface to the liquid of 227 square inches.

At 15 r.p.m. of the paddle wheels, a minimum velocity of 1·7 feet per second is set up in the aeration tank channels.

The installation covers an area of less than ·5 acre, and the cost of the work, carried out departmentally, was £12,000.

Apart from the machinery, the three sludge outlet valves at the settling tanks are the only valves requiring attention.

Mr Haworth describes the action of the aeration tank as resembling a river containing a very large number of oxidising organisms, capable of purifying putrescible matters. To this river or stream sewage is added in such volume as it is able to purify continuously. A portion of the liquid is continually being taken from the stream at a point remote from the inlet and equal in volume to that of the sewage which is being added. This portion passes to the settling tanks, where the purified liquor and sludge are separated.

The aeration tank of the installation was filled with sewage on November 4th, 1920, 40 tons of sewage sludge and humus collected from contact beds, etc., being thrown in. After some 21 days circulation, the sludge became matured.

On November 26th, 1920, sewage was admitted, and since then the plant has operated continuously.

The sludge allowed to accumulate in the tank amounts to from 25 per cent. to 30 per cent., any excess being discharged to a land filter.

From November 26th, 1920, to February 18th, 1921, Tinsley sewage only was treated, the dry weather flow being about 250,000 to 350,000 gallons a day, one-third of this consisting of trade wastes from large steel works.

All the sewage up to three times the dry weather flow, was passed through this plant. Before entering the aeration tank the sewage was passed through two small detritus and screening chambers, and through roughing tanks of 20,000 gallons capacity to remove the heavier solids.

The following figures of analysis refer to the sewage treated, and the effluent leaving the settling tanks after treatment.

November 26th, 1920, to February, 1921.

Tinsley Sewage being treated.

	Sewage			Effluent		
	Worst	Best	Av.	Worst	Best	Av.
Suspended solids	52·0	11·0	27·23	less than 3·0		
Oxygen absorbed in 4 hrs.	9·22	1·58	5·90	1·23	·39	·76
Free and saline N. ...	5·16	1·06	3·37	5·70	·70	3·30
Albuminoid N.	1·62	·29	·62	·27	·04	·14
Nitric N.	—	—	—	·03	·54	·16
Dissolved oxygen taken up in 5 days at 65° F. ...	—	—	—	2·20	·13	1·0

(62 samples)

Results stated in parts per 100,000.

Subsequently strong Sheffield sewage was tried, which had passed catchpits and tanks, the daily volume treated being about 500,000 gallons. The results obtained are given below.

February 22nd, 1921, to April 2nd, 1921.

Sheffield Sewage being treated.

	Sewage			Effluent		
	Worst	Best	Av.	Worst	Best	Av.
Suspended solids	267·4	21·6	77·42	less than 3·0		
Oxygen absorbed in 4 hrs.	45·56	5·0	13·93	3·02	·50	1·39
Free and saline N. ...	9·06	3·27	5·09	5·87	3·20	4·41
Albuminoid N.	2·57	·73	1·22	·31	·12	·19
Nitric N.	—	—	—	·05	·20	·10
Dissolved oxygen taken up in 5 days at 65° F. ...	—	—	—	2·17	·52	1·30

(33 samples)

Results stated in parts per 100,000.

Later results obtained from the Tinsley sewage are given in the following table.

February 1st, 1921, to December 31st, 1921.

Tinsley Sewage entering the tank.

	Sewage			Effluent		
	Worst	Best	Av.	Worst	Best	Av.
Suspended solids	101·0	11·0	56·0	less than 3·0		
Oxygen absorbed in 4 hrs.	10·76	2·5	6·63	2·02	·37	1·2
Free and saline ammonia	6·8	·70	3·8	5·8	1·9	3·9
Albuminoid ammonia ...	1·38	·23	·81	·4	·05	·23
Nitric nitrogen	—	—	—	·05	·37	·21
Dissolved oxygen taken up in 5 days at 65° F.	—	—	—	3·2	·16	1·34

Results expressed in parts per 100,000.

January 1st, 1922, to June 30th, 1922.

Tinsley Sewage entering the tank.

	Sewage			Effluent		
	Worst	Best	Av.	Worst	Best	Av.
Suspended solids	1·50	6·8	78·4	less than 3·0		
Oxygen absorbed in 4 hrs.	13·15	·84	7·0	1·02	·35	·69
Free and saline ammonia	8·04	·73	4·39	4·71	·77	2·74
Albuminoid ammonia ...	2·04	·21	1·13	·27	·06	·17
Nitric nitrogen	—	—	—	·03	·91	·47
Dissolved oxygen taken up in 5 days at 65° F. ...	—	—	—	1·89	·09	·99

Results expressed in parts per 100,000.

Mr Haworth observes that the H.P. required to treat a given volume of sewage depends upon the strength of the sewage, and that for a sewage of great strength probably 50 H.P. per million gallons per day would be required: for a weak sewage probably half of this.

It was found that a velocity of 1½ feet per second was necessary to keep the bacterial sludge in complete suspension. The water content of the sludge produced is 98–99 per cent.

At Sheffield, as elsewhere, difficulty in dewatering the sludge is recognised.

The sludge can be satisfactorily dealt with where ample land is available, and later experiments show that by the use of specially prepared ash drying beds, the sludge can be dewatered in a few days to a condition in which it can be removed with a shovel, if the layer of wet sludge applied is not more than 6 to 10 inches deep.

The foregoing description is adapted from a paper compiled by Mr Haworth, which will be found in the *Proceedings of the Institution of Municipal and County Engineers*, for June, 1921.

The present scheme for dealing with the whole sewage of Sheffield (dry weather flow 15,000,000 gallons a day) will be modelled on the installation which has been described. The main features of the scheme are given below.

Sheffield Bio-aeration Extension Scheme.

Consists of 12 units for d.w.f. of 15 million gallons, or 1¼ million gallons each.

Consists of 12 units for w.w.f. of 45 million gallons.

Four units are now in operation[1].

Single Unit.

Capacities.

Circulating Tank 840,000 gallons.

No. 9 Settling Tanks 351,000 gallons.

Power provided.

35 B.H.P. per million gallons, including sludge pumping.

Paddles.

Diameter—10 feet. Blade area 205 sq. ins. per double arm.
R.P.M. 15.

Paddle Power House.

Each Power House will serve 4 units and will contain
four 50 B.H.P. Motors direct coupled to paddle shafts through
double helical double reduction gears.

Sludge Pump House.

Each Pump House will serve 8 units and will contain six 9 inch
centrifugal pumps for circulating sludge and two 4 inch centrifugal
pumps for evacuating surplus sludge. Pumps will work intermittently and by automatic control.

Transformer House.

Current will be supplied at extra high tension on a maximum
demand rate of charge. The Transformer House will contain
the transformers 11000/350 volts and the necessary high and
low tension switch gears, and condensers for improving the
power factor.

The author is indebted to Mr John Haworth for perusing
the proofs relating to his process, and also for permission to
reproduce Fig. 58.

THE "SIMPLEX" SURFACE AERATION PROCESS.

In this method, devised by Mr Joshua Bolton, simplicity of
action, economy in power, and maximum purification are
aimed at. To activate the sludge it has been customary to blow
air under pressure into the sludge at the bottom of the tank.

---

[1] These four units are treating 5 million gallons per diem. Eight other
units are under construction, two of these being nearly completed.

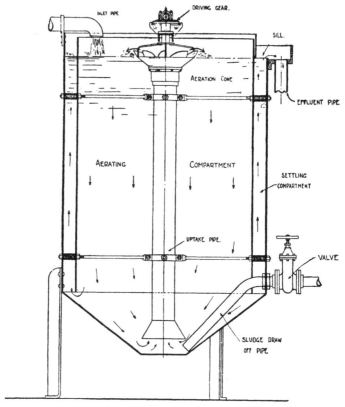

INLET PIPE

DRIVING GEAR.

SILL.

AERATION CONE

EFFLUENT PIPE

AERATING COMPARTMENT

SETTLING COMPARTMENT

UPTAKE PIPE.

VALVE

SLUDGE DRAW OFF PIPE

SECTIONAL ELEVATION

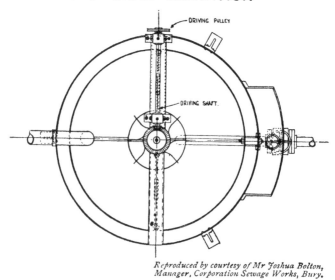

DRIVING PULLEY

DRIVING SHAFT.

Reproduced by courtesy of Mr Joshua Bolton,
Manager, Corporation Sewage Works, Bury.

PLAN

Fig. 59. J. Bolton's "Simplex" Surface Aeration Process.

In the Simplex process mechanical means provide the agitation and exposure to the atmosphere for aeration, the liquid being kept constantly agitated and circulated: mechanical means furnishes the necessary amount of oxygen required for purification purposes.

The tank is arranged with a conical bottom and a central tube, coned at the lower end, and fixed a few inches from the bottom of the tank, the top portion terminating in a dish, the outer edge of which is raised about half an inch above the top water level. Inside the dish a revolving cone with suitably formed vanes is suspended by means of a vertical shaft running on ball bearings, and rotated by shafting and bevel wheels.

Fig. 59 shows a plan and section of the plant.

When the cone is in motion, the liquid is thrown out in the form of a film wave, the liquid and sludge then rises in the central tube to replace the liquid thrown out by the revolving cone. The vanes of the cone are arranged to throw the liquid off so as to strike the surface of the main volume of liquid in the tank in such a manner as to induce a circular motion which causes the liquid to sink in the form of a spiral to the bottom of the tank to be re-circulated.

To obtain the necessary amount of agitation and aeration, the contents of the tank are circulated once in twenty minutes, or three times an hour; the H.P. absorbed is about 15 H.P. per 24 hours per million gallons.

The time taken for purification depends upon the strength and composition of the sewage, and the standard of purification required, but, generally, about eight hours' treatment in the tank is ample.

A plant on Mr Bolton's system is now in course of construction at the Bury Corporation sewage works. This plant, when completed, will deal with a sewage flow in dry weather of 1,250,000 gallons per 24 hours. The Bury sewage is of average strength, containing trade waste waters from tanneries, fellmongers, wool scouring, bleaching and dyeworks.

The process can be seen working at Bolton, Bury, Birmingham and Macclesfield.

THE BIRMINGHAM DEODORISING AND PARTIAL PURIFICATION PLANT.

At Birmingham, the constant increase in filtration area, rendered necessary to keep pace with augmented sewage flow, led Mr J. D. Watson, then Engineer of the Drainage Board, to instal an experimental station, for the purpose of trying out the activated sludge and bio-aeration processes.

Three plants were constructed, each capable of treating 10,000 gallons per 24 hours: they were as follows:

    (1)   Activated sludge plant (air blowing),
    (2)   Bio-aeration (mechanical agitation),
    (3)   Percolating filters.

Research work on these plants, carried out by Mr F. R. O'Shaughnessy, the Board's Chemist, demonstrated that the Birmingham sewage could be treated either by air blowing, or by agitation.

It was also shown that a tank liquor was a better subject for purification than a crude sewage, and that efficient flocculation of tank liquor for one hour removed 60 per cent. of its impurities, whilst eliminating its objectionable smell.

Lastly, and most important of all, it was found that the flocculation of the tank liquor for one hour produced a liquid which might be oxidised at more than twice the usual rate on the percolating filters.

It was also ascertained that eight parts per 100,000 of visible suspended matter, together with ten parts of colloidal sludge, were sufficient to provide the medium essential for the required organisms.

The experiments, therefore, showed the possibility of at one and the same time eliminating smell, and greatly increasing the purifying power of the existing percolating filters, by interposing a deodorisation and partial purification plant between the settlement tanks at Saltley and the percolating filters at Minworth, and a unit of the proposed scheme, on the lines suggested by the experimental work has now been constructed, and brought into operation.

This plant is divided into three sections—flocculation, settlement and re-aeration.

The tank liquor will remain in the flocculating channels for one hour, the rate of motion through them being one foot per second; it will then pass to the separating tanks, provided to remove the exhausted sludge, which will then be passed to a re-aeration chamber, and agitated until re-vivified, and ready for mixing with the incoming sewage.

The following figures of analysis show the character of a typical sample of the Birmingham sewage:

	Parts per 100,000
Oxygen absorbed in 4 hours	26·34
Free and saline ammonia	4·06
Albuminoid ammonia	1·52
Chlorine	18·90
Total suspended matter	57·70

COST OF ACTIVATED SLUDGE PROCESS.

As regards the cost of the activated sludge process, there is, at the present time, scarcely a sufficient number of installations in use under varying conditions, to enable accurate cost data to be given, but it may be remarked that the Ministry of Health, in their *Fourth Annual Report*, appear to indicate that the capital outlay needed for the treatment of a dry weather flow of one million gallons per diem of domestic sewage of average strength, and three times this volume in wet weather, would average approximately £30,000, the annual working cost being from £1200 to £1400. The quality of effluent which would be produced, however, is not stated, and this is an important factor.

As to which system should be adopted in a particular instance, local conditions, *e.g.* configuration of site, must enter largely into deciding the question.

THE CLIFFORD INLET.

This apparatus is intended to dissipate the energy of the inflowing stream of sewage in continuous flow sedimentation tanks.

In tanks of the vertical flow type, with central inlet, a cylindrical flat bottom bucket of a suitable size, is placed under the inlet orifice, and is surrounded by a light sheet iron or wood partition, which extends from a few inches above the water level to the level of the inlet orifice.

The action may be described as follows:

The inflowing liquid strikes the bottom of the bucket, curls on itself in rapid eddies, and issues in a vertical direction; the upward movement continues until the surface of the water is reached, but with a much diminished velocity.

The water surface, with the surrounding partition, acts as an inverted bucket where slow eddy movements take place near the surface; the direction now becomes vertically downwards with an almost imperceptible movement.

The sediment in fact falls faster than the liquid, provided, of course, that the tank and inlet are designed to give time for the sediment to deposit.

With horizontal flow tanks, the eddy bucket may be either horizontal or vertical, and the surrounding chamber is modified accordingly.

This inlet was designed by Mr William Clifford, A.M.Inst.C.E., Manager and Chemist of the Wolverhampton Sewage Works: it is shown in plan in the drawing of the Hale Works (Fig. 57).

SLUDGE DIGESTION.

In the deep double-storied Imhoff tank, the sludge is stored in the lower storey of the tank, where it undergoes fermentation, the fresh settled sewage passing through the upper storey.

At Birmingham, the hot year of 1911, led Mr J. D. Watson to abandon the septicising of the sewage and sludge, and to utilise some of the existing settling tanks as a substitute for the lower storey of the Imhoff tank.

The object of this procedure was to separate the sewage and sludge treatment, fresh settled sewage being forwarded to the filters and treated before it became septic and liable to cause nuisance, whilst the sludge was dealt with separately.

As a first step, an installation of 20 tanks was employed, sixteen of these having a combined capacity of 4,539,000 gallons;

the combined capacity of the other four was 2,750,000 gallons, or 7,289,000 gallons for the 20 tanks. These tanks were provided with the usual arrangements for filling and emptying.

The capacity of the 20 tanks proved insufficient, and further tanks were improvised, by embanking certain areas of land with ash banks, bringing the total tank capacity up to 350,000 cubic yards, and this is the total capacity in use at the present time (1924), being equal to about $6\frac{1}{2}$ months' production of wet sludge, equivalent, under working conditions, to a five months' digestion period.

The digestion process is divided into two parts: (1) Primary digestion, and (2) Secondary digestion. Primary digestion is carried on in tanks having a capacity of 190,000 cubic yards, a tank capacity of 160,000 cubic yards being used for secondary digestion.

This method of dividing the process into two parts was adopted in 1912, since it was found to induce vigorous fermentation, and tank space was saved by pumping from one tank to another. At the present time (1924), with a total tank capacity equal to six months' storage, it is still found necessary to pump twice.

Mr Watson finds that the sludge digestion process is remarkably free from nuisance, and, in 1922, when the author examined the process, it was certainly markedly free from smell.

It should be noted that at Birmingham, it has been found that small tanks are better adapted to the digestion process than large.

The total estimated capital outlay on the plant has been as follows:

Estimated capital value of tanks	£70,000
Capital in drying bed area	20,000
Value of land (150 acres at £150 per acre)... ...	22,500
Total capital cost	£112,500

Interest on capital outlay at 5 per cent.	5,600
Annual cost of pumping, drying, etc.; less value of sludge	19,600
Total annual cost	£25,200

The actual working of the process is as follows:

The sludge is pumped from a settlement tank to five or six of the digestion tanks: simultaneously part of the ripest sludge is pumped into the same pumping main, in the proportion of 1 of ripe sludge to 4 of raw, thus seeding the raw sludge with the necessary microbes of fermentation.

This seeding or inoculation of the raw sludge with ripe was found to speed up the fermentation process. In cold weather steam is injected into the delivery main to raise the temperature of the sludge.

The average figures of analysis of the sludge are as follows:

	1915 to 1918 inclusive		1919 to 1922 inclusive
Water	92·5	per cent.	92 per cent.
Dry solid matter	7·5	,,	8 ,,
Specific gravity:			
wet sludge ...	1·0256	,,	8 ,,
dry solid matter	1·50	,,	8 ,,

Average analysis of dry solid matter.

Matter volatile at red heat	...	...	58·5 per cent.
,, non-volatile	...	...	...	41·5	,,
Total nitrogen ...	...	...	...	2·71	,,

The digested sludge is pumped to drying beds covering a total area of 60 acres, divided into ½ acre plots, all these being levelled, covered with engine ashes, and underdrained with 4" agricultural tiles, laid herring-bone fashion, and connected up to a master drain. This last drain leads the bed drainage to a well, whence it is lifted to a percolating filter.

The drying beds are formed by surrounding land with embankments two feet high, and the sludge is deposited to a thickness of some 18 inches, subsequently drying and shrinking to 6–7 inches. The time occupied in drying varies, but it has been found inadvisable to attempt more than two fillings per annum.

The dried sludge is removed by means of light railways to storage sheds, which cover an area of about 7 acres, where it is taken over by a contractor.

The sludge is then broken up and spread thinly over the

floors of the sheds: when sufficiently dry, it is gathered and ground into a fine meal, and fortified with sulphate of ammonia, bone phosphates and sulphate of potash.

Mr Watson states that the present cost (1924), including working expenses and interest on capital, amounts to 9·6d. per cubic yard of wet sludge, having an average water content of 92 per cent.

It should be observed that the digestion process destroys some 30 per cent. of the dry sludge, and also that the digested sludge is almost entirely free from grease.

For further particulars regarding the sludge digestion process as carried out at Birmingham, the reader is referred to a paper read by Mr J. D. Watson at a meeting of the Association of Managers of Sewage Disposal Works, on November 22nd, 1923, held in connection with the Public Works, Roads and Transport Congress, from which paper the foregoing abstract has been compiled.

It may be mentioned that sludge digestion with a purely domestic sewage has been in use for some years at Carshalton, Surrey, but the storage there is only equal to about three months' sludge production.

At Baltimore, U.S.A., there is a large installation, only recently completed, using this process.

The author is adopting this process at Royton, Lancashire, the sewage here being purely domestic. Here, however, it is intended to apply steam in cold weather to the sludge as it is circulated through the digestion tanks, and it is proposed to pass the sludge through a series of eight long and narrow tanks, after which it will pass to a storage tank, and be pumped to specially prepared drying beds.

STRAW FILTERS[1].

This interesting process was originated by Messrs H. B. Hutchinson and E. Hannaford Richards with a view to utilising the fertilising content of sewage, or other nitrogenous solutions, for breaking down and transferring the fertilising constituents to such materials as straw, thereby converting such materials

[1] *Inst. Civ. Eng. Proceedings of the Engineering Conference*, June, 1921. Section VI. Waterworks, Sewage and Gasworks.

into a valuable manure, with a nitrogen content exceeding that of farm yard manure. The process originated with laboratory experiments at the well-known Rothamsted Experimental Station, and subsequently a large scale plant was erected at Wainfleet, and the process fully tried out. The laboratory experiments, very briefly, consisted in passing a solution of ammonium carbonate equal in strength to a very strong sewage, through a percolating filter of wheat straw at a rate of 250 gallons per cubic yard of straw per day. On the first day 5 per cent. of the nitrogen passed on to the filter was removed, this amount increasing steadily up to the twentieth day when only 1 per cent. of the nitrogen in the artificial sewage was found in the effluent, the remaining 99 per cent. being held in the filter. The filter was then mature and continued to remove practically all the nitrogen applied to it, until the saturation point was reached. On dismantling the filter, it was found that the straw had retained 86 per cent. of the nitrogen contained in the original ammonia solution, 20 per cent. of the straw had disappeared in the process of fixation. The effluent was brown in colour, but non-putrefactive.

The straw, or other material, when saturated with nitrogen can be removed from the filter, and stored, when the fermentation occurring improves its physical condition.

The Wainfleet installation, which was designed by Mr M. G. Weekes, M.Inst.C.E., consisted of a filter 20 feet long × 10 feet wide × 7 feet 6 inches deep, placed over a sloping concrete floor. Two false floors of gas piping were provided in the filter, so that the ripest straw could be easily removed when required without disturbing the remainder, the pipe flooring being easily pulled out when and where required.

Distribution of the sewage (obtained from a camp of some 300 navvies) was effected by means of troughs, the sewage being pumped to the top of the filter.

The time taken for the straw to become thoroughly activated is some 14 days, the optimum temperature being about 35° C., with a temperature of 60° F. to 70° F. the period was 16 days. Straw, it may be added, consists of some 10 per cent. of starch and about 80 per cent. of other carbohydrates, chiefly pentosans and cellulose.

Artificial manures, as is well known, contain little or no humus, which forms one of the most valuable constituents in farmyard manure, and is present to a marked degree in the artificially produced manure.

It will be seen that the process lends itself to the utilisation of straw and other similar material containing sufficient carbohydrate, and to the production therefrom of a most useful m'anure. Sewage by itself contains insufficient carbohydrate and an excess of nitrogen.

It is probable that the process could be most usefully employed in rural districts, nor is it essential that sewage should be the vehicle for the nitrogen, since any of the usual nitrogenous fertilisers can be used. The best results are obtained by means of a special reagent containing the phosphate required by the active organisms. Sewage, of course, supplies phosphate as well as nitrogen.

BIBLIOGRAPHY.

Ardern, Edward, M.Sc. *Activated Sludge plant, Withington Sewage Works, Manchester*.

Bolton, Joshua. *Elasticity of the Activated Sludge Process*.

Clifford, Wm, A.M.Inst.C.E. *Friction of Sewage Sludge in Pipe Lines*.

Fowler, Prof. Gilbert J. *Activated Sludge Process in India and the East*.

Hatton, T. Chalkley, M.A.M.Soc.C.E. *Sewage Disposal plant for the City of Milwaukee*.

Hurd, Chas. H. *Spiral Circulation in the Activated Process*.

Kadish, Victor H. *Investigations of the Fertilising Value of Activated Sludge*.

McVea, John C. *Operation of Activated Sludge Plant, Houston, Texas*.

Pearse, Langdon. *Experience in dewatering Activated Sludge from the Sanitary District of Chicago*.

Wilson, Arthur. *Colloid Chemistry as applied to Activated Sludge*.

(The preceding ten papers were read at the International Conference of Sanitary Engineers, held in London, July, 1924, and can be obtained from the Secretary, Institution of Sanitary Engineers, 120, Victoria Street, Westminster, S.W. 1.)

Haworth, John, F.I.C. *Sewage disposal in Sheffield*.
    A paper prepared for the Annual Meeting of the Institution of Municipal and County Engineers in London, June, 1924.

Martin, A. J., M.Inst.C.E. *The Bio-Aeration of Sewage. Proc. Inst. C.E.*, Vol. XVII. pt. I. (1923–4).
    (This paper contains a very complete bibliography on the subject.)

Porter, J. G. *The Activated Sludge process of Sewage treatment*. A bibliography of the subject. General Filtration Co. Inc. Rochester, N.Y.

Richards, Éric Hannaford, B.Sc., and Michael George Weekes, M.Inst.C.E. *Straw Filters for Sewage Purification. Proc. Inst. of Civil Engineers, Engineering Conference*, Section I. 30 June, 1921.

Watson, J. D., M.Inst.C.E. *Works of the Birmingham Tame and Rea District Drainage Board*. Engineer's Office, July, 1923.

SUBJECT INDEX

INDEX OF AUTHORS

INDEX OF PLACES CITED

www.ingramcontent.com/pod-product-compliance
Ingram Content Group UK Ltd.
Pitfield, Milton Keynes, MK11 3LW, UK
UKHW040659180125
453697UK00010B/273